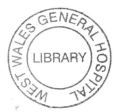

Accident and Emergency Nursing

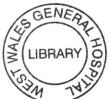

Accident and Emergency Nursing

Edited by

STUART TOULSON

BSc(Hons), RGN, DPSN, PGCHSCE, A&ECert
Clinical Training and Quality Manager, NHS Direct,
Bedfordshire & Hertfordshire

W
WHURR PUBLISHERS
LONDON AND PHILADELPHIA

© 2001 Whurr Publishers Ltd
First published 2001
by Whurr Publishers Ltd
19b Compton Terrace
London N1 2UN England and
325 Chestnut Street, Philadelphia PA 19106 USA

British Library Cataloguing in Publication Data

A catalogue record for this book
is available from the British Library.

ISBN 1 86156 190 3

Printed and bound in the UK by Athenaeum Press Ltd,
Gateshead, Tyne & Wear.

Contents

Dedication

This book is dedicated to my wife, Alison,
and my children, Sarah and Jack.
Thanks for all your patience and encouragement.

Contributors

Lynn Beun, BA(Hons), RGN, PGCHSCE, OND, Diploma in Professional Studies in Nursing, Integrated Care Facilitator, Royal Sussex County Hospital, Brighton, Sussex.

Andrew Carter, RGN, Assistant Nurse Director – Training and Education, Accident and Emergency Department, The Lister Hospital, Stevenage, Herts.

Julie Dight, RN (Adult), DipHe, Senior Staff Nurse, Accident and Emergency Department, St George's Hospital, London.

Nancy Fontaine, BA(Hons), MSc, PGDipHE., Consultant Nurse, Accident and Emergency Senior Lecturer, King George's Hospital, London.

Melanie Gunstone, BSc (Critical Care), RGN, OPSn (Critical Care), Sister/Emergency Nurse Practitioner, Accident and Emergency Department, Lister Hospital, Stevenage, Herts.

Jean Haire, MSc, RGN, National Projects Manager, Emergency Services Programme, Leicester.

Melanie House, EN(g) RGN, Resuscitation (UK) Council Instructor, Lead Practitioner, Nuffield Hospital, Guildford, Surrey.

Helen Markham, BSc(Hons), RGN, Senior Staff Nurse, Accident and Emergency Department, Royal Sussex County Hospital, Brighton.

Helen Murdoch, RSCN, RGN, Diploma in Professional Studies One (Scotland), Resuscitation Council (UK) ALS and PALS Instructor, ITU Outreach Sister, Royal Sussex County Hospital, Brighton, Sussex.

Anne O'Loughlin, MSc, BSc(Hons), RGN DipN, Charge Nurse, Accident and Emergency Department, University College London Hospital.

Janet Parker, BA(Hons), RGN, Sister, Accident and Emergency Unit, Wycombe General Hospital, High Wycombe, Bucks.

Katherine Power, BA(Hons) Health Studies, RGN, NHS Clinical Assessment System (CAS) Trainer.

Andrew Rideout, MPhil, BA(Hons) Nursing Studies, RGN, DipN, RN (Children), Emergency Nurse Practitioner, Accident and Emergency Department, Royal Sussex County Hospital, Brighton.

Judith Smith, RGN, Senior Staff Nurse, Accident and Emergency Department, Warwick Hospital.

Kathy Steward, Dip HE (Nursing), ALS, Sister, Accident and Emergency Department, Royal Sussex County Hospital, Brighton, Sussex.

Tina Marie Stokoe, BSc(Hons), RGN, Clinical Manager, Accident and Emergency Department, Barnet Hospital, Hertfordshire.

Stuart Toulson, BSc(Hons), RGN, DPSN, PGCHSCE, A&E Cert, Clinical Training and Quality Manager, NHS Direct (Beds & Herts).

Ellen Turner, SRN, ENP, Senior Sister, Accident and Emergency Department, Lister Hospital, Stevenage, Herts.

Liana Wakeford, RGN, RN(Child), Senior Staff Nurse, Accident and Emergency Department, Royal Sussex County Hospital, Brighton, Sussex.

Jeanette Welsh, BSc(Hons), RGN, Cert Ed, Practice Development Sister, Accident and Emergency Department, Russells Hall Hospital, Dudley, West Midlands.

Jacqueline Willan, BA(Hons), RMN, RGN, A&E Cert, DipN, RCNT, Cert Ed, RNT, Senior Clinical Nurse, Accident and Emergency Department, Leicester Royal Infirmary.

Yvonne Wimbleton, BSc (Hons), RGN, FAETC, Assistant Nurse Director, Guys and St Thomas's NHS Hospital Trust, London.

Preface

This book has been written by practising nurses to give an overview of the changing and challenging world of accident and emergency (A&E) nursing. It has been written with the underlying assumption that readers already possess basic nursing and interpersonal skills. Since it is clearly impossible to include all associated aspects within such a text it is also assumed that nurses, as accountable professionals, will consult other specific works to develop topics as required.

This book is aimed at general nurses of all levels, especially those who may be considering a career within the speciality or who are undertaking a period of relevant academic study. It is subsequently hoped that the book will become a key addition to any reading lists for both level 2 and level 3 study.

In summary, this book has been written by nurses, for nurses. Its aims are equally simple: to highlight the pivotal role of the A&E nurse with rationale for current practice. It is recognized that the culture of accident and emergency nursing is changing progressively and the book attempts to address this by highlighting a number of current professional issues which are seen as being of relevance for the development of innovative practice into the next millennium.

The book has been written by many friends and colleagues who are all advocates of high standards of nursing care. It is subsequently hoped that their enthusiasm is apparent and that it will inspire others to view the speciality in a new and favourable light.

Stuart Toulson
July 2001

Introduction

It has been difficult to create a book on accident and emergency (A&E) nursing which encompasses all the important aspects of care whilst attempting to avoid excessive overlap and repetition. The chapters of the book, therefore, have been written using a standard approach, enabling them to be read either in isolation or in conjunction with others. In using such an approach it is hoped that readers of the book will find it easy to use and will learn how to find relevant information both quickly and easily.

It has also been difficult to decide on the best way of sequencing chapters as certain topics may be seen to fit under a number of chapter headings. The book has consequently been divided into two distinct sections and covers both clinical and professional issues that are seen as relevant for both current and future A&E practice.

The first section of the book addresses clinical conditions commonly seen within the 'majors' side of accident and emergency and continues with those conditions commonly seen within the 'minors' side of departments. Certain chapters are highlighted as falling between the two classifications and therefore cover all spectrums of injury presentation. The second section of the book addresses a number of professional issues and initiatives that are relevant to the practising A&E nurse and which demand attention within such a specialized text. Nurses who are both passionate and enthusiastic about their specialist subject area have compiled the chapters.

The layout of the chapters aims to ensure that all relevant information is covered using a standard format. The chapters highlight the prevalence of specific conditions by outlining relevant aetiology and incidence. Brief mention is made of associated basic anatomy and physiology although it is taken as implicit within the book that readers will consult more detailed texts if further detail is required. All chapters give an overview of common presenting signs and symptoms and outline nursing assessment, intervention and nursing care that may be required, with the associated rationale.

The book covers all information that is deemed necessary to ensure safe practice within A&E and emphasizes the central role of the clinical nurse within the speciality. The philosophy of the book is that all nurses, despite any external financial or manpower restrictions, still believe in delivering the highest standards of holistic nursing care using informed assessment skills to prioritize workload. All chapters have been written by confident and competent practising nurses and are therefore both topical and typical of current clinical practice. All contributing nurses have worked within various A&E departments and objectivity of clinical and professional information should ensure that the book is subsequently characteristic of national A&E practice.

Editing this book has been both a challenging and gratifying experience and it is hoped that the reader will find it just as enjoyable!

Chapter 1
Advanced Trauma Life Support

Stuart Toulson

> In the days of Mother Goose, putting Humpty Dumpty together again couldn't be done: but today, with trauma specialists (pre-hospital personnel, surgeons, nurses) who function on the principle of the 'Golden Hour' (the first hour post-injury during which the shock process must be reversed if the patient is to be saved), it often happens. (Ward, 1985, p. 1)

Introduction

In the United Kingdom, approximately 25,000 people are killed every year as a direct consequence of trauma whilst a further 50,000 sustain major injuries (Robertson and Redmond, 1991). In the under-35 age group, the total number of fatalities due to such injuries exceeds the combined total for deaths caused by both cardiovascular disease and cancer (Irving, 1990). As with most critical illnesses, the quality of the initial assessment and management of the severely injured patient influences the final outcome. An organized, aggressive and consistent approach to trauma management therefore results in optimum patient care (Davies et al., 1992; American College of Surgeons 1993).

This chapter does not aim to be an exhaustive account of trauma resuscitation but offers a basic overview of the standard advanced trauma life support (ATLS) approach to patient care and the subsequent role of the accident and emergency (A&E) nurse. It will highlight why the need for trauma training exists for nursing staff and will stress the importance of a team approach within trauma management.

1

Overview of ATLS Principles

Deaths due to trauma follow three distinct patterns:

(1) The first peak occurs within seconds to minutes after injury, often
    due to lacerations of the brain, brain stem, high spinal cord,
    heart, aorta or other large vessels.
(2) The second death peak happens within minutes to a few hours
    after injury – referred to as the 'Golden Hour'. These deaths are
    due to potentially preventable conditions including subdural or
    extradural haematomas, haemopneumothorax, ruptured spleen,
    lacerations of the liver, pelvic fractures or other multiple injuries
    associated with a significant loss of blood.
(3) The final group dies several days to weeks after injury, usually as a
    result of sepsis and organ failure (American College of Surgeons,
    1993).

It is the protection of life within this first hour following injury that
ATLS training addresses as it is deaths within this time frame that are
viewed as potentially preventable. A team approach to resuscitation
of the trauma patient therefore involves a rapid initial assessment with
subsequent restoration of the body's vital functions. A thorough and
orderly evaluation is then performed to ensure that less obvious
injuries are not overlooked. The underlying principle is to presume
that serious injuries are present until proven otherwise and detracts
from the old style approach of treating only visible symptoms.

Patient management includes:

• a primary survey;
• subsequent resuscitation phase;
• a secondary survey;
• a definitive care phase.

Mechanism of injury

A thorough history in respect of the injury-producing mechanism is
a useful tool in the diagnosis of resultant injuries and the paramedics
are especially competent at providing and relaying such information
to the A&E team. Such injury types are classified according to the
direction and amount of force involved: the energy wave extending
away from the point of impact in blunt trauma and laterally from the
missile pathway in penetrating trauma.

Mechanisms of injury that should alert the A&E nurse to the possibility of significant underlying injury include:

- falls of 20 feet or more;
- patient ejection from a vehicle;
- patient involved in a vehicle 'rollover';
- death of a same-vehicle occupant;
- impacts greater that 20 mph without restraint or 30 mph with restraint;
- pedestrian hit at 20 mph or greater;
- patient in close proximity to an explosion;
- 30 degree deformity of car;
- passenger compartment intrusion – 18° on patient side or 24° on opposite side.

In addition to these criteria the nurse should calculate a patient's overall trauma score and should alert the trauma team/request senior medical assistance immediately should the score be anything less than the maximum 12 (see Table 1.1).

Table 1.1 Revised trauma score

Glasgow coma scale (GCS)	Systolic blood pressure	Respiratory rate	Trauma score
13–15	>89	10–29	4
9–12	76–89	>29	3
6–8	50–75	6-9	2
4–5	1–49	1–5	1
3	0	0	0

The respective injuries that differing mechanisms of injury may cause are highlighted in Table 1.2.

The mnemonic 'AMPLE' is used to highlight key areas of information that the nurse should elicit alongside those relating to the mechanism of injury:

A – allergies;
M – medications;
P – past medical history;
L – last time ate or drank;
E – events/environment (injury mechanism).

Table 1.2 Mechanisms of injury and potential injury patterns

Mechanism of injury	Suspected injury patterns
Frontal impact: • Bent steering wheel • Knee imprint in dashboard • Bull's-eye fracture of windshield	• Cervical spine fracture • Anterior flail chest • Myocardial contusion • Pneumothorax • Transection of aorta (decelerating injury) • Fractured spleen or liver • Posterior fracture/dislocation of hip and/or knee
Side impact to vehicle	• Contralateral neck sprain • Cervical spine fracture • Lateral flail chest • Pneumothorax • Traumatic aortic rupture • Fractured spleen or liver (depending on side of impact) • Fractured pelvis or acetabulum
Rear impact vehicle collision	• Cervical spine fracture
Ejection from vehicle	Such a mechanism can result in virtually all mentioned injury patterns and mortality is significantly increased
Pedestrian	• Head injury • Chest and abdominal injuries • Fractures of lower extremities

Source: American College of Surgeons (1993).

The Primary Survey

This is designed to identify all life-threatening conditions to enable subsequent medical/nursing intervention to commence. The survey involves a rapid examination of the patient by an experienced ATLS-trained doctor. The author would stress that any ATLS-trained nurse should also be prepared to adopt this role if required until senior medical help arrives and may therefore have to guide junior medical colleagues in the principles of the primary survey. The survey is an adaptation of the well-established ABCs of cardiac resuscitation and utilizes all history as obtained from the accident scene. The following criteria are assessed/performed in strict order:

A – airway maintenance with cervical spine control;
B – breathing and ventilation;
C – circulation with haemorrhage control;
D – disability or dysfunction;
E – exposure/environmental control.

It cannot be over-stressed that it must be assumed that all trauma patients have sustained a cervical spine injury and that neck immobilization be maintained, even during emergency airway interventions, until such an injury has been categorically excluded by senior medical staff. This is a prime nursing role and the recommended technique of cervical spine (c-spine) immobilization is with proficient application of a stiff-neck collar with sandbags placed either side of the head and strong tape applied across the patient's forehead prior to fixation to the trolley or spinal board.

Resuscitation Phase

During this phase shock management is initiated, management of patient oxygenation reassessed and haemorrhage control re-evaluated. Any life-threatening conditions identified in the primary survey are constantly reassessed as management is continued.

Secondary Survey

This involves a comprehensive head-to-toe examination, including the recording of all vital signs. Each region of the body is examined individually and in an orderly sequence to ensure that no injury is missed – the 'tubes and fingers into every orifice' philosophy. Standard trauma X-rays of c-spine, chest and pelvis are ordered at this stage. Strict log-rolling techniques with total spine immobilization must be maintained when examining the patient's back at the end of this survey as moving the patient's back incorrectly may result in an unstable spinal injury causing permanent paralysis. Good nursing care dictates that any spinal board should be removed at this point for patient comfort should his/her medical condition allow and that any fragments of glass etc. are removed.

The secondary survey does not begin until the primary survey has been completed and the resuscitation of life-threatening conditions has begun.

Definitive Care Phase

All of the patient's injuries are managed including fracture stabilization, wound dressing, tetanus immunization and any necessary operative interventions that are not immediately life-threatening. The patient may subsequently be transferred at this stage to either a ward or a specialist unit.

The following will highlight the assessment and associated medical/nursing intervention required for all potentially life-threatening conditions identified within the primary survey.

Airway

The nurse should expect either actual or potential airway obstruction in any patient presenting following injury, and assisting in establishing and maintaining a patent airway (whilst maintaining c-spine control) is therefore the first priority. Partial or complete airway compromise may occur unexpectedly following trauma, and definitive airway intervention aims to protect the patient from airway obstruction and aspiration, allowing adequate oxygenation and ventilation. Assessment and continuous reassessment of the patient is therefore essential.

During the initial assessment of the airway the nurse must observe for signs of current or impending airway obstruction and must intervene accordingly.

Assessment will include:

- Is the patient agitated (suggesting hypoxia)?
- Is the patient drowsy (suggesting hypercarbia)?
- Is the patient using accessory muscles of ventilation?
- Is the trachea midline?
- Are there any abnormal breath sounds (e.g. gurgling/stridor/crackles/wheezing/snoring)?

Airway obstruction may present as a result of foreign bodies (teeth, gastric contents etc.) or obstruction by the tongue in the semi-conscious patient, and clearing the airway is an obvious nursing prerequisite to the more complex techniques of airway management.

Basic Airway Intervention

- *Chin lift and jaw thrust*: The chin lift manoeuvre is performed by placing two fingers of one hand under the mandible and gently lifting upward to position the chin anteriorly. The jaw thrust is performed by manually elevating the angles of the mandible to obtain the same effect.
- *Oropharyngeal airway*: This is a mechanical adjunct to the manoeuvre described above and its use should be familiar to the A&E nurse.
- *Nasopharyngeal airway*: These are better tolerated in the semiconscious patient and carry a lesser risk of causing vomiting. Their use is contraindicated in patients with suspected skull fractures.
- *Endotracheal intubation*: This is viewed as the 'gold standard' for airway protection and must be performed with strict in-line cervical spine immobilization and may require nurse assistance to perform cricoid pressure. Indications for endotracheal intubation include apnoea, respiratory insufficiency, upper airway obstruction (actual or potential) and protection of the lower airway from foreign bodies.
- *Nasotracheal intubation*: This is again contraindicated in patients with suspected facial or basilar skull fractures.

Inability to intubate the patient indicates an immediate need for advanced surgical airway intervention.

Advanced Airway Intervention

- *Cricothyroidotomy*: This is indicated in any patient who has a strong indication for intubation but in whom the trachea cannot be intubated. It has become the procedure of choice over the traditional tracheostomy as the trachea resides deeper in the neck and involves a highly vascular surrounding area.
- *Needle cricothyroidotomy*: This can provide up to 45 minutes of extra time so that intubation can be completed, and involves a large-bore needle being inserted into the trachea lumen through the

cricoid membrane. The plastic cannula is then connected to a high-flow oxygen source and intermittent insufflation commenced. This is a last resort, however, and merely buys time.

Nursing intervention must include ensuring that 100% oxygen is administered to the patient since maintaining oxygenation (and so preventing hypercarbia) is an essential goal in trauma resuscitation.

Breathing

The nurse should observe and record:

- respiratory rate;
- presence of chest symmetry/tracheal deviation;
- obvious open sucking chest wounds;
- use of accessory muscles;
- patient colour/pallor;
- mental status.

Life-threatening chest injuries to exclude include:

- *Tension pneumothorax*: Any patient presenting with respiratory distress, tracheal shift, distended neck veins, dullness to chest percussion, hypotension and tachycardia should alert the nurse to the probability of a tension pneumothorax and the associated need for immediate decompression. This occurs owing to the presence of a one-way valve air leak from the lung or through the chest wall. Air is subsequently forced into the thoracic cavity and becomes trapped, resulting in complete collapse of the affected lung and eventual shift of internal organs. This is an emergency clinical diagnosis and should not wait for X-ray confirmation.
- *Open pneumothorax*: This results in an open sucking chest wound causing an imbalance between intrathoracic and atmospheric pressures. Ventilation is impaired and subsequent hypoxia develops. Management includes the application of a sterile three-sided dressing (allowing air out but not in) and chest tube insertion.
- *Large haemothorax*: This involves significant blood loss into the chest cavity (>1500 ml) resulting in both hypotension and hypoxia.

Initial treatment in A&E involves adequate fluid replacement and decompression of the chest cavity by chest tube insertion.

- *Flail chest*: This occurs when a segment of the chest wall loses bony continuity with the rest of the thoracic cage and causes hypoxia owing to disruption of normal chest wall movement. Treatment usually involves intubation and controlled ventilation.

Circulation

Shock can be defined as inadequate organ perfusion and tissue oxygenation. It is important to note that blood loss is the most common remedial cause of morbidity and mortality following trauma, and all types of shock may present (although hypovolaemia is the most common). The first priority in the evaluation of the trauma patient, therefore, is to recognize the presence of shock; this is based on clinical findings and a high sense of suspicion on the part of the nurse rather than on any laboratory results.

It is important for the nurse to realize that the compensatory mechanisms of shock may prevent a fall in systolic blood pressure until the patient has lost up to 30% of his or her blood volume. Early signs of tachycardia and peripheral vasoconstriction are therefore important and, as a golden rule, any patient who is cool and tachycardic should be presumed to be in shock until proven otherwise. Nurse assessment indicating early signs and symptoms of hypovolaemic shock (which reflects underlying physiology) include:

- hypotension (due to hypovolaemia with possible subsequent myocardial insufficiency);
- skin pallor (vasoconstriction due to catecholamine release);
- tachycardia (due to catecholamine release);
- confusion, aggression, drowsiness and coma (due to cerebral hypoxia and acidosis);
- tachypnoea (due to hypoxia and acidosis);
- general weakness (due to hypoxia and acidosis);
- thirst (due to hypovolaemia);
- reduced urine output (due to reduced perfusion) (Baskett, 1991).

Subsequent fluid resuscitation involves the insertion of two large-bore cannulae (size 14 or 16) and use of blood-giving sets (without use of air inlets because of the associated high pressure involved) to ensure a rapid fluid transfusion. Use of a level one blood-warming system is advised to allow rapid transfusion of warmed fluids.

There is a continuing debate regarding which fluid to use in the initial resuscitation of the hypovolaemic patient until type-specific blood or O Rhesus negative packed cells can be obtained. The choice centres around crystalloid fluids such as Hartman's solution and colloid fluids such as Haemaccel. The former has the advantage of being isotonic, so will permeate both the depleted intravascular system and subsequently the depleted extracellular fluid. The latter, however, remains within the circulation, resulting in a more rapid improvement of the patient's haemodynamic status. In practice a combination of both seems to give the best results although isotonic electrolyte solutions are now advocated during the initial fluid resuscitation phase (American College of Surgeons, 1993) with two litres given stat and further fluid replacement being based upon the subsequent response.

In summary, circulatory assessment/intervention centres around:

- control of external bleeding – this is generally controlled by paramedics prior to arrival in A&E but may be continual and significant in quantity. Direct pressure should be used and tourniquets considered only in the most severe circumstances;
- the efficiency of the cardiac pump – empty or collapsed neck veins should alert the nurse to the presence of hypovolaemia whilst distended neck veins suggest the presence of underlying pump failure. It is also important to note that these two conditions may coexist;
- the volume status (degree of shock) - see Table 1.3.

During the primary survey, several absolute emergencies must be recognized and treated:

(1) *Cardiac arrest*: This will follow the standard resuscitation guidelines although may be heavily dependent upon fluid replacement. Subsequent emergency thoracotomy within the A&E department may provide the best chance of survival for the following conditions:

- to control great vessel and cardiac bleeding;
- to release cardiac tamponade;
- to optimize cardiac output;
- to redistribute the available blood to vital organs by cross-clamping the descending aorta.

(2) *Cardiac tamponade*: This causes impairment of the heart action due to blood within the pericardium following injury and may result from blood loss as small as 30 mls. Any patient who is shocked with distended neck veins, cool extremities and no tension pneumothorax should be suspected of having a cardiac tamponade that will require rapid medical aspiration.

(3) *Myocardial contusion*: This may occur following deceleration injuries or crush injuries to the chest and may rapidly result in cardiac arrhythmias.

(4) *Myocardial infarction*: Underlying infarction may have been the cause of the accident or a result of subsequent coronary under-perfusion.

Table 1.3 Classification of hypovolaemic shock according to blood loss

	Class 1	Class 2	Class 3	Class 4
Blood loss (ml)	Up to 750	750–1500	1500–2000	>2000
Blood loss (%)	Up to 15%	15–30%	30–40%	>40%
Pulse rate	<100	>100	>120	>140
Blood pressure	Normal	Normal	Decreased	Decreased
Pulse pressure	Normal or increased	Decreased	Decreased	Decreased
Respiratory rate	14–20	20–30	30–40	>35
Urine output (ml)	>30	20–30	5–15	Negligible
Mental state	Slightly anxious	Mildly confused	Anxious Lethargic	Confused

Disability

A rapid assessment of cerebral function is performed using the AVPU method with associated recording of pupillary response:

- Is the patient Alert?
- Does he/she respond to Verbal stimuli?
- Does he/she respond to Painful stimuli?
- Is he/she Unresponsive?

Exposure

All the patient's clothing is removed to allow a thorough front and back assessment of the patient, with the nurse remembering the basics of patient warmth and dignity.

The Trauma Team

The multiply injured patient has, by definition, multiple problems and adequate treatment necessitates a team approach. Trauma teams must be organized appropriately and work well in a well-equipped resuscitation room (Driscoll and Skinner, 1991) and research has highlighted that a structured organized team, with predetermined roles and responsibilities for both nursing and medical staff, has a direct positive bearing on patient outcome (Lomas and Goodall, 1994). The ATLS system is designed such that a single doctor or nurse can safely and systematically assess the treatment priorities of the multiply injured patient until help arrives, because tasks are performed in sequence, one after the other. In reality, this 'vertical' approach is rarely needed and the 'horizontal' team approach is practised with a significant reduction in resuscitation times. Team members may vary, but the following are advocated for optimal team performance and patient care:

- team leader (the most experienced member of the A&E team);
- anaesthetist (of senior level, with assistant – nurse or ODP);
- general surgeon (of senior registrar level or above);
- orthopaedic surgeon (of senior registrar level or above);
- A&E SHO;
- two nurses (or three if no ODP to assist anaesthetist);
- radiographer;

- scribe (nurse/doctor);
- porter (outside the resuscitation room ready to transfer bloods etc).

Roles and responsibilities may also vary between departments, but it is advocated that predetermined action cards are provided for all staff with regular trauma scenarios to clarify roles and to enhance team-building, respect and understanding between team members. It is also advised that team members meet on a monthly basis to discuss any trauma calls and any problem areas in need of address.

Nurse Training in Trauma Care

The arrival in A&E of a critically injured patient is potentially one of the most difficult situations that can confront a nurse, especially as several patients can be brought in simultaneously from the same incident (Walsh, 1985). A nurse is usually the first member of the hospital personnel to meet injured patients within the A&E setting, and must have the skills to assess the injuries quickly and accurately and decide upon the urgency with which they will be treated (Hamilton, 1993). Incorrect care or lack of intervention may result in death, further disability or irreversible damage to the brain or spinal cord (Jones, 1986) and the goal of doing the patient no harm requires total immobilization of the spine until injury has been excluded (Tippett, 1993).

In a survey of A&E nurses, Hamilton (1991) concluded that half lacked knowledge in caring for the multiply injured patient. The author reported that 66% of junior nurses had received no formal training in trauma care despite the fact that 81% may have been left in charge of a trauma patient. It was clear that both nursing and medical staff should share a common core of knowledge because a coordinated and well-rehearsed approach to trauma patient care, where all assessment and interventions are performed simultaneously, is essential for quality care (Castille, 1991). The ATLS working party concurred that nurses were very much equal partners in team management of trauma care and should have access to the same theoretical training as their medical colleagues (Skinner, 1991). The high rate of self-funded places by nurses on such courses has previously highlighted that a strong motivation to improve knowledge exists (Eyre, 1993) whilst formal nurse training using an abbreviated ATLS model has also demonstrated measurable improvement in both thought and action priorities (Gautam and Heyworth, 1994).

Indeed, many doctors now agree that the widespread introduction of ATLS courses and trauma teams has significantly improved the initial management of severely injured patients (Nolan, 1995).

Conclusion

Advanced trauma life support has now become well established throughout the world as the gold standard for trauma care. Gone are the days of nurses and doctors treating only what the eye could see by applying pressure to a bleeding wound whilst failing to recognize that the patient is apnoeic. The systematic and standardized nature of ATLS enables a nurse to enter any A&E department and become a safe and valuable member of the trauma team. It has resulted in the two professions of medicine and nursing working side by side as an efficient and coherent team, with the common goal of saving lives and with mutual respect for the role that each speciality plays.

Suggested Further Reading

American College of Surgeons (1993) The Advanced Trauma Life Support Course. Chicago: American College of Surgeons.

British Medical Journal (1991) ABC of Major Trauma. London: British Medical Journal.

References

American College of Surgeons (1993) Advanced Trauma Life Support Course. Chicago: American College of Surgeons.

Baskett PJF (1991) Management of hypovolaemic shock. In Skinner D, Driscoll P, Earlam R (Eds) ABC of Major Trauma. London: British Medical Journal.

Castille K (1991) Trauma training for nurses. Nursing 4(32): 22–3.

Davies S, Hill P, Wood L, Maryosh J (1992) Assessing trauma. Nursing Times 88(17): 54–7.

Driscoll P, Skinner D (1991) Initial assessment and management. In Skinner D, Driscoll P, Earlam R (Eds) ABC of Major Trauma. London: British Medical Journal.

Eyre G (1993) Shock treatment. Nursing Times 89(34): 30–3.

Gautam V, Heyworth J (1994) The value of the abbreviated ATLS course for accident and emergency nurses. Accident and Emergency Nursing 2(2): 100–2.

Hamilton A (1991) Trauma training. Nursing Times 87(2): 43–4.

Hamilton A (1993) Trauma: initial assessment skills. Accident and Emergency Nursing 1(4): 183–98.

Irving M (1990) Foreword. In Skinner D, Driscoll P, Earlam R (Eds) ABC of Major Trauma. London: British Medical Journal.

Jones G (1986) Learning to Care in the A&E Department. London: Hodder & Stoughton, p 86.

Lomas GA, Goodall O (1994) Trauma teams vs non-trauma teams. Accident and Emergency Nursing 2(4): 205–10.

Nolan JP (1995) Resuscitation of the trauma patient. Care of the Critically Ill 11(6): 222–6.

Robertson C, Redmond AD (1991) The Management of Major Trauma. Oxford: Oxford University Press, p 5.

Skinner DV (1991) The Advanced Trauma Life Support (ATLS) Course in The Royal London Hospital Emergency Medical Service. Herts: Saltdatore, p 46.

Tippett J (1993) Spinal immobilisation of the multiply injured patient. Accident and Emergency Nursing 1(1): 25–33.

Walsh M (1985) Accident and Emergency Nursing: A New Approach. London: Heinemann Nursing, p 55.

Ward JM (1985) Foreword. In Cardona VD (Ed) Trauma Nursing. New Jersey: Medical Economics.

Chapter 2
Cardiac Emergencies

KATHY STEWARD AND HELEN MURDOCH

Introduction

Any nurse working within the field of accident and emergency (A&E) will be familiar with patients displaying the symptoms of a potential cardiac-related problem; chest pain, collapse and shortness of breath. It is therefore essential that the A&E nurse is able to identify such signs and symptoms and know treatment patterns for cardiac emergencies to ensure that patients are cared for safely and effectively within the busy A&E environment. This chapter seeks to explain why cardiac problems occur, how they commonly present and to outline the care that patients subsequently require.

The Heart

The main function of the heart is to supply constant circulation of blood throughout the body. The heart is a sophisticated pump with four chambers: two atria and two ventricles. It lies in the thoracic cavity in the mediastinum between the lungs and its tissues consist of three layers:

- the pericardium, which is made up of two layers – an outer fibrous sac and a double layer of serous membrane;
- the myocardium – specialist muscle cells that are found only in the heart. As a heartbeat is initiated it very quickly spreads across the myocardium owing to the nature and arrangement of these cells;
- the endocardium – a smooth lining to the inside of the heart chambers that continues from the lining of the blood vessels.

16

Blood Flow through the Heart

Initially blood enters the right atrium via the inferior and superior venae cavae. The blood then passes through the atrioventricular valve into the right ventricle. The deoxygenated blood flows into the pulmonary artery where it is carried round the lungs for gaseous exchange to take place. The now oxygenated blood flows via the pulmonary veins into the left atrium and then into the left ventricle. The left ventricle, the most muscular part of the heart, then expels the blood through the aorta and around the body. The heart obtains its own blood supply via the left and right coronary arteries that branch from the aorta immediately after the aortic valve.

The Conduction System of the Heart

The conduction system of the heart is intrinsic (i.e. no nerve impulse is required from the brain). However, the nervous system can stimulate or depress this intrinsic system. The initiation and conduction of an impulse is carried out by groups of specialized cells. The sinoatrial node (SA node), located in the right atrium, is the pacemaker of the heart. The atrioventricular node (AV node), situated near the atrial septum, can be thought of as the gateway to the ventricles and is stimulated by a wave of impulses passing though the atria. The impulse is then carried by the bundle of His across the fibrous ring separating the atria and the ventricles. The fibrous ring acts to delay the impulse in order to allow for ventricular filling. The bundle of His then separates into the right and left bundle branches. These eventually divide into fine fibres, called the Purkinje fibres, which effect a wave of contraction to sweep up though the ventricles. It is important to note that there are many areas of the heart capable of initiating impulses and all conductive tissue of the heart has an inherent rate. The SA node, being the fastest, is the normal pacemaker. However, if this slows down then another area may take over.

The approximate intrinsic rates are:

• sinoatrial node 70-75 bpm;
• atrioventricular node 60 bpm;
• bundle of His 50-55 bpm;

- Purkinje fibres 30-45 bpm ;
- myocardium 15-30 bpm.

Nerves from the cardiac centre in the brain also influence the myocardium. The vagus nerve supplies the SA and AV nodes, reducing the rate of impulses, whilst the sympathetic drive tends to increase the rate and force of the heartbeat. The catecholamines also have a similar effect on the heart with adrenaline stimulating and noradrenaline depressing the heart's activity. An increased heart rate can occur due to temperature, exercise, anxiety, smoking, thyrotoxicosis, myocardial infarction, heart failure, toxic shock, adrenaline or atropine. Heart rate may decrease due to myxoedema, myocardial infarction, obstructive jaundice, increased parasympathetic tone (vagal stimuli), raised intracranial pressure, digoxin or beta-blockers. It is normally slowed during sleep.

The Cardiac Cycle

Cardiac cycle is the term used to describe the contraction and relaxation of the heart. It lasts for approximately 0.8 seconds and involves a period of atrial systole (contraction), ventricular systole and then complete cardiac diastole (relaxation). By attaching the patient to an electrocardiograph (ECG) a picture of the cardiac cycle can be seen.

The ECG is an invaluable tool when assessing and monitoring patients with potential and real cardiac problems. It reflects the voltage change produced on the surface of the body as a result of electrical activity in the heart. The complex pattern seen on the ECG paper represents a full cycle of cardiac events of the heart and is labelled P, Q, R, S, T, and U.

Each labelled section represents part of the cardiac cycle as follows:

- P wave – atrial activity (depolarization);
- P-R interval – short period of impulse delay within the AV node;
- QRS complex – the conduction of an impulse through the ventricles (depolarization);
- ST segment – the end of ventricular depolarization to the beginning of ventricular repolarization;

- T wave – repolarization of the ventricles (N.B. atrial repolarization happens simultaneously and is therefore hidden);
- U wave – repolarization of the Purkinje fibres (rarely seen).

An ECG is always recorded at the same speed, 25 mm per second; therefore on ECG paper a small square will equal 0.04 seconds, a large square equals 0.2 seconds and five large squares equals one second of the heart's activity. Each stage of the cardiac cycle can be expected to be completed within a certain time on a normal ECG and any deviation from this indicates an abnormality.

The timings are as follows:

- P-R interval 0.12–0.20s (3–5 small squares);
- QRS complex 0.08–0.11s (2–2.5 small squares);
- ST segment 0.27–0.33s;
- QT interval 0.35–0.42s.

When the electrical activity of the heart flows towards an electrode this is shown as a positive deflection and where it flows from an electrode it is a negative deflection. Each deflection should return to the isoelectric line.

A rhythm strip gives one view of the heart, whereas a twelve-lead ECG provides a multidimensional representation. When interpreting an ECG it should be approached in a systematic manner. Quinn and Jones (1996) advocated that the nurse should ask these questions when interpreting an ECG:

- What is the rate?
- Is the QRS regular?
- Is there evidence of atrial activity?
- Is the atrial activity related to the QRS complex?
- Is the QRS normal?

This will give enough information to detect abnormalities, even on a rhythm strip, allowing the nurse to establish treatment priorities. Remember: always judge an ECG in conjunction with the patient's clinical condition and history.

When Things Go Wrong: Ischaemic Heart Disease

The most common cause of unstable angina, myocardial infarction and sudden death is ischaemic heart disease (IHD). Ischaemic heart disease is an umbrella term used to describe the disease process of reduction, interruption or cessation of blood supply to the heart muscle caused mainly by atheroma or atherosclerosis of the coronary arteries (Thompson and Webster, 1992).

Despite a steady decline since the 1970s, IHD still accounts for 25% of all deaths in the United Kingdom. The Office for National Statistics (OFNS, 1997) suggested in its conclusions that prevention is better than cure and that the decline of IHD is due to better education that has resulted in a reduction of smoking and an improvement in diet. Although prevention is better than cure, hospital emergency teams still have a vital role to play since sudden death has been shown to be the first manifestation in 20% of myocardial infarctions. The role of thrombolysis as part of the hospital treatment has not, as yet, conclusively been labelled as a major factor in the reduction of deaths from IHD. However, receiving thrombolysis immediately after myocardial infarction has been seen to reduce the risk of mortality by 25%. A recent study cited in OFNS (1997) demonstrated that mortality in a Minneapolis hospital had declined by 41% between 1985 and 1990 in the 25–74 age group as a result of new treatment strategies, namely thrombolytic drugs. This is mentioned to demonstrate its usefulness in the reduction of overall deaths rather than in the prevention of the disease, and these figures clearly show that the work carried out in A&E departments has a significant contribution to make.

Who does and does not acquire IHD is a matter subject to intense research and analysis. Many factors are thought to influence the incidence of IHD and it can be tempting, based on the long list of risk factors, to form a stereotype of the kind of patient who would be expected to present with symptoms suggestive of IHD. It must be remembered, however, that stereotypes can prevent an objective patient assessment because a person with one or none of the known risk factors may still present with a life-threatening form of IHD.

Risk Factors for Ischaemic Heart Disease

- Lipoproteins
- Obesity
- Culture
- Cigarette smoking
- Diabetes
- Alcohol
- High blood pressure
- Lack of physical activity
- Stress

(Thompson and Webster, 1992)

Progression to Angina and Myocardial Infarction

When the coronary arteries become diseased, the symptom of angina pectoris can occur. To produce symptoms the stenosis of the vessel lumen usually exceeds 75% and compromises blood flow, especially on increased demand. In 90% of cases this narrowing is caused by athero-sclerosis although other less common causes include spasm, embolism, thrombus, dissection or aneurysm (Thompson and Webster, 1992). Atherosclerosis is characterized by an accumulation of smooth muscle cells and lipid within the intima of large and medium arteries.

When the endothelium is damaged, atheroma (plaques) are formed. Injury is caused by numerous factors including lipoprotein levels, haemodynamic forces and chemicals (e.g. tobacco). Minor endothelial damage will heal, causing a slight thickening of the intima, whilst repeated or long-lasting injury leads to further plaques being formed. As the disease progresses, the lumen of the artery is narrowed and there is a greater risk of the plaque rupturing.

The heart, unlike other muscles, cannot sustain oxygen debt as it relies on aerobic metabolism. It extracts oxygen from the coronary artery blood, so that to increase oxygen to the heart an increased coronary artery blood flow is required. This relies on the coronary arteries being able to increase their diameter and as the lumen of diseased vessels is narrowed by atheroma the arteries are unable to perform this function adequately. The pain experienced in angina pectoris and unstable angina is a symptom of, in part, that supply and demand imbalance where coronary artery disease is present. The pain is also due to a metabolic process that occurs when the heart experiences hypoxia. Normal cardiac function is dependent on an adequate supply of high-energy phosphate compounds, especially adenosine triphosphate (ATP), and these are metabolized using oxygen. Where a lack of oxygen occurs, oxidative phosphorylation is inhibited and there is a shift to anaerobic metabolism that is less efficient. The now ischaemic and hypoxic heart produces lactic acid and other metabolites that, as they accumulate, cause the pH to fall. Anaerobic metabolism is inhibited and production of high-energy compounds halts. Ischaemia (inadequate blood flow) therefore causes pain and decreased myocardial function.

In angina pectoris, the ischaemia is transient and reversible. The discomfort produced is identified by four factors:

* location;
* character;
* relation to exercise;
* duration (Julian and Cowan, 1992).

It is not related to myocardial necrosis.

Patients who present to A&E with angina are usually those with new angina or those in whom the angina has become unstable. Angina is considered unstable when existing angina is uncontrolled owing to reduced effectiveness of the present treatment caused by disease progression. To the patient this can mean increased severity or frequency of angina attacks.

Julian and Cowan (1992) stated that it is helpful for health professionals to see ischaemia, injury and infarct (and therefore angina and myocardial infarction) as being on a continuum rather than as separate events, because all are caused by the same underlying disease process. However, it is also important to note the differences that exist between these conditions.

Within approximately 30–40 minutes of total ischaemia the myocardial cells are permanently damaged. Infarction is the necrosis of a proportion of the myocardium and is irreversible. In most acute myocardial infarctions (MI) atheroma fissure through their fibrous caps allowing blood to flow into the plaque, resulting in thrombus formation. This thrombus causes muscle infarction when complete obstruction of the coronary artery takes place for 20 minutes or more. The body can thrombolyse such clots, although this occurs over days or hours and so depending upon the length of time taken the person will experience either resolution of symptoms or become acutely unwell. Acute myocardial infarction is therefore characterized by myocardial necrosis but will also cause areas of ischaemia and injury.

The necrosed area will eventually become scar tissue, reducing the effective functioning of the heart. Prognosis of patients with acute myocardial infarction is directly related to the quality of surviving myocardium and much of the nursing care is related to improving this quality.

Assessment of a Patient With Chest Pain

When a person arrives in A&E with chest pain a rapid assessment is essential in order to establish whether or not the pain is of cardiac origin and whether or not the pain is a symptom of a myocardial infarction. As necrosis of the myocardium occurs within 30–40 minutes of total ischaemia, 'time is muscle', and any delays in diagnosis and treatment can affect patient prognosis (Julian, 1990). Studies such as ISIS-2 (1988) have shown early thrombolytic therapy can reverse the advancement of cell death and reduce morbidity and mortality. McMurry and Rankin (1994), in their summary of advances in healthcare, stated that the earlier treatment is given the better. With this in mind the initial assessment need only be a brief outline of data, enough to establish 'does this patient need thrombolysis?'.

The initial assessment should include an ECG, a brief investigation into the pain – its nature, intensity, and duration (Quinn, 1997), a short past medical history, observation of the patient's general condition and his/her vital signs. General observations of the patient should include heart rate, respiration rate, blood pressure and oxygen saturation in addition to observing the patient's skin colour for pallor or cyanosis. It is also important to note whether the patient is nauseated or vomiting and the current level of consciousness.

These observations will:

• establish a baseline for subsequent observations;
• indicate the possible presence of complications (e.g. shock, arrhythmias);

- complete the picture of ECG findings or, if the ECG is inconclusive, these observations will help build up a clinical picture that can aid diagnosis.

Following this rapid assessment the ECG and clinical findings should be shown to a clinician who can interpret ECGs and is able to prescribe thrombolysis.

When assessing pain it is important that accurate and comprehensive information is obtained, despite the rapid nature of the assessment, as one of the most important functions of a nurse is to alleviate suffering. Pain is a complex phenomenon and why some people experience what is thought to be more pain than others is influenced by many variables. Cooper (1994) described these as:

- sociocultural (a person's background and upbringing);
- emotional state (anxiety has been found to increase pain);
- previous experience (found to increase or decrease pain);
- significance of pain (what the pain means to the patient);
- distraction (what attention he/she gives to the pain);
- duration and intensity (acute pain is threatening, chronic pain is wearing).

These factors do not increase or decrease pain but affect a person's reaction to it (Scholfield, 1995). Often a person's chief complaint when having an acute myocardial infarction is chest pain (Akyrou et al., 1995, O'Connor, 1995). Pain relief is therefore essential, as after the patient arrives in A&E the pain no longer serves a useful purpose (Tanabe, 1995).

Despite the importance to the patient of pain assessment and relief, nurses have consistently been found to assess pain inaccurately and to give inadequate analgesia as a result (O'Connor, 1995; Tanabe, 1995). O'Connor (1995) reported that nurses underestimated pain in 46% of patients with acute myocardial infarction and documented only half of the information representative of a complete pain assessment. Nurses were found to document pain from their own perspective, including only site and verbal report of pain, leaving out quality, intensity and duration. If these aspects are omitted from assessment and documentation then care may be compromised as these are the very factors that help determine whether or not the pain is of cardiac origin. Pain assessment is insufficient when it is subjective, unrecorded and does not incorporate the patient's actual pain experience.

Many authors recommend having a formal pain assessment tool as part of assessment and history taking (Cooper, 1994, Akyrou et al., 1995, O'Connor, 1995, Tanabe, 1995). Of all the different types of objective pain assessment tools, visual analogue scales (VAS) have been found to best measure intensity. However, chest pain assessment should include onset, possible cause (e.g. past medical history or mechanism), site, the patient's description of the pain and relieving and/or aggravating factors. For this reason such scales have been found to be inadequate when used in isolation (Scholfield,1995).

McGill's Pain Questionnaire is an example of a more comprehensive assessment tool, allowing for all the different aspects of pain and influences to be considered. However, in an acute setting it can become too complicated and time consuming. Indeed, there are a number of other pain tools and by focusing on just these two it is easy to see that both have advantages and disadvantages related to the setting in which they are to be used. It may be said, therefore, that no single tool is the solution to pain assessment and that tools serve only as a basis of an assessment that relies on good communication and health professionals believing the patient's description of his/her pain (McCaffery and Beebe, 1989/1994).

A&E nurses may further improve their assessment skills through knowledge of the characteristics of cardiac chest pain. These characteristics are demonstrated in Table 2.1.

Table 2.1 The characteristics of cardiac chest pain

Angina	*Myocardial infarction*
Gradual building onset	Sudden or gradual onset
Heavy or crushing pain lasting for 5 to 10 minutes	Severe heaviness/constriction lasting for more than 20 minutes
Patient often clenches the fist over the sternum	Retrosternal and radiating down the arms
Retrosternal radiating to jaw, arms, shoulders and neck	Associated with nausea, weakness, pallor, syncope, dyspnoea
Often occurring after meals, stress, sexual activity or dream-sleep	With or without history of IHD
Associated with dyspnoea and weakness	Not related to exercise
Often relieved by rest	Patients may also experience an impending sense of doom

Source: Green (1992).

As part of the initial assessment the ECG is one of the most important tools in diagnosing and evaluating a patient with cardiac problems. Therefore, whilst it is essential for the treating clinician to see and act upon the ECG, it is also important that nurses have a certain skill in interpretation to enable them to prioritize care.

Damage to the myocardium, either permanent in the case of infarct or reversible in the case of ischaemia, can be differentiated according to the changes that present on the ECG. It can also be used to show the location of myocardial damage, allowing for prediction of complications. This is made possible as the electrodes are always placed in the same anatomical position and so always correspond to a specific area of the heart (Figure 2.1).

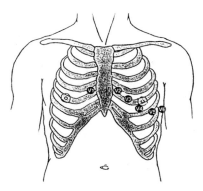

V1 – 4th intercostal space right sternal edge
V2 – 4th intercostal space left sternal edge
V3 – Halfway between V2 &V4
V4 – 5th intercostal space in the midclavicular line
V5 – anterior axillary line level with V4
V6 – midaxillary line level with V4

Figure 2.1 Position of ECG electrodes.

The ECG representation of the areas of the heart can be summarized as follows:

- extensive anterior I, aVL and V1–V6;
- anteroseptal I, aVL and V1–V4;
- anterolateral I, aVL and V4–V6;
- inferior II–III and aVF.

The ECG Criteria of Ischaemia

Ischaemia is usually transient, but may be more prolonged when it is representative of an ischaemic area surrounding an injured/ infarcted area. The ECG will show inverted T waves and/or ST segment depression in the leads facing the affected area. The T wave inversion is symmetrical and pointed. ST depression occurs when an ST segment dips 1 or 2 mm or more below the isoelectric line for 0.08 seconds. Ischaemia should also be suspected where a flat or depressed ST segment makes a sharp angle when joining the T wave.

The ECG Criteria of Injury

The sign of myocardial injury has been called the 'hallmark of an MI' (Gonce-Morton, 1996). In injury the ST segments elevate greater than 1 mm in standard (limb) leads and 2 mm in the precordial (chest) leads. The ST segment tends to have a concave or cove shape and merges with the T wave. This will be in leads facing the affected area.

The ECG Criteria of Infarction

Infarction occurs when acute injury persists. The infarction process passes through three stages: the hyperacute phase, fully evolved phase and finally resolution (Thompson and Webster, 1992). The hyperacute phase occurs within the first few hours of onset of acute myocardial infarction, the transition to the fully evolved stage taking up to 24 hours. For this reason the hyperacute stage is often missed. ECG markers are an elevated ST segment with a tall and widened T wave. In the fully evolved stage the ECG shows myocardial necrosis, reflected in a broad and deep Q wave in the leads facing the necrosed area. The necrosed tissue is inert and cannot depolarize/ repolarize and this area becomes a window, so that any electrode placed over this window will show activity of other muscles.

The phase of resolution occurs within the following weeks. The ST segment gradually returns to the baseline and the T waves return to normal (although this can take many months) and the only evidence of the MI is pathological Q waves. Old copies of ECGs should therefore be kept within the A&E notes so that any abnormalities in an ECG can be compared with previous recordings.

After the initial assessment, serial ECGs should be taken because, as stated earlier, ischaemia, injury and infarct are part of a continuum, and changes need to be detected early and treatment initiated.

The changes found on an ECG can be summarized as follows:

- T wave changes – ischaemia;
- ST segment changes – injury;
- Q wave changes – infarction.

Once the diagnosis is made, treatment will follow one of four pathways:

- fast track, where evidence of myocardial infarction exists and the patient quickly receives thrombolysis;
- slow track, where myocardial infarction is suspected but further investigations are required;
- there is evidence of ischaemia but no suspicion of infarct and the patient is treated for unstable angina;
- the patient is found to have a non-cardiac cause for his/her pain and is diagnosed and treated accordingly.

Ongoing Care and Treatment

Care of the Patient with Unstable Angina

The main complication of unstable angina is progression to a myocardial infarction (MI) which occurs in between 10% and 20% of patients (Julian and Cowan, 1992). The patient's primary complaint on admission is usually chest pain of unusual presentation for him/her or that has not been relieved by his/her normal medications. Treatment is therefore aimed at alleviating pain and also preventing progression to a MI.

Pharmacological treatment may involve nitrates, aspirin and heparin. Nitrates are given as they act to dilate the coronary arteries and so alleviate pain that has been caused by the narrowed intima of the coronary arteries and the subsequent hypoxia. Initially, buccal glyceral trinitrate may be used but if this is ineffective and the patient's blood pressure is above 100 mmHg systolic then a nitrate infusion may be commenced. Aspirin is given to prevent platelet aggregation. Heparin, an anticoagulant, may also be given as it has been found to reduce risk of progression to MI. Oxygen is given to ensure a high circulating concentration of oxygen to aid in the prevention of hypoxia.

Nursing considerations include frequent assessment of the patient's pain, vital signs and repeated ECGs. This is especially important when pain is unresolved or becomes more severe, because it is essential that changes to the patient's condition and ECG are detected early. The patient should be encouraged to rest, especially in the acute stages of the illness, as activity increases myocardial demand for oxygen and therefore may worsen myocardial ischaemia. These patients can be extremely anxious and information, explanation and reassurance are essential.

Care of a Patient with Acute Myocardial Infarction

Myocardial infarction is an acute life-threatening disorder. The care of a patient with an acute myocardial infarction (AMI) should therefore be treated with the same urgency as a cardiac arrest (Rawles, 1996) and the care of such patients is similarly a team effort involving both medical and nursing staff. After rapid assessment and diagnosis these patients require oxygen, intravenous cannulation, blood tests (including cardiac enzymes), aspirin, analgesia and thrombolysis if no contraindications exist.

Fear is a common feature of acute myocardial infarction (Rowe, 1995) and therefore information and reassurance are important nursing considerations. A helpful mnemonic for remembering treatment priorites is to use the TPA or STREP abbreviations:

T = thrombolysis	S = stop occlusion
P = pain relief OR	T = treat pain
A = anxiety relief	R = rapidly
	E = ease anxiety
	P = pass on information

The use of thrombolysis has transformed the care of the patient with acute myocardial infarction. In the 1980s several large studies (GISSI, 1986; ISIS-2, 1988) highlighted that early use of thrombolysis could reverse the advancement of myocardial cell death and reduce morbidity and mortality. That time is muscle has already been

emphasized and this is especially true in the administration of thrombolysis. When given 4–6 hours after onset of symptoms, approximately 25 lives per 1000 treated are saved; when given in the second
to third hour, 27 lives per 1000 treated are saved; and when given in
the first hour, 65 lives per 1000 treated are saved (Weston et al., 1994).
Therefore a dramatic improvement in a patient's prognosis can be
seen when thrombolysis is given early. Although the greatest benefit is
gained within the first six hours, some benefit is gained up to 12 hours
after onset and so it is routinely given to patients up to 12 hours after
onset of symptoms (McMurry and Rankin, 1994; Why, 1994).

How does thrombolysis work? The body has its own clot-dissolving
system (intrinsic fibrinolytic system) which is balanced with the clotting cascade to ensure that clotting does not occur in the general
circulation. Thrombolysis enhances the effect of this fibrinolytic
system so that lysis exceeds clot formation.

As delay in drug administration has a devastating effect on the
outcome for the patient, in both length and quality of life, much
work has been done to study where the cause of any delay may lie
and what can be done to reduce this. The different stages where
delays can occur can be summarized as follows:

- time of onset of symptoms to the call for help;
- call to hospital (door);
- door to diagnosis;
- diagnosis to drug therapy.

The Health of the Nation document recommended a door-to-needle
(drug therapy) time of 30 minutes (Quinn and Jones, 1996) and the
British Heart Foundation stated that the call to thrombolysis time
should be less than 60 minutes and no more than 90 minutes
(McMurry and Rankin, 1994; Weston et al., 1994).

Patient delay from onset of symptoms to the call for help
remains a big problem as this is the least controllable area. Many
patients do not recognize their symptoms as being of cardiac origin
and believe that their symptoms are not severe enough to be
considered a serious problem. Even patients with known IHD,
who make up 30% of those who suffer acute myocardial infarction,
do not present any earlier (Leitch et al., 1989). Mass media
campaigns educating patients as to the possible signs and symptoms of an AMI have been shown to be effective but only for a

short time (Herlitz et al., 1989) and it is apparent that further research into this area is required.

The delays that occur in stage two, the call-to-door time, often depend upon local practices. In the majority of cases the ambulance service is the most appropriate service to call in cases of chest pain of probable underlying cardiac origin. However, in the GREAT study (1992) a trial was undertaken to assess the safety and efficacy of thrombolysis given at home by general practitioners within a rural setting. It was found that GPs gave rapid high-quality care that improved the outcome for the patient, especially where thrombolysis was given within two hours of onset of symptoms. Delays in time to thrombolysis can also be reduced at this stage by a call to inform the A&E team of an incoming patient with a possible MI, and by the ambulance crew undertaking cannulation, and administration of oxygen therapy and aspirin where protocol allows.

The A&E team plays a vital role in reducing the door-to-diagnosis and drug therapy time. Morris (1997) subsequently suggested that definition of roles for a fast track MI team be implemented to further speed up the delivery of thrombolytic therapy. The following roles were advocated:

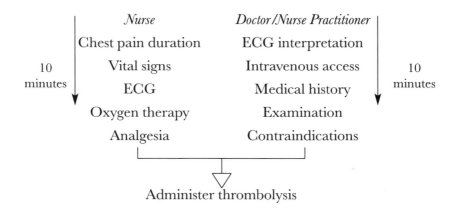

The only acceptable delay is where diagnosis is not clear and when cardiac enzyme results are needed. This slow-track approach should also be treated with a sense of urgency and the laboratory should be informed accordingly. When any muscle is damaged, enzymes are released. Creatinine kinase and its isoenzymes MM, MB and BB are found in skeletal muscle, myocardial tissue and brain tissue respectively. CK-MB is cardiospecific and a rise can be diagnostic of an MI. Cardiac enzymes and other biochemical tests are of limited usefulness in the initial stages of the treatment of a MI as they are not immediately available. However, the test results can play an important role in cases where diagnosis from the history and ECG are unclear. They are also important for the medical team in the assessment of patient progress.

Clear guidelines for the administration of thrombolysis should be available. For example:

- 30 minutes or longer history of pain typical of a MI;
- ECG changes, namely ST segment elevation in two or more leads, 0.1 mV in the limb leads and 0.2 mV in the precordial leads, or new left bundle branch block.

Unfortunately, not all patients are suitable for thrombolytic therapy as certain contraindications exist. However, few of these contraindications are absolute and at all times the risk of treatment should be measured against the benefits to the patient (Hendrick, 1994; Flisher, 1995). The main complications of thrombolysis are haemorrhage, allergic reaction, hypotension and reperfusion arrhythmias. A patient may also experience further pain if the therapy has been ineffective or if there is further artery occlusion.

Contraindications to thrombolytic therapy include:

- known allergy to streptokinase;
- recent streptococcal infection;
- previous CVA (within the last year);
- active peptic ulceration;
- recent surgery (within the last six days);
- possible aortic dissection;
- pregnancy;
- anticoagulation therapy;
- recent central or arterial line insertion;
- diastolic pressure above 110 mmHg. (Flisher, 1995, p. 565).

Those most at risk from haemorrhage are those of advanced age, patients with low body weight and those with hypertension. Hypotension and allergic reaction are most common with streptokinase as it is a natural bacterium. In each case the problem is treated symptomatically. In hypotension STREP can be stopped or slowed to allow BP to recover.

The blood returning to the affected and previously jeopardized area of the heart may causes reperfusion arrhythmias. The most common arrhythmias are bradycardia and idioventricular rhythms. These usually resolve spontaneously and are of no harm to the patient. Further pain should not be ignored as it may indicate reocclusion of an artery. A 12-lead ECG should be performed and compared with previous ECGs, and pain relief should be given accordingly. Unresolving or worsening pain can represent unresolving or worsening infarct. In these cases different thrombolysis is given or patients may be transferred for urgent angioplasty.

The benefit of aspirin in conjunction with thrombolysis has been proven in clinical trials (Wyllie and Dunn, 1994). It works by inhibiting platelet aggregation and prevents a partly lysed thrombus building up again. It should subsequently be given to all patients who have suffered a myocardial infarction as it significantly reduces the risk of reinfarction (Bhagat, 1994). A delay in giving aspirin to patients has not been found to reduce its benefits (Deeks et al., 1995).

Oxygen is a supportive therapy given to reduce hypoxia. In the majority of cases high-flow oxygen is indicated although this should be reassessed after the initial resuscitation. Oxygen therapy dries mucous membranes and so humidified oxygen is preferable and frequent mouth care is essential. Heparin is given in some cases after thrombolysis to prevent reocclusion of the reperfused artery, although the evidence that heparin reduces mortality rates is not clear-cut.

Pain relief is a major component of the care of a patient with acute myocardial infarction. As discussed earlier this may be the patient's main complaint, although the nurse should be aware that acute myocardial infarction can occur with no pain at all. Pain is detrimental to the patient as it may increase blood pressure, heart rate and stroke volume, compromising the coronary circulation further and so increasing myocardial oxygen demand and infarct size (Rowe, 1995).

Nitrates are often given in the initial stages of treatment as part of the pain-relief strategy. However, the usual pharmacological treatment for pain caused by acute myocardial infarction is diamorphine. This should be given intravenously as this is more effective against pain and will not interfere with enzyme results if non-cardiospecific enzymes are taken. Diamorphine also has a euphoric effect that can be useful in reducing stress levels. Reduction of anxiety reduces the body's stress responses such as tachycardia, which in turn alleviates the work of the heart. Information given to the patient and his/her family can relieve anxiety and pain and should also be considered as the start of a patient's rehabilitation. Pain relief in all its forms should be addressed at all stages and patients should be made aware of the need to inform their nurse should further pain occur.

Inferior Infarctions

Special considerations are required for those patients who suffer from an AMI in the inferior area of their heart. A right-sided ECG should be taken and if there is right ventricle involvement, IV fluids are required.

Potential Complications of Angina and Myocardial Infarction

Complications can include progression to myocardial infarction, heart failure, cardiogenic shock, arrhythmias and sudden death. Early detection and treatment are therefore essential.

Following a myocardial infarction, certain complications can be predicted as being more likely to present owing to the specific part of the heart affected. These are summarized in Table 2.2 and can aid the A&E nurse in anticipating potential problems.

Table 2.2 The complications of myocardial infarction

Area of infarction	Affected artery	Complication
Anteroseptal	Left anterior descending artery	Cardiogenic shock, bundle branch block
Anterolateral	Left circumflex artery	SA node dysfunction and associated arrhythmias
Inferior	Right coronary artery	Bradycardia and heart block

Heart Failure

Heart failure may be an acute event caused by myocardial infarction or a chronic condition caused by disease and old age. As a chronic condition it affects 3–5% of those aged over 65 and in severe cases the prognosis is poor (Pascual, 1993). It is when the condition becomes acute or presents as a complication following myocardial infarction that patients require A&E intervention.

Heart failure is pump failure. The heart ceases to supply the body tissues adequately with blood and oxygen, and blood flow through the heart is hindered giving rise to breathlessness due to pulmonary oedema and eventual hypoxia. Stroke volume is the volume of blood ejected from the heart with every beat. The causes of heart failure may be grouped according to which component of stroke volume they subsequently affect.

Stroke volume is made up of:

- preload – venous filling pressure of the heart;
- afterload – resistance to cardiac emptying;
- contractility – force of the heart contracting.

Heart failure can also be caused by conditions in which circulatory demand is increased beyond the heart's ability to respond.

Causes of Cardiac Failure

- Decreased preload due to mitral stenosis, ineffective filling (e.g. in atrial fibrillation) or restricted filling (e.g. pericarditis or tamponade).
- Increased afterload due to hypertension, aortic or mitral valve regurgitation, fluid or salt retention.
- Decreased myocardial contractility due to recent MI, IHD, cardiomyopathy, hypoxaemia, negative inotropic effects (e.g. acidosis), antidysrhythmic drugs and pericardial disease.
- High-output states (e.g. intracardiac shunts, thyrotoxicosis, severe anaemia, Paget's disease, vitamin B deficiency or septicaemic shock) (Leyden, 1992; Why, 1993).

Cardiac failure is a vicious circle of physiological events that eventually become counter-productive and lead to death.

The right and left sides of the heart can fail individually, resulting in varying signs and symptoms of differing degrees of severity. However, since the sides of the heart are so closely linked, the unaffected side will also fail over time.

Assessment of a Patient with Suspected Cardiac Failure

On arrival in A&E the patient may display a range of symptoms from fatigue and peripheral oedema to breathlessness, hypotension and severe confusion. The aim of the nursing assessment is therefore to establish the extent of the heart failure, obtaining a baseline estimation of his/her condition and planning care accordingly.

A thorough nursing history should be obtained, using relatives as a resource where the patient is unable to communicate. Vital signs including blood pressure, heart rate, respiratory rate, temperature and oxygen saturation should be recorded and an ECG performed to aid diagnosis of the underlying cause. Assessment of the skin may reveal clamminess or pallor that occurs due to increased sympathetic drive. Peripheral and central areas should be observed, noting any cyanosis and/or oedema. Any presence of cough should be recorded, including a description of any sputum that is produced; in left-sided heart failure, where pulmonary oedema is present, sputum is often frothy and white with blood staining. Noting consciousness level will reveal whether cerebral perfusion is adequate and should include observation for lethargy, agitation or confusion.

Chest pain may be present due to a pleural effusion or underlying myocardial infarction. Pain in the hypochondrial area may be a sign of right heart failure. Pain is an important area of assessment and adequate assessment will go some way to ensuring that adequate pain relief is administered.

Reduction of urinary output is an important indicator of cardiac failure, although this is difficult to assess in the initial stages. In severe cases a catheter should be inserted to gain a clearer assessment of renal perfusion and function.

Goals of Care

- Support the heart by maintaining cardiac output.
- Relieve pulmonary congestion.
- Provide comfort.
- Reduce anxiety.
- Assist in the treatment of underlying causes.

Treatment

All patients should have oxygen administered, using an oxygen mask with a reservoir bag plus nasal cannula, to give 100% oxygen concentration. The physiological changes that occur during cardiac failure lead quickly to hypoxia and post MI this may increase the infarct size (Perrett, 1990). Arterial blood gases are used to assess the efficiency of oxygen therapy. The patient should be sat upright and, where possible, the legs should be lowered to reduce preload. Severely dyspnoeic patients rapidly become tired and leaning on a table may help. Activity should be restricted to reduce myocardial expenditure and skeletal muscle demand for oxygen. Rest also increases renal blood flow that initiates diuresis in an oedematous patient.

Patients with heart failure are at high risk of pressure sore development as a result of restricted mobility, oedema and reduced capillary blood flow. Patients should have small but frequent position changes and some form of pressure-reducing mattress and excessive trolley waits for transfer to a hospital bed should be avoided.

During the acute phase patients can be extremely anxious and the nurse can help the patient by explaining all nursing and medical treatments. Sedation may be given where necessary. Morphine is often used for analgesia as it reduces respiratory rate and also aids in decreasing venous return and therefore preload (Fowler, 1995). The drug may also reduce anxiety. Respiratory rate should be monitored carefully as an overdose of an opiate can lead to respiratory arrest.

Comfort and personal hygiene are important but this should be balanced with the need for rest and removing sweat-soaked clothes may be all that is initially required. The patient should be on fluid restriction and it is essential that good nursing records of all input and output are maintained. As discussed previously, catheterization is recommended for the acutely unwell patient to ensure accurate fluid balance monitoring and to alleviate the effort of using a bedpan or commode that may cause stress and symptom exacerbation. (Williams, 1993).

Whilst in A&E the patient should be monitored and observations repeated regularly and compared with the baseline assessment.

Pharmacological Management

The three main pharmacological approaches used are:

- diuretics;
- vasodilators;
- inotropic agents.

Vasodilators lessen preload by reducing venous return and systemic vascular resistance. A fall in blood pressure often results but cardiac output is often increased enough to prevent an extreme hypotensive event. The force of cardiac contractility is not increased but the efficiency of the myocardium improves owing to reduction of afterload. Nitroglycerine is commonly used as a general vasodilator to lower filling pressures but should be used with caution in patients with inferior MIs or hypotension. Nitroglycerine also improves renal perfusion, allowing any diuretics to have greater effect. Diuretics are often given in the treatment of left ventricular failure to decrease intravascular volume, lower left atrial pressure and relieve pulmonary oedema. Frusemide is commonly used and drugs are given intravenously because of their rapid action.

Inotropic agents are given to increase the force of cardiac contractions and therefore increase cardiac output by increasing cardiac contractility. However, cardiac oxygen demand is increased which, in the case of a myocardial infarction, may further increase infarct size (Tritschler, 1993). These drugs may be given to patients when the first-line treatments of reducing circulating volume and preload (and therefore afterload) have been ineffective or where low circulating volume already exists. The three main categories used are digitalis, beta-adrenergic antagonists (dopamine/dobutamine) and non-adrenergic positive inotropic agents. The most commonly used are dobutamine and adrenaline, which have varying degrees of inotropic effect. The choice is usually dictated by haemodynamic measurement (e.g. Swann-Ganz monitoring) and these agents should be commenced after transfer from the A&E department.

Arrhythmias

An arrhythmia is any abnormality of the heartbeat and occurs when there is a disruption to the normal formation or conduction of an impulse. Diseased or damaged hearts are more likely to exhibit arrhythmias and they are commonly seen in patients with ischaemic heart disease. The need for treatment is based on the actual and potential effects of the arrhythmia and not merely on the fact that a rhythm strip deviates from normal parameters.

Assessment

Patients may present with a variety of different complaints including collapse, lethargy, shortness of breath or palpitations and the main aim of any nursing assessment is to establish the effect that the arrhythmia is having on the patient.

Initially the patient should be attached to a cardiac monitor and have a 12-lead ECG performed. Certain arrhythmias may require immediate medical involvement to ensure prompt treatment. Baseline nursing observations will indicate whether the patient's cardiac output is compromised and a more detailed history, including relevant past medical history and current medication, should be undertaken if the patient's condition allows.

Aims of Treatment/Nursing Intervention

- Ensure safety through stabilization of the patient by treating the underlying causes of the arrhythmia.
- Alleviate anxiety and pain if present.
- Observe for reduction in cardiac output by frequent observation of vital signs.
- Assist with the administration of prescribed medication.

Specific Features and Treatment of Cardiac Arrhythmias

Sinus Bradycardia

Any heart rate of less than 60 bpm is considered a bradycardia. This may be normal for a person who is an athlete or for some people when they are asleep. Bradycardia can also occur as a result of drug therapy (e.g. beta-blockers), altered metabolic states or acute myocardial infarction. Ageing can cause scarring to the SA node and this also can lead to bradycardia.

Bradycardia may result in decreased cardiac output causing a fall in blood pressure, fainting and heart failure due to the congestion of blood flow through the heart. However, bradycardias are usually treated only where evidence of ensuing failure exists. Atropine is often used as a first-line treatment as it blocks the effect of the vagus nerve. When this is ineffective temporary pacing may be required.

Sinus Tachycardia

Any heart rate greater than 100 bpm is considered a tachycardia. Sinus tachycardia is normal and expected during exercise, whilst at rest it is a normal response to anxiety and pain. It is also part of the body's compensatory mechanism in high-output states such as septicaemia or hypovolaemia. In myocardial infarction it is thought to occur due to increased catecholamine activity. Drugs, hypothyroidism, electrolyte imbalance and pericarditis are other causes. Treatment, if necessary, involves identification and treatment of the underlying cause.

Supraventricular Tachycardia (SVT)

Myocardial infarction, ischaemic heart disease, thyrotoxicosis and mitral valve disease can all cause supraventricular tachycardia. It can also occur as a result of Wolff-Parkinson-White syndrome.

SVT is a fast spontaneous impulse arising from the atria over-riding the heart's natural pacemaker. The patient may experience chest pain, breathlessness or palpitations. They may also present at A&E in a collapsed state due to low blood pressure resulting from associated reduction in cardiac output. The arrhythmia may be self-limiting or the patient may require rapid treatment. The increased myocardial oxygen demand increases the risk of heart failure.

Treatment

Treatment consists of three tiers. Vagal manoeuvres are often tried in the first instance. These include carotid massage, stimulating the gag reflex and breath-holding. Such manoeuvres stimulate the vagus nerve, inhibiting the SA node firing and subsequent AV node conduction, which may slow or terminate the arrhythmia. If these treatments are unsuccessful then antiarrhythmic drugs are administered. These include adenosine, amiodarone or flecainide. In certain cases the patient will have to undergo electrical cardioversion. Cardioversion involves a timed electrical shock to the heart and is carried out under sedation. The defibrillator is synchronized to reduce the risk of producing ventricular fibrillation.

Atrial Fibrillation

This rhythm is most commonly seen in patients with ischaemic heart disease and can affect patients who have had a myocardial infarction, rheumatic valve disease, thyrotoxicosis, heart failure or hypertension.

Atrial fibrillation is a rapid and uncoordinated impulse originating from one or more foci within the atria. The rate is often so rapid that the ventricles cannot conduct all the impulses and are only stimulated by a small percentage of the strongest stimuli. This results in an irregular pulse, and an apex and radial pulse deficit may be felt. The atria are unable to contract fully and therefore unable to empty. In fast rates the cardiac output will fall rapidly as the ventricles are unable to respond adequately and the patient can quickly develop congestive cardiac failure. There is also a risk of thromboemboli forming as the blood pools due to congestion of blood flow through the heart.

Treatment

Treatment very much depends upon the condition of the patient. The most common treatment for symptomatic patients is intravenous digoxin, although if the arrhythmia causes severe compromise then cardioversion may be required. Anticoagulant therapy is often given to prevent or dissipate thromboemboli.

Atrial Flutter

This rhythm is the rapid and regular fluttering of the atrium originating from a single focus within the atrium other than the SA node. It is characterized by sawtooth flutter waves. Treatment is the same as for atrial fibrillation.

Ventricular Ectopic Activity

For some people ventricular ectopic activity is normal, but in a diseased heart it may result in something more sinister. Causes of premature ventricular complexes (PVCs) include myocardial infarction, digoxin, tricyclic drugs or adrenaline. Smoking, caffeine or alcohol can also provoke the condition.

Pacemaker foci within the ventricles normally have an intrinsic rate of 30–40 bpm. Occasionally these foci fire early causing a premature ventricular complex. These are often followed by a pause as the atrial beat may not be conducted through the junctional tissue.

The following are terms used when referring to certain types of premature ventricular complexes:

- BIGEMINY – every other beat is a PVC; this is a common result of digoxin toxicity;
- TRIGEMINY – every third beat is a PVC;
- UNIFOCAL – PVCs all originate from the same ectopic focus;
- MULTIFOCAL – PVCs of different ectopic sites (a sign of a very irritable ventricle);
- COUPLETS – two PVCs in succession;
- SALVOS – more than two PVCs in immediate succession;
- R on T – this is where the R wave of the ventricular ectopic beat occurs on the T wave of the normal preceding sinus beat. The likelihood of ventricular fibrillation is increased with this arrhythmia.

Treatment

Ventricular ectopic beats are always treated if they are multifocal, frequent in number/occurrence or where the R on T phenomenon is seen. If the cause is drug related, for example in the case of digoxin, then the drug will be stopped or changed. For other causes an anti-arrhythmic drug, such as lignocaine, may be used.

It should be noted that in bradycardia complexes that look like PVCs may be seen. However, these are actually ventricular escape beats that are part of the body's compensatory mechanism to maintain adequate cardiac output. In such situations the administration of atropine will usually raise the heartbeat sufficiently, eliminating the need for further escape beat production.

Ventricular Tachycardia

This potentially lethal arrhythmia is most commonly seen when there is severe ventricular dysfunction, for example following an MI. The entire rhythm consists of ventricular beats at a rate of >100 bpm. This rhythm originates from ectopic foci within the ventricles and can quickly lead to a reduced cardiac output with patients becoming pulseless.

Treatment

Initially a sharp blow to the sternum or asking the patient to cough may stimulate the heart back into a normal rhythm. If the patient is tolerating the rhythm well then an anti-arrhythmic drug such as lignocaine may be tried. If the patient is more severely compromised or the anti-arrhythmic drug has been ineffective then electrical cardioversion is performed. Should the rhythm result in cardiac arrest then resuscitation should be commenced using the standard ALS algorithm.

Complete Heart Block

Heart block refers to a block in the conduction pathways of the heart. Although other degrees of heart block may also be seen within the A&E setting, complete heart block poses the most serious threat to life.

The ECG will show a regular P-P interval but no association between P waves and the QRS complex (AV dissociation) and the rate of the P waves is faster than the QRS complex.

Some patients may have an adequate escape rhythm that will maintain their blood pressure whilst others will require urgent medical/nursing intervention. If the condition persists, patients will require urgent transfer to a coronary care unit for pacemaker insertion. In extreme cases, external temporary pacing within the A&E department will be required. Complications of complete heart block are ventricular tachycardia, ventricular fibrillation, heart failure, pulmonary oedema and ventricular standstill.

In summary, it is important when treating any patient with an abnormal ECG that nurses treat the patient and not the arrhythmia, looking at the overall condition. This ensures patient safety and prompt and appropriate treatment to avoid progression to more sinister arrhythmias.

Transfer

Patients who have been treated for any cardiac emergency should be a priority for transfer as they require one-to-one nursing observation and a quiet environment, both of which are difficult to achieve within the busy A&E environment. It is essential that emergency equipment is taken on transfer, including a defibrillator and airway adjuncts, and that the transfer nurse is trained to use it.

Cardiopulmonary Resuscitation

Introduction

A cardiac arrest is an event that demands instant recognition and immediate intervention to allow a patient to have the optimum chance of survival. A nurse in the A&E department is likely to see a cardiac arrest that has occurred in the department itself or out of hospital, with subsequent delivery to the department by a paramedic crew. The latter is often telephoned ahead by the ambulance staff, giving the A&E nurse time to prepare for the patient's arrival.

Cardiopulmonary resuscitation (CPR) has developed over decades and is still developing today. Initial records of resuscitation being performed date back as far as biblical times. These methods were very crude by today's protocols, but nonetheless resuscitation was being attempted in some form. The late 1950s and early 1960s saw the development of closed-chest compressions in conjunction with mouth-to-mouth ventilation. These methods are the basis of resuscitation today. The Bresus study (Tunstall-Pedoe et al., 1992) was a large 4000-patient study in the United Kingdom that rated immediate survival from cardiopulmonary arrest at 39%, 24 hours post-arrest at 28% and patients from initial arrest to discharge at 12.5%. The Bresus study also clarified that speed is of the essence in recognition and treatment of cardiac arrest. This is complemented by a witnessed event of short duration. These will all contribute to the likelihood of patient survival.

Reasons for Advanced Life Support

Advanced life support (ALS) is more often than not preceded by basic life support (BLS), even within the A&E department where there is immediate access to advanced life support equipment and personnel. Basic life support has its place in an environment with no access to ALS equipment or trained people to use it, but BLS is only a holding procedure for a rapidly deteriorating situation. The purpose of BLS is to maintain adequate ventilation and circulation until measures can be instituted to reverse the underlying cause of the arrest; it is therefore a 'holding operation' only.

Effective basic life support will provide ventilation and circulate the blood to the vital organs. Performing effective external chest compressions and ventilation aims to preserve cerebral and myocardial perfusion. The sooner that ALS is used in conjunction with BLS the more the probability of survival increases.

Priorities of Care

The 'chain of survival' (Cummins et al., 1991) is a concept and term now widely referred to in cardiopulmonary resuscitation. This concept should be known by, and used in, the community as well as the A&E department, although each area obviously has very different levels of resuscitation skills and availability of equipment to offer. Reflecting on this, Handley (1997) documented that 70% of all arrests happen out of the hospital environment, and the paramedic crew will bring many of these patients into the A&E department.

Early Access

The first link of the 'chain of survival' is early access. On recognition of the patient collapsing, the nurse assesses that the patient is unresponsive by a gentle 'shake and shout' (both physical and verbal stimulus is necessary as the patient may be profoundly deaf). If alone, the nurse must then shout for assistance. Before establishing whether or not the patient is breathing the airway must be made patent: the tongue, vomit, or broken/loose dentures or teeth may cause occlusion. The head-tilt chin-lift manoeuvre is used to achieve an open airway. Vomit must be removed with suction, or finger sweeps if no suction is readily at hand. Only ill-fitting dentures should be removed. The first responder must then take up to 10 seconds to look, listen and feel for breath sounds. If no breath sounds are present the hospital emergency number must be called to activate the cardiac arrest team. If the nurse is still on his/her own at this point he/she must leave the patient to initiate the call. Once this call is made the first important link of the chain of survival has been initiated: early access to the emergency medical services or the 'crash team'.

Early Basic Life Support

There should be no delay in commencing BLS within the A&E department as there should be adequate staff members to initiate two-person CPR. Instituted early, BLS can sustain life for a period of at least 12 minutes in a heart in ventricular fibrillation (Bossaert, 1997). This length of time far exceeds the arrival of the cardiac arrest team at an A&E department. As the emergency call is being made, BLS continues. Two ventilations should be given, preferably with a pocket mask device delivering supplementary oxygen.

Circulation must now be assessed. The nurse should feel for a major pulse, either carotid or femoral, for no longer than 10 seconds. At the same time she is looking at the patient's colour, assessing for movement, swallowing or any signs of life. Should there be no signs of circulation and the arrest was a witnessed or monitored collapse, a precordial thump is administered with a further 10-second circulation check thereafter. With help on its way BLS is commenced as a two-person technique, one at the airway and the other performing chest compressions at a rate of 100/min with a ratio of five chest compressions to one ventilation.

The ideal sequence of events, particularly in an acute area such as A&E, is the assessment of *A a*irway, *B b*reathing and *C c*irculation simultaneously, in one 10-second check, then an immediate move to *D d*efibrillation. This obviously requires the nursing personnel to be trained in defibrillation. Eastwick-Field (1996) reported that because the nurse is usually the first responder, he/she is the ideal person to deliver ALS treatment without delay before medical personnel arrive.

Early Defibrillation

With early access initiated and early BLS under way, to have defibrillation delayed at this stage in the chain of events will significantly reduce the patient's chance of survival. The patients who are most salvageable from a cardiac arrest are those with a shockable rhythm, namely ventricular fibrillation (VF) or pulseless ventricular tachycardia (VT) (Bossaert, 1997). Defibrillation is the definitive treatment for these rhythms and the sooner that it is administered the more likely it will be successfully reverted to a rhythm with a cardiac output. If defibrillation is delayed for even a few minutes the amplitude or coarseness of the VF becomes finer and finer. After about four minutes of fibrillation the success rate of reversal by defibrillation falls enormously, and eventually after approximately 15 minutes will be indistinguishable from asystole (Basket, 1993). Once asystole is present the situation is far more desperate and even less likely to have a successful outcome (Robertson, 1997b).

It is clear that the A&E nurse should be trained in ALS and therefore initiate defibrillation if it is indicated, before the hospital cardiac arrest team arrives. Survival from cardiac arrest to discharge from an American source was between 5% and 15%. In 1997 the author's hospital determined a 30% survival rate from arrest to discharge from in-hospital cardiac arrests (Coady, 1998). Stewart (1993) concurred that programmes to teach staff nurses how to use defibrillators can improve survival after in-hospital arrests. For successful defibrillation 75-90% of the fibrillating myocardium must be depolarized simultaneously. By achieving this, the natural pacemaker of the heart (the sinoatrial node) is then given the chance to resume control after a brief refractory period. The SA node can then initiate a normal sinus beat and therefore restore spontaneous circulation with a cardiac output. In the A&E department (and particularly within the resuscitation bay) there should be defibrillators available for use and people trained to use them. Whelan (1997) reported that often there is availability of defibrillators in areas where nursing staff are untrained to operate them.

Having nurses trained in rhythm recognition and defibrillation is an achievable and realistic goal. Multidisciplinary courses in ALS training, such as the Resuscitation Council (UK) courses, are run nationwide. Having successfully completed a Resuscitation Council ALS course is an achievement, but is only the first step in ensuring safe practice is maintained. It is well documented that the skills of performing resuscitation are notoriously poorly retained (Conaghan, 1995). This applies equally to medical and nursing staff. The resource of Resuscitation Training Officers (RTO), who are now commonplace in most hospitals as recommended by the Royal College of Physicians' report of 1987, can keep a rolling programme of update sessions for ALS training after completion of an ALS course. Practice-simulated cardiac arrests are a method of keeping ALS skills up to date for both nursing and medical staff. However, to have each and every nurse complete an ALS course is financially not practical (Conaghan, 1995). 'In house' education on rhythm recognition and manual defibrillation could be an option to train nurses in greater numbers and with less expense. Ultimately the aim must be for the nurse to pick up the defibrillator paddles and have the ability and confidence to recognize a shockable cardiac arrest rhythm and treat it appropriately, quickly and safely.

Defibrillation Threshold

The defibrillation threshold is the term used to describe the minimum amount of electrical energy required to successfully revert ventricular fibrillation. The existing recommendation of energy levels is 200 Joules, 200 Joules and 360 Joules for the third and subsequent shocks. Should ventricular fibrillation recur after a return of spontaneous circulation then the energy may be returned to 200 J from 360 J. This is because the second episode of ventricular fibrillation is being treated as a 'new' VF, where 200 J may be successful (Jakobsson, 1989). There must, however, be a balance of delivering enough energy, as too little will be ineffective and too much will cause myocardial tissue damage (Bossaert, 1997). The sequence of Joules as outlined above is used within the European Communities.

Transthoracic Impedance

The speed of delivery of the defibrillation is a priority, but there are also other important practical aspects to take into consideration when performing the task. Transthoracic impedance is the resistance to the current of electricity through the chest wall before it actually reaches the mass of the myocardium. There are certain hindrances to the flow of that current, primarily the skin, bones and lungs in the thoracic cavity since these are all poor conductors of electricity. The transthoracic impedance will be reduced by several actions:

(1) The appliance of jelly impregnated pads over the area of the paddle position, which is below the right clavicle to the right of the sternum and the left apex of the heart (at the position of V4 and V5 of a 12-lead ECG). Jelly smeared on the chest is less satisfactory as the jelly tends to spread and run across the chest and can lead to the electricity arcing. This can have safety implications

for the operator. The anterior-posterior paddle position is an alternative or ideal if the patient has an implantable defibrillator or permanent pacemaker *in situ* (Bossaert, 1997). Jelly pads also reduce the risk of burns to the chest wall.

(2) Application of pressure to the paddles being held on the chest wall is required.

(3) The paddle size of defibrillators is fairly standard and should be between 8 cm and 13 cm in diameter for adults. Actual body size should not be of relevance (Advanced Life Support Group, 1996). Another poor conductor of electricity is air and the shock should therefore be delivered at the end of expiration during ventilation.

Defibrillation Safety

Safety is of prime importance. A defibrillator is a potentially danger-ous piece of equipment if used by an untrained person or used care-lessly without respect by one who is trained. Direct contact with the casualty or indirect contact via the bed/trolley, drip stand or intra-venous fluid bag connected to the patient must be avoided, as all will transfer the electric current. The whole resuscitation team must therefore receive a verbal warning that defibrillation charging and shock delivery is about to occur: 'Stand clear, I am charging. Stand clear, I am about to shock.'

This is the responsibility of the person who delivers the shocks. The verbal warning is accompanied by a visual sweep around the patient area, with a final look at the monitor to confirm the shock-able rhythm. This safety sequence is repeated each and every time that a shock is given. The oxygen supply to the airway, whatever method is employed, should also be either turned off at source or removed from the patient's chest vicinity to prevent combustion of the oxygen during defibrillation.

If present for whatever reason, water is an obvious potential danger when a casualty requires defibrillation. The rescuer should always ensure the environment is safe for him/her to enter to carry out the necessary treatment to help the patient. As long as the patient's chest area is adequately dried and there are no pools of water in contact with both the patient and rescuer, then defibrillation is safe. Nitrate patches should be removed from the chest prior to defibrillation as they are explosive in nature.

Familiarization with the defibrillator is essential. Daily checks of the equipment and its operation will prevent user error when it has to be operated in an emergency situation (Bossaert, 1997).

There are now many different models of defibrillator on the market. The standard manual defibrillator relies on the operator to have rhythm recognition skills to make the correct rhythm diagnosis and therefore follow the appropriate advanced life support protocol. This obviously requires an ALS trained person to be the first responder. In reality the event may occur in a non-acute area with staff inexperienced in ALS. To overcome this there are defibrillators called 'AEDs' or advisory external defibrillators, with large self-adhesive pads that are stuck to the patient's chest in the usual positions. After pressing an 'analyse' button the machine will make a rhythm assessment and give written and/or verbal instructions. The operator then presses 'charge' and 'shock' buttons as per the instructions. No rhythm recognition skill is required. Some AEDs will be fully automatic such as used by ambulance crews, some general practices and dental surgeries. These require much less training to operate and it is hoped they will enable the first responder, not trained in ALS, to quickly defibrillate the patient when indicated. In an A&E department this would generally not be the type of machine used as nurses are more likely to be ALS trained (Liddle, 1997-98). The AEDs often have the facility to simply override the advisory mode. They can then be used in a hospital setting by both ALS and non-ALS trained personnel. This has a positive financial implication for the purchaser as one defibrillator will suffice for all levels of skill but still provides a piece of equipment for quick defibrillation without necessarily having to wait for ALS-trained personnel to arrive.

Early Advanced Life Support

The final link in the 'chain of survival' is early ALS. Unfortunately early BLS and defibrillation will together not always achieve a successful outcome in a resuscitation attempt (Cummins et al., 1991). Further advanced life support interventions are more often than not also necessary. Figure 2.2 shows the European Resuscitation Council 1998 'Advanced Life Support Algorithm'. Unfortunately there is not worldwide uniformity of this algorithm although there are common core points with variations in only some aspects.

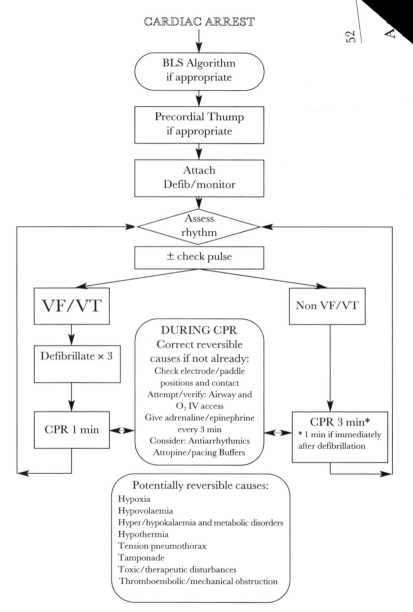

Figure 2.2 The 1998 European Resuscitation Council guidelines for adult advanced life support.

Source Resuscitation (1998) 37: 81-90. ALS algorithm reproduced by permission of Prof. L. Bossaert, Executive Director, European Resuscitation Council.

group formed in 1992, the 'International Liaison Committee on Resuscitation' (ILCOR), strives to achieve accord to ensure world-wide standardisation of resuscitation practice.

The ALS algorithm has a simple layout with a flow-chart appearance. The starting point in the algorithm will depend on the situation of the arrest. Ideally basic life support will have already been commenced and, if appropriate, a precordial thump should be administered while awaiting the attachment of the defibrillator for the assessment of the rhythm. When the paddles are placed onto the chest in the standard positions the manual defibrillator will produce a rhythm on the screen. ECG leads should be attached as soon as possible after the procedure has been completed. The rhythm seen is then interpreted, concurrently taking into account the clinical presentation of the patient.

VF or Pulseless VT

The left-hand side of the algorithm is followed if the interpretation is of a shockable rhythm. There is a pulse check only if the operator sees a rhythm he/she would normally associate with a cardiac output. In between shocks there is no pulse check if the rhythm remains in VF. The three shocks must be delivered within a maximum period of one minute. If VT presents on the screen there must be a pause of no longer than 10 seconds to check for a pulse. VT can potentially have a cardiac output and to prevent inappropriate shocking a pulse check should be made. If the morphology and the rate of the pulseless VT remain constant a pulse check is not necessary (Working Party on ALS, 1998).

If a shockable rhythm remains after the third shock the paddles are placed back in the defibrillator. A period of one minute of CPR commences to maintain cerebral and myocardial perfusion. When one minute has passed there is a reassessment of the rhythm and further shocks are given as indicated. This loop is repeated until restoration of a cardiac output is achieved. In normal circumstances, while a patient remains in a shockable rhythm, which is a potentially reversible state, resuscitation should continue.

Stunning of the myocardium may occur after it has received 200 or 360 Joules of electricity. As a result of this, the immediate post-shock rhythm on the monitor may well present as a non-shockable rhythm. This can be the stunned myocardium slowly recovering from the shock and it may well revert to a rhythm compatible with a cardiac output, given a short period of time. This should be taken into consideration before assuming the rhythm as a non-shockable one and treating it as such. The 1998 European Guidelines recommend that following a DC shock, if a non-shockable rhythm appears on the screen for more than one sweep of the screen, one minute of CPR is commenced with no medication and then the rhythm reassessed. If the non-shockable rhythm remains on reassessment, the right-hand side of the algorithm is followed by commencing another two minutes of CPR to complete the loop. Reassessment may reveal a return of spontaneous circulation or return of a shockable rhythm.

The activities occurring during CPR are common to both sides of the algorithm and will be discussed after looking at the treatments for the non-VF and non-VT side.

Non-VF /VT

The right-hand side of the algorithm is the treatment for patients who are either asystolic or in electro-mechanical dissociation (EMD). If asystole is thought possibly to be fine VF then a shock should be delivered to exclude this. Asystole and EMD have a less favourable outcome (Robertson, 1997a) although there can be specific contributory causes that result in these arrest rhythms. Once a non-shockable rhythm is diagnosed the defibrillator paddles are placed back in the machine and a period of up to three minutes of CPR is commenced. After no more than the three minutes has elapsed the rhythm is reassessed and the appropriate side of the algorithm is followed.

ALS Procedures

During the periods of CPR on both sides of the algorithm there are certain ALS procedures the team must perform:

- The position of the paddles/electrodes and their contact should be checked.
- Airway security must be achieved with intubation by the anaesthetist, taking care not to spend longer than 30 seconds at one single attempt before re-oxygenation. The laryngeal mask airway may be used in some areas.
- Intravenous access should be gained.

- Epinephrine 1 mg should be administered once during each cycle of CPR.
- Other drug therapy must be considered, such as atropine, antiarrhythmics and sodium bicarbonate.

There are eight potentially reversible causes of cardiac arrest. These are grouped into the Four 'H's' and Four 'T's'. The cardiac arrest team leader should take into consideration these eight causes and exclude each as the cause for the arrest, regardless of which cardiac arrest rhythm the patient is in.

- *h*ypoxia;
- *h*ypovolaemia;
- *h*yper/hypokalaemia and metabolic disorders;
- *h*ypothermia;
- *t*ension pneumothorax;
- *t*amponade;
- *t*oxic/therapeutic disturbances;
- *t*hromboembolic/mechanical obstruction.

Drugs used in Cardiac Arrest

Drug therapy in resuscitation is a contentious issue. Because of the obvious logistical problems of research in humans, animal research predominates. How applicable this is to humans continues to produce conflicting views (Vincent, 1997).

Epinephrine (Adrenaline)

Owing to the nature of its properties, epinephrine is the first drug of choice in any rhythm of cardiac arrest. Primarily, due to stimulation of the alpha receptors, peripheral vasoconstriction occurs with the effect of improving diastolic pressure. This in turn will increase cerebral and myocardial blood flow. The dose of 1 mg is given intravenously. A dose of 5 mg may be considered in the non-shockable rhythms after three loops of the algorithm have been completed.

Atropine

Atropine will block vagal tone, thereby increasing the conductivity and the automaticity of the sinoatrial and atrioventricular nodes. Its benefit in an asystolic patient is more than likely minimal but worth considering in such cases after epinephrine (Vincent, 1997). The dose is 3 mg, given only once.

Antiarrhythmics

These groups of drugs can be considered after two to four loops of the algorithm where VF and/or pulseless VT are persistent. The drug of choice is 100 mg of lidocaine (lignocaine). Bretylium and lidocaine are two antiarrhythmics subject to a clinical trial which is running both nationally and internationally. The CALIBRE study is looking at these drugs in a double-blind trial along with a placebo, and the results eagerly awaited.

Sodium Bicarbonate

Acidosis will develop during a cardiac arrest as a result of anaerobic metabolism. Establishing a secure airway is a priority, to eliminate carbon dioxide accumulation. Sodium bicarbonate is therefore best reserved for a prolonged arrest with an established airway. The ALS Resuscitation Council (UK) recommends its use with arterial blood gases showing a pH of 7.10 or less and a base excess of less than -10. 50 mmol of 8.4% is given and repeated according to the arterial blood gases (ABGs). Administration via central access is recommended as extreme irritation and necrosis can occur if given peripherally.

Calcium

A patient with a known overdose of calcium channel blockers or high potassium merits the administration of calcium during resuscitation.

Endotracheal Drug Administration (ETT)

Epinephnine, atropine and lignocaine may be administered via the ETT by doubling the recommended dose if intravenous access is not possible. Calcium and sodium bicarbonate must not be administered this way.

The Nurse's Role during a Cardiac Arrest

Each hospital will vary in the composition of the cardiac arrest team but the principles of the roles remain the same. Before the medical team arrive there must be a nurse at the airway to provide oxygenation and ventilation. This can be administered via a pocket mask, laryngeal mask airway or a bag-valve-mask device. A second nurse should be commencing chest compressions and, if appropriately trained, defibrillating if indicated. In anticipation, a third nurse should be preparing the drugs and fluids for administration. This nurse is also responsible for documentation of the sequence of events such as the timings and drug administration. The nurses should have clearly defined roles during an arrest, which they should have allocated themselves before the team arrives. The importance of teamwork and communication between the team is vital to produce an organized resuscitation attempt.

When the medical team arrive, communication once again is of prime importance. The doctors will probably not know the patient. They will need to receive information initially on the rhythm the patient is in and later on the history. The most senior doctor usually assumes the role of team leader although any person who is ALS trained can undertake this role. The junior doctor or nurse can establish intravenous access and administer the drugs. The anaesthetist will attend to the security of the airway.

The nurse's responsibilities or role may well vary from arrest to arrest. A nurse trained in ALS is able to be the team leader, but in practice when the medical team arrives the senior doctor will take over the running of the arrest. The nurses in many areas will assume many of the remaining roles such as defibrillation, chest compressions, gaining intravenous access, drug administration and documentation of the events.

A role that will also very often be carried out by a nurse is accompanying a relative who wishes to observe the resuscitation attempt. If such a request is made it must not be disregarded as unreasonable. Provided there is a senior nurse available to be a companion to a relative throughout the duration of the attempt, it may be acceptable. The people who perceive this as a negative experience for the relative are often the medical and paramedical team. It is more often than not the thought of being watched in this situation that makes nurses and doctors quite uncomfortable (Williams, 1996). Relatives often find it of benefit to visualize what has happened, and therefore understand and accept the situation better. This is true even if the patient dies as a result of the event (Resuscitation Council (UK), 1996). Keeping an open mind regarding such a potential situation will reduce the surprise element if a relative asks to be present.

Summary

Resuscitation is an area of ongoing advancement and change. Every A&E nurse must accept personal responsibility to maintain a high standard in his/her practical skills and knowledge in basic and advanced life support. This will allow him/her to deliver confidently optimum care, from recognition of cardiopulmonary arrest to early defibrillation and advanced life support.

Conclusion

Patients with cardiac emergencies present a challenge to accident and emergency nurses. On the one hand efficient and speedy care is required whilst on the other time is needed to care for and reassure a group of people who are frightened and often in pain. Greater understanding of the disease processes and treatment pathways will enable nurses to prioritize care, allowing them to fulfil the need for both efficient and competent care.

Recommended Further Reading

Basket P et al. (1996) Advanced Life Support Manual, 2nd edn (with revisions). England: Resuscitation Council (UK).

Basket PJ (1993) Resuscitation Handbook, 2nd edn. London: Wolfe Publishing.

Hampton J (1980) The ECG Made Easy. Edinburgh: Churchill Livingstone.

Resuscitation Council (1998) Advanced Life Support Course Provider Manual, 3rd edn. London: Resuscitation Council.

Safer P (1996) On the history of modern resuscitation. Critical Care Medicine 24(2, Suppl.): S3–S11.

Skinner DV, Vincent R (1993) Cardiopulmonary Resuscitation. New York: Oxford University Press.

Thompson DR, Webster RA (1992) Caring for the Coronary Patient. Oxford: Butterworth-Heinemann.

References

Advanced Life Support Group (1996) Advanced Life Support Manual, 2nd edn (with revisions).

Akyrou D et al. (1995) Pain assessment in acute myocardial infarction patients. Intensive and Critical Care Nursing 11(5): 252–5.

Basket PJ (1993) Resuscitation Handbook, 2nd edn. London: Wolfe Publishing.

Bhagat K (1994) Aspirin. Nursing Standard 8(49): 52.

Bossaert L (1997) Fibrillation and defibrillation of the heart. British Journal of Anaesthesia (79): 203–13.

Brunner LS, Suddarth DS (1993)The Lippincott Manual of Medical-Surgical Nursing, 2nd edn. London: Chapman & Hall.

Coady E (1998) Audited results of in hospital cardiac arrests during 1997 at the Royal
    Sussex County Hospital, Brighton. Unpublished.
Conaghan P (1995) A cause for concern! Emergency Nurse 3(1): 23–25.
Cooper AD (1994) Pain assessment in accident and emergency. Accident and
    Emergency Nursing 2:103–7.
Cummins RO (1989) From concept to standard-of-care? Review of the clinical experi-
    ence with automated external defibrillators. Annals of Emergency Medicine 18:
    1269–75.
Cummins RO et al. (1991) Improving survival from sudden cardiac arrest: the 'chain of
    survival' concept, American Heart Association Statement. Circulation 83(5):
    1832–47.
Deeks J et al. (1995) Aspirin and acute myocardial infarction: clarifying the message.
    British Journal of General Practice 45(Aug.): 395–6.
Eastwick-Field P (1996) Introducing nurse-initiated management of cardiac arrest.
    Nursing Standard 10(26): 46–48.
Flisher D (1995) Fast track: early thrombolysis. Following a myocardial infarction.
    British Journal of Nursing 4(10): 562–5.
Fowler JP (1995) From chronic to acute when cardiac heart failure turns deadly. Nursing
    95(Jan.): 54–5.
GISSI (1986) Gruppo Italiano per lo Studio della Streptochinzsi nell'Infarto
    Miocardico. Effectiveness of intravenous thrombolytic treatment in acute myocar-
    dial infarction. Lancet 1: 397–402.
Gonce-Morton P (1996) Using the 12-lead ECG. To detect ischaemia, injury, and
    infarction. Critical Care Nurse 16(2): 85–94.
GREAT group (1992) Feasibility, safety, and efficacy of domiciliary thrombolysis by
    general practitioners: Grampian Region Early Anistreplase Trial. British Medical
    Journal 305: 548–53.
Green E (1992) Solving the puzzle of chest pain. American Journal of Nursing January:
    32–7.
Handley AJ (1997) Basic life support. British Journal of Anaesthesia 79: 151–8.
Hendrick JA (1994) The challenge of myocardial infarction in accident and emergency
    nursing. Accident and Emergency Nursing 2(3):160–6.
Herlitz J, Hartford M, Holberg S, Blohm M, Luepkar R, Karlson BW (1989) Effects of a
    media campaign on delay and ambulance use in suspected acute myocardial infarc-
    tion. American Journal of Cardiology 64(1): 90–93.
ISIS-2 (1988) Second International Study of Infarct Survival Collaborative Group.
    Randomised trial of intravenous streptokinase, oral aspirin, both, or neither
    amongst 17,187 cases of suspected acute myocardial infarction. Lancet 2: 349–60.
Jakobsson J et al. (1989) Energy requirement for early defibrillation. European Heart
    Journal 10: 551–4.
Julian DG (1990) Time as a factor in thrombolytic therapy. European Heart Journal
    11(Suppl. F): 53–5.
Julian DG, Cowan JC (1992) Cardiology. London: Ballière Tindall, pp 116–37.
Leitch JW, Birbara T, Freedman B et al. (1989) Factors influencing the time from onset
    of chest pain to arrival at hospital. Medical Journal of Australia 150(1): 6–10.
Leyden C (1992) Acute cardiac failure. In Ashworth PM, Clarke C. Cardiovascular
    Intensive Care Nursing. London: Churchill Livingstone, pp 67–89.

Liddle R (1997–98) Defibrillation: a new way forward. Health Care Risk Report December/January: 16–17.

Lieberman KS (1995) Markers of reperfusion after thrombolytic therapy for acute myocardial infarction. Journal of Emergency Nursing 21(2): 112–15.

McCaffery M, Beebe A (1989/1994) Pain: A Clinical Manual for Practice. Toronto: CV Mosby.

McMurry J, Rankin A (1994) Cardiology-I: treatment of myocardial infarction, unstable angina, and angina pectoris. British Medical Journal 309(19 November).

Morris N (1997) Door to needle times in Brighton, an examination of factors that may affect delay. As part of the postgraduate diploma in cardiology, Trafford Centre for Graduate Medical Education and Research. University of Sussex, unpublished work.

O'Connor L (1995) Pain assessment by patients and nurses, and nurses' notes on it, in early acute myocardial infarction, Part one. Intensive and Critical Care Nursing 11: 183–91.

O'Connor L (1995) Pain assessment by patients and nurses, and nurses, notes on it, in early acute myocardial infarction, Part two. Intensive and Critical Care Nursing 11: 283–92.

OFNS (1997) The Health Of Adult Britain 1841–1994, vol. 2. Eds Charlton J, Murphy M. Cardiovascular Diseases. London: Office for National Statistics, ch. 18, pp 60–76.

Pascual J (1993) Managing cardiac failure. Care of the Elderly 5(11): 427.

Perrett EM (1990) Acute heart failure in myocardial infarction: principles of treatment. Critical Care Medicine 18(1): 26–9. [In Ashworth PM, Clarke C. Cardiovascular Intensive Care Nursing. London: Churchill Livingstone, pp 67–89.]

Quinn T (1997) Assessment of the patient with chest pain in the accident and emergency department. Accident and Emergency Nursing 5: 65–70.

Quinn T, Jones C (1996) Electrocardiography, knowledge for practice. Nursing Times Development Supplements. Nursing Times 92(18): 9–14.

Rawles J (1996) Magnitude of benefit from earlier thrombolytic treatment in acute myocardial infarction: new evidence from the Grampian Region Early Anistreplase Trial (GREAT). British Medical Journal 312(7025): 212–215.

Resuscitation Council (UK) Advanced Life Support Manual, 2nd edn. London: Resuscitation Council.

Robertson CE (1997a) Advanced life support guidelines. British Journal of Anaesthesia 79: 172–7.

Robertson CE (1997b) The 1997 Resuscitation Guidelines for use in the United Kingdom. London: Resuscitation Council (UK).

Rowe K (1995) Care study: nursing a person who had suffered a myocardial infarction. British Journal of Nursing 4(3): 148–54.

Royal College of Physicians (1987) Resuscitation from cardiopulmonary arrest: training and organisation. Journal of the Royal College of Physicians of London 21(3): 175–81.

Scholfield P (1995) Using pain assessment tools to help patients in pain. Professional Nurse 10(11): 703–6.

Stewart JA (1993) Why not let staff nurses defibrillate? American Journal of Nursing 93(12): 7.

Tanabe P (1995) Recognising pain as a component of the primary assessment: adding D for discomfort to the ABCs. Journal of Emergency Nursing 21: 299–304.

Thompson DR, Webster RA (1992) Caring for the Coronary Patient. Oxford: Butterworth-Heinemann.

Tritschler I (1993) Drug therapy: drugs used in cardiogenic shock. Nursing Standard 8(8): 52.

Tunstall-Pedoe H et al. (1992) Survey of 3765 cardiopulmonary resuscitations in British hospitals (the BRESUS study): methods and overall results. British Medical Journal 304: 1347–51.

Vincent R (1997) Drugs in modern resuscitation. British Journal of Anaesthesia 79: 188–97.

Weston CFM, Penny WJ, Julian DG on behalf of the British Heart Foundation Working Group (1994) Guidelines for the early management of patients with myocardial infarction. British Medical Journal 308: 767–71.

Whelan Y (1997) Cardiac arrest: the skills of the emergency nurse practitioner. Accident and Emergency Nursing 5: 107–10.

Why H (1993) Modern management of cardiac failure. Nursing Standard 7(18): 52–4.

Why H (1994) Thrombolysis (thrombolytic therapy for acute myocardial infarction). Nursing Standard 31 August (Suppl. 8): 50–2.

Williams A (1993) A case for emotional support and human contact: management of cardiogenic shock. Professional Nurse 8(8): 520–3.

Williams K (1996) Witnessing resuscitation can help relatives. Nursing Standard Oct 9 (11): 3.

Working Party on Advanced Life Support (1998) A Statement from the Working Party on Advanced Life Support, and approved by the executive committee of the European Resuscitation Council. The 1998 European Resuscitation Council Guidelines for adult advanced life support. Resuscitation 37: 81–90.

Wyllie HR, Dunn FG (1994) Pre hospital opiate and aspirin administration in patients with suspected myocardial infarction (research). British Medical Journal 308 (19 March): 760–1.

Chapter 3
Nursing Care of Patients with Acute Respiratory Conditions

ANNE O'LOUGHLIN

Introduction

Emergency assessment of every patient begins with the airway, followed by his/her breathing. An adequate airway and functioning respiratory system are vital to life. An assault on either can rapidly lead to cell death through oxygen starvation.

This chapter aims to reflect the key role of A&E nurses in caring for patients with acute respiratory conditions from recognition and brief ABC assessment to more thorough assessment and intervention based on sound decision making. A collaborative approach to care is promoted. The common presenting conditions that are covered are asthma, pulmonary embolism, lower respiratory tract infection and chronic obstructive pulmonary disease. Anaphylaxis is included because it is potentially life threatening, involving the respiratory system.

Asthma

Asthma is a chronic inflammatory disease of the airways. It is characterized by an inflamed tracheobronchial tree that is hyper-responsive to various stimuli. Subsequent bronchoconstriction causes coughing, wheezing, chest tightness and dyspnoea. It may result in bronchospasm. The airway narrowing is largely reversible, sometimes without intervention. There is often nocturnal deterioration in symptoms.

Prevalence

Asthma was the registered cause of 1439 deaths in Great Britain in 1997 (Office for National Statistics, 1998). A large proportion of

61

these may have been avoided with aggressive medical intervention. The National Asthma Campaign (NAC) has estimated that there are more than 1.9 million adults with asthma living in Great Britain (NAC, 1998). This included the highest prevalence among young adults (20–44 years old) in Europe (European Community Respiratory Health Survey, 1996).

Aetiology

Asthma can be classified as either allergic or idiopathic asthma.

Allergic asthma

The causative stimulus can be identified in around 50% of people with asthma. This is described as allergic asthma. Common allergens include house dust mites and various pollens. Skin testing can identify the allergen: the patient will have raised titres of the specific immunoglobulin (IgE) antibody to the allergen. Allergic asthma may be seasonal, reflecting the cause (e.g. pollen). It may be associated with a familial history of other allergic conditions such as eczema.

Idiopathic asthma

When it has not been possible to identify an allergen using the usual tests, the asthma is described as idiopathic. This group includes people with exercise-induced asthma, those who react to non-steroidal anti-inflammatory drugs and occupation-related asthma (e.g. 'baker's asthma'). There may be common stimuli but as yet no identifiable allergen.

The National Asthma Campaign has estimated that up to 2000 people develop occupational asthma every year (NAC, 1998). Many others find their asthma is exacerbated by work and/or working conditions.

The parasympathetic and adrenergic nervous systems control airway smooth muscle tone. The airway smooth muscle contains vagal receptors, cholinergic irritant receptors and beta-adrenergic receptors. Stimulation of the vagal and irritant receptors, for example by histamine or upper respiratory tract infection, causes reflex bronchoconstriction via the vagus nerve. Stimulation of the beta-adrenergic receptors includes activation of the enzyme adenylate cyclase to produce cyclic AMP. This has a bronchodilator effect and inhibits the release of anti-inflammatory agents from mast cells. Beta blockers prevent this action causing bronchoconstriction.

Allergens cause bronchoconstriction through the inflammatory response. The inhaled allergens connect with IgE molecules in the mast cells of the mucosa and submucosal layer. This releases histamine and other mediators of inflammation that act directly on the smooth muscle. They also stimulate cholinergic irritant receptors.

Airflow Obstruction

The resistance to airflow within the lung is calculated using various physiological measurements. Briefly, it reflects the frictional resistance between airflow and airway wall and between airflow and tissues, reflecting the viscosity of lung parenchyma. Any reduction in the diameter of the airway increases the resistance to airflow. Peak expiratory flow rate (PEFR) measurements assist in assessing the patient's large airway obstruction. Spirometry gives more information using forced maximal expiration. The forced vital capacity, forced expiratory volume in one second (FEV1) and their ratio, the maximal expiratory flow rate (MEFR) and maximal mid-expiratory flow rate (MMFR) are obtained. The MMFR is sensitive to small airway obstruction whereas the MEFR and PEFR reflect large airway obstruction. As large airway obstruction is more rapidly reversible than small airway obstruction, the MEFR and PEFR will return to normal much earlier than the MMFR after an acute episode.

Management

The British Thoracic Society (BTS, 1993) produced guidelines for the management of severe, acute asthma and chronic, persistent asthma. These were endorsed by the British Association for Accident & Emergency Medicine (BAAEM, 1993) in their subsequent guidelines for the treatment of acute asthma in A&E.

The aims were as follows:

(1) to prevent death;
(2) to restore the patient's clinical condition and lung function to their best possible levels as soon as possible;
(3) to maintain optimal function and prevent early relapse (BTS, 1993, Suppl., p. 12).

Signs and Symptoms

The patient will usually present with dyspnoea at rest, audible wheezing and may be cyanosed. He/she may not be able to finish a sentence in one breath. Breathing will require increased effort, using accessory muscles and chest distension. The immediate intervention is to administer high-flow oxygen. It is important to remember that an absence of wheezing and reduced effort of breathing can be signs of exhaustion. This is a serious deterioration and requires rapid medical and nursing intervention.

Nursing Assessment

While speed is of the essence in assessing the asthmatic patient (the BAAEM, 1993 stated five seconds) it must not be at the expense of reassurance. A chaotic, excitable resuscitation room can exacerbate the rising panic in a patient unable to breathe. A calm, firm voice explaining all investigations and interventions will reassure the patient and build rapport and trust between nurse and patient.

Whilst talking to the patient the nurse can assess his/her colour and ability to talk. Vital sign recordings will include heart rate, respiratory rate, PEFR and oxygen saturation by pulse oximetry. If the patient is unable to complete sentences in one breath, the history may be obtained from any other available source such as partner or parent. The BAAEM (1993) guidelines advised administration of a B2 agonist nebulizer, salbutamol being the most common in use. Levels of severity were devised, dividing patients into four categories: life-threatening, severe, moderate and mild (Table 3.1).

Patients in the life-threatening and severe categories should have their blood gases checked during resuscitation. Patients in the lower three categories can be clinically assessed while on oxygen prior to further intervention.

Blood Gas Analysis

Patients in life-threatening and severe categories should have their blood gases checked during resuscitation. The markers of respiratory acidosis include a low pH with a normal to high $PaCO_2$. These markers and the level of hypoxia indicate the severity of the asthma attack (Anderson, 1990).

Table 3.1 Presenting symptoms of acute asthma

	Life-threatening	Severe	Moderate	Mild
Ability to talk	Unable	Cannot finish sentence	Can finish sentence	Can talk normally
Heart rate	Bradycardic < 56	Tachycardic >110	Normal	Normal
Resp. rate	Bradypnoeic 10	Tachypnoeic >25	Normal	Normal
PEFR	Unable or <33%	33–50% of expected	50–75% of expected	>75% of expected

Source: Adapted from BAAEM (1993).

Further Nursing Assessment and History

It is important to note the context of this attack: when it started, when symptoms started deteriorating, what treatment the patient has self-administered or has been administered by ambulance personnel *en route*, his/her regular medication (e.g. if he/she is already taking steroids or theophylline), his/her previous asthma history (is this attack worse than before? Has he/she been intubated before?). Old notes and/or A&E records should be obtained where possible.

Brittle Asthma

While most patients' symptoms deteriorate over a few days or even weeks there are some whose attacks occur in minutes and with little warning. This is known as brittle asthma. It is a severe, life-threatening form of asthma and must be treated aggressively and promptly. Patients with brittle asthma should always carry B2 agonist inhalers and prednisolone. Some have home oxygen and nebulizers. The life-threatening care pathway should be followed.

Treatment and Monitoring

Following nursing/clinical assessment the nurse should continuously monitor respiratory rate, heart rate and rhythm, pulse oximetry (aiming for > 92%) and blood pressure. PEFR should be recorded before and 15–30 minutes after each nebulizer use.

A chest X-ray may be indicated to exclude pneumothorax. Blood gases should be taken initially and within two hours of commencing treatment. Urea and electrolytes and theophylline levels, where appropriate, may be taken. The patient with severe acute asthma is at high risk of serious hypokalaemia following treatment with B2 agonists. Their effect is potentiated by concomitant corticosteroid and methylxanthine preparations and by hypoxia (British National Formulary, 1998).

Patients with a PEFR of 50% or less than their expected level (see Table 3.2) will need to be admitted. A patient with severe asthma will receive further nebulized B2 agonists and possibly anti-cholinergic medication plus oral or intravenous corticosteroids. Subsequent intervention may include an intravenous bronchodilator such as aminophylline.

Table 3.2 Peak expiratory flow rate in men and *women* (l/min)

Height (ft/ins)	20		30		40		50		60	.
					Age (yrs)					
5'3"	572	*433*	560	*422*	548	*401*	512	*380*	488	*539*
5'6"	597	*459*	584	*448*	572	*427*	534	*406*	509	*385*
5'9"	625	*489*	612	*478*	599	*457*	560	*436*	533	*415*
6'0"	654		640		626		585		558	

Source: Adapted from Sprigings et al. (1995).

Drug Therapies

In 1995, 54 million prescriptions were dispensed in the UK for respiratory medicines, most of them for asthma (NAC, 1998). These drugs can be described logically using the five-step approach of the BTS (1993) guidelines for the treatment of chronic asthma:

(1) occasional use of bronchodilators – inhaled B2 agonists (e.g. salbutamol);
(2) twice-daily use of inhaled anti-inflammatory agents – low-dose steroids (e.g. beclomethasone) or cromoglycate or nedocromil sodium;

(3) high-dose inhaled steroids – 800-2000 mcg/day via spacer;
(4) high-dose inhaled steroids and regular bronchodilators – possibilities include:
  • long-acting inhaled B2 agonists (e.g. salmeterol);
  • sustained release oral theophylline;
  • inhaled ipratropium bromide;
  • long-acting oral B2 agonist (e.g. salbutamol);
  • cromoglycate/nedocromil sodium;
(5) regular oral corticosteroids (e.g. prednisolone)

Bronchodilators: Beta Agonists

Stimulation of the beta-adrenergic receptors causes bronchodilation through activation of adenylate cyclase, which produces cyclic AMP. There are many beta receptor agonists currently available. Salbutamol is the nearest to a pure B2 agonist so it has fewer side-effects than those that stimulate all adrenergic receptors, such as epinephrine. Because of B2 receptors in the central nervous system (CNS) and in skeletal muscle, tremor and CNS excitation do occur with salbutamol administration. Beta agonists may be administered orally, intravenously or by inhalation. Inhalation offers a rapid therapeutic effect by direct action of a relatively small dose of the B2 agonist on the airway smooth muscle. This is also associated with fewer side-effects.

Anti-cholinergic Agents

These drugs, of which inhaled ipratropium bromide is the most common, block the cholinergic receptors in the airway smooth muscle. This halts the bronchoconstrictive action of the irritant receptors, which is mediated by the vagus nerve.

Methylxanthines

These are drugs that inhibit the enzyme phosphodiesterase which is responsible for breaking down cyclic AMP. This results in bronchodilation. Methylxanthines are available in oral (theophylline) and intravenous (aminophylline) preparations. All patients given IV aminophylline infusions should have cardiac monitoring throughout, as side-effects include tachycardia and arrhythmias may occur.

Corticosteroids

The exact action of corticosteroids in the treatment of asthma is yet to be confirmed. They are thought to increase the effect of bronchodilators as well as reducing inflammation. Inhaled steroids, including beclomethasone and budesonide, have a local effect so dosage is small and side-effects rare. Their role is largely prophylactic in steps two, three and four of chronic asthma management. Oral and intravenous preparations are reserved for chronic severe asthma and acute episodes, owing to the undesirable side-effects. Prednisolone is the most commonly used oral preparation while methylprednisolone and hydrocortisone are administered intravenously (IV). The effect of oral or IV corticosteroid will be noticeable 12–24 hours following administration.

Discharge

A patient should have recovered at least 75% of his/her expected PEFR before discharge is considered. Ideally he/she should not be returning home alone and his/her inhaler technique should be checked. The patient should have his/her own peak flow meter and should be encouraged to use it, recording the measurements to monitor his/her own condition. A plan of self-treatment should be agreed with clear instructions regarding where and when to seek medical intervention. Some A&E departments have asthma advice sheets that can be used for this purpose and these are advocated by the author.

The patient should be advised to see his/her GP for follow-up within 36 hours of discharge and have out-patient follow-up within four weeks, either with his/her physician or at a nurse-led asthma clinic. If the patient returns to A&E with a relapse within 24 hours he/she should be admitted.

Pulmonary Embolism

A pulmonary embolism (PE) is the partial or total blockage of a pulmonary artery. It is potentially life threatening: the size of the embolus determines the severity of the patient's condition. A total of 5322 people in England and Wales died from pulmonary emboli in 1997 (ONS, 1998).

Aetiology

Blood clots are the most common emboli, usually arising from a deep vein thrombosis (DVT) in the legs or pelvis. Factors increasing the risk of developing DVTs and PEs include:

(1) previous DVT/PE;
(2) heart disease, including:
  • heart failure;
  • atrial fibrillation;
  • patients with prosthetic valves;
(3) pregnancy;
(4) obesity;
(5) malignant disease;
(6) oral contraceptive (high oestrogen) pills, HRT;
(7) family history of PE/DVT;
(8) immobilization
  • surgical patients in the operating theatre for a long time;
  • bedrest or similar, often secondary to illness or injury;
  • long plane/car journeys, 'economy class syndrome';
  • application of lower limb plaster cast or splint.

Lack of movement subsequently leads to poor venous return. The stagnant condition of the blood promotes clot formation. An embolus is formed when part of the clot detaches into the circulation, passes through the right side of the heart and enters the pulmonary artery.

Fat emboli are found following long bone fractures. There is also a possibility of amniotic fluid entering the maternal circulation during delivery causing embolus formation and any foreign material injected intravenously has the potential to become a PE, for example air, coagulated or incompletely dissolved medication, or impurities in illicit drugs.

Deoxygenated blood leaves the right side of the heart by the pulmonary trunk. This divides into the left pulmonary artery which enters the left lung and the right pulmonary artery which enters the right lung. The pulmonary arteries divide further into arterioles and capillaries. An embolus will be carried to the right side of the heart by large veins and by the inferior vena cava.

On leaving the right side of the heart the embolus will occlude the artery or arteriole in which it lodges (this will depend upon the size of the clot). The occlusion will cause infarction and will increase pulmonary vascular resistance. A deadspace is created by the embolized portion of lung. The entire cardiac output is forced through the remaining pulmonary circulation, reducing the ventilation:perfusion ratio. This results in hypoxia and right heart strain. The patient's blood pressure may subsequently fall and his/her jugular vein may become distended.

Signs and Symptoms

The pulmonary infarction may produce:

- sharp, pleuritic chest pain – often lateral, sometimes central;
- cough and haemoptysis;
- cyanosis;
- dyspnoea.

At one extreme a large embolus will occlude one of the pulmonary arteries causing sudden, severe chest pain, respiratory distress, collapse and almost certain death. If a much smaller vessel is blocked there may be little or no pain, mild dyspnoea and possibly haemoptysis.

Nursing Assessment and Intervention

A patient presenting with a sudden onset of severe shortness of breath and pleuritic chest pain should be managed as a suspected PE until proven otherwise. Accompanying haemoptysis and hypotension are further indications. The patient should be transferred to the resuscitation room, the airway secured and high-flow oxygen administered. Baseline vital signs should be recorded with subsequent regular observations. The patient will require pulse oximetry, an electrocardiogram (ECG) and cardiac monitoring. Hypoxia can be expected but oxygen saturations > 95% do not rule out a minor embolism. Sinus tachycardia will be seen initially. The patient may develop atrial fibrillation or atrial flutter. An ECG should be recorded for two reasons: to rule out myocardial infarction and to identify right heart strain.

If analgesia is necessary, opiates such as morphine sulphate should be used. A chest X-ray will be required to rule out other diagnoses such as a pneumothorax or pneumonia. It may show a dilated pulmonary artery or focal shadowing. Blood gases should be taken to establish the severity of hypoxia and hypercapnia. The percussed chest will be dull in the embolized area and auscultation will detect absent breath sounds. The patient will usually have at least one of the risk factors mentioned earlier.

Treatment

A life-threatening pulmonary embolism may be treated surgically by embolectomy (rare) or medically by anticoagulation and thrombolysis. The patient should receive a loading dose of IV heparin 5000u-10000u, depending upon the severity of the embolism. IV colloid should be administered to support the cardiac output, aiming for a systolic blood pressure above 90mmHg (Sprigings et al., 1995).

If a life-threatening PE is clinically certain and there are no contraindications, thrombolytic therapy should be commenced. Fibrinolytic drugs are employed for thrombolysis. These are plasminogen activators. Plasmin degrades fibrin thus breaking up the clot. The drugs used include streptokinase, urokinase and alteplase (TPA). They are administered by intravenous infusion. TPA is given as a bolus, immediately followed by infusion. Side-effects include nausea, vomiting and bleeding, and close monitoring is required.

Non life-threatening pulmonary emboli are treated with intravenous and oral anticoagulant therapy, usually heparin and warfarin. This is to prevent further emboli as well as to dissolve the presenting one. A standard heparin IV infusion of 1000u–2000u per hour is given for up to five days. The activated partial thromboplastin time (APTT) should be checked six hours into treatment. Warfarin will be started concomitantly at around 10mg/day and takes 48–72 hours for full effect. Heparin will be discontinued when the patient's international normalized ratio (INR) is more than 2.0 (BNF, 1998).

Health Education

Patients presenting with DVT or PE should be sensitively informed about predisposing risks and may be assisted in identifying their own risk factors and exploring solutions, should their condition allow.

Patients being discharged from A&E with conditions causing or requiring immobilization should also be informed of the risk factors of DVT/PE. They should be alert for signs and symptoms and take steps to reduce unnecessary immobility, e.g. regular lower limb exercises.

Patients on long-term anticoagulant therapy – three months after first DVT/PE and indefinitely after subsequent DVT/PE – need to know that they are at risk of haemorrhage. They need to understand the importance of taking their medication at the same time each day and of having their INR checked regularly. They must also be told to seek medical attention after epistaxis, haematuria or similar minor bleeds.

Respiratory Infections

The lower respiratory tract infections pneumonia and tuberculosis (TB) will be discussed in this section. Infective exacerbations of chronic obstructive pulmonary disease (COPD) will be covered in the next section. Non-emergent upper respiratory tract infections (URTI) such as the common cold, otitis media, sinusitis, pharyngitis, and epiglottitis will not be discussed. Respiratory infections in immunocompromised adults are more appropriately addressed within the relevant speciality, e.g. HIV and AIDS. However, emergency nursing care of the acutely breathless patient would be largely the same.

Pneumonia: Aetiology

Pneumonia is the inflammation of lung tissue caused by bacterial or viral micro-organisms or inhaled toxins. The alveoli in the infected tissue become engorged with blood and filled with pus. This reduces and may prevent gaseous exchange. It is described as consolidation. Blood vessels may be damaged by engorgement leading to small haemorrhages that colour the sputum. Pneumonia can range in severity from mild infection in an otherwise healthy adult, which is easily treated at home, to overwhelming disease with associated respiratory distress and septic shock. Pneumonia was registered as the underlying cause of 56,719 deaths in 1997 (ONS, 1998).

Classification

Pneumonia can be classified by its anatomical location and/or by where it was most likely contracted:

- Bronchopneumonia refers to multiple areas of infection at the ends of one or both bronchi.
- Lobar pneumonia refers to an infection contained in one or more distinct lobes of lung tissue. The inflammation may also involve the pleural membrane. If more than one lobe is involved there is an increased risk of death (BTS, 1987).
- Hospital-acquired pneumonia refers to the disease infecting a patient after at least a short stay in hospital or other care environment. It is often preceded by invasive treatment or investigations or by immunosuppression. The pathogens responsible are resident at the hospital and may be resistant to some antibiotics. They are sometimes called nosocomial pathogens, methicillin resistant staphylococcus aureus (MRSA) being the one to cause greatest concern (Amyes, 1998). While it is less likely to see hospital-acquired pneumonia in the A&E department than elsewhere in the hospital, the nurse needs to be aware of the possibility in early readmissions and transfers from care homes from an infection control point of view.
- Community-acquired pneumonia refers to the same disease but is caused by different pathogens, and is often secondary to a viral URTI (cold). This distinction is helpful when the doctor is deciding on antibiotic therapy in the absence of a sputum gram stain. The most common micro-organism is streptococcus pneumoniae, which was identified in over three-quarters of cases by Macfarlane et al. in 1982.

Predisposing factors to community-acquired pneumonia:

- upper respiratory tract infection (URTI);
- age > 60 years;
- malnutrition;
- acute or chronic systemic illness;
- other lung disease;
- alcohol:
- impaired mucociliary clearance system;

- reduced consciousness increasing the risk of aspiration;
- congenital abnormality (Sawicka and Braithwaite, 1987).

Signs and Symptoms

The patient usually presents with breathlessness, fever and weakness. Some or all of the following may be present:

- difficulty in breathing, using accessory muscles, may be sudden in onset;
- respiratory rate > 30/min is a marker of severity;
- exhaustion, including inability to talk in long sentences;
- hypoxia, indicated by confusion and/or cyanosis;
- sepsis, indicated by spiking temperatures and rigors, tachycardia, possibly arrhythmia and hypotension; BP <60 mmHg diastolic is a marker of severity;
- chest pain: pleuritic indicates inflammation of the pleura, pain may be secondary to coughing;
- cough may be dry but if productive sputum may be purulent or rust coloured;
- dehydration.

Nursing Assessment and Intervention

The ABC airway, breathing and circulation assessment will give enough information to move the patient with severe pneumonia to a high-dependency area. Respiratory rate and volume, oxygen saturation, heart rate and blood pressure should be recorded regularly. In the absence of chronic irreversible lung disease, high-flow oxygen should be administered. If oxygen saturations are below 92% then blood gases should be taken. PaO_2 <8kPa despite 60% oxygen is another marker of severity usually requiring intensive care (Sprigings et al., 1995).

The patient's pain should be assessed for location, nature and severity. Non-steroidal anti-inflammatory drugs are the preferred analgesia of choice rather than opiates, which may depress respiration. Positioning may ease pain and aid respiration. Recording an ECG should be considered if there is an equivocal history. The patient's temperature should be recorded and anti-pyretics given as necessary. A sputum sample should be obtained before the administration of antibiotics. The patient may require assistance with expectoration. The sample should be sent for gram stain and culture.

An urgent X-ray should be organized to identify consolidation, which appears opaque on the film. Consolidation in one or more lobes indicates lobar pneumonia while fluffy, snow-like consolidation in many areas identifies bronchopneumonia. The X-ray will also show or rule out cavitation, a pneumothorax and a pleural effusion which, if present, would then require aspiration. The aspirate would subsequently be sent for gram stain and culture.

Apart from arterial blood gas analysis, venous blood should be collected for full blood count, urea and electrolytes, and culture and sensitivity.

Markers of severity are:

- WBC > 20 or <4 x 109/l;
- urea > 7mmol/l;
- albumin <35g/l. (BTS, 1987)

Treatment

The medical diagnosis will be made from the history and the chest X-ray, with blood results and nursing observations marking the severity of the disease. Sputum specimens and blood cultures will later identify the causative micro-organism. The patient will need high-flow oxygen, antibiotics and chest physiotherapy. The severely ill patient will require IV antibiotics, possibly intravenous fluids and high-dependency care.

The choice of antibiotic will depend on local policy, the patient's age and concomitant disease. Generally, penicillin or erythromycin in penicillin allergy and a first- or second-generation cephalosporin are given for community-acquired pneumonia. Third-generation cephalosporins and aminoglycosides are used in hospital-acquired pneumonia. The antibiotic therapy should be reviewed after two days to assess response, and gram stain/cultures reviewed as they become available.

Tuberculosis: Aetiology

Pulmonary tuberculosis is a notifiable infectious disease. It is caused by the inhalation of mycobacterium tuberculosis, which is spread by droplet infection from other infected individuals. Predisposing factors to tuberculosis include malnutrition, overcrowded living accommodation, poverty, extremes of age and concomitant illness. The incidence dropped in the 1960s but started to rise again in the late 1980s. There were 4156 notifications of respiratory tuberculosis in 1996 and 304 deaths with this disease named as the underlying cause (ONS, 1997). This may only be the tip of the iceberg, with diseases going undiagnosed and untreated.

The inhaled bacteria enter the lungs and form a primary tubercle. This spreads to the nearest lymph nodes. The primary focus, inflamed lymph nodes and lymph vessels together are called the primary complex. The infection usually starts in the upper lobes. A tubercular abscess may form which breaks down diseased tissue into a cheese-like mass called caseation. This is expectorated as sputum, leaving lung tissue with thick fibrosed walls.

Mycobacterium tuberculosis is virulent: most people in contact with it become infected. Cell-mediated immunity is sufficient in around 95% of cases to contain the disease. Affected individuals will be lifelong carriers at risk of reactivation of tuberculosis at any time (Kryger, 1995). About 1% of those infected develop serious primary tuberculosis, which spreads systemically causing miliary tuberculosis. The remainder develop less serious symptomatic pulmonary tuberculosis, or 'open TB'.

Signs and Symptoms

Tuberculosis does not usually present as an emergency illness. There is a gradual onset of worsening symptoms, including swinging temperatures, night sweats, weight loss, productive cough and sometimes haemoptysis. If the pleura is involved there will be pain and possibly a pneumothorax. Inner-city A&E departments are more likely to see tuberculosis amongst homeless, immigrant and poor communities.

Nursing Assessment and Intervention

Any difficulty in breathing should be noted. Respiratory rate and volume should be recorded. Raised metabolic rate and fever as a marker of infection should also be noted. The presence of a cough, its nature and sputum production and appearance should be documented. There may be haemoptysis. Early-morning sputum specimens should be collected for culture and sensitivity. The weak patient will need rest and may need food and fluid supplements.

Treatment

Patients recovering from TB need convalescence, which will possibly require social services input. Treatment advised by the Joint Tuberculosis Committee of the British Thoracic Society (BNF, 1998) is by antituberculous drugs in two stages. The initial stage is usually triple therapy for about two months with daily isoniazid, rifampicin and pyrazinamide. Ethambutol or streptomycin are sometimes added where isoniazid resistance is suspected. Triple therapy aims to rapidly reduce the presence of myocobacterium tuberculosis and prevent drug resistance. The second or continuation stage is daily treatment with isoniazid and rifampicin. It lasts at least four months.

Health Education

The biggest hurdle in the treatment of tuberculosis is non-compliance amongst patients unable or unwilling to take their medication daily. Supervised regimens exist for tri-weekly administration, possibly by a TB health visitor or practice nurse. Patient education and support is vital to a successful outcome. Patients should be aware of the possibility of liver damage secondary to tuberculosis treatment and should subsequently be observed for signs such as jaundice and vomiting. Patients should be informed that TB drugs cause a reduction in the effectiveness of oral contraceptive pills and should be advised about their options. Patients should also be told that their bodily fluids will be coloured orange-red by rifampicin.

Chronic Obstructive Pulmonary Disease (COPD)

COPD describes a collection of progressive diseases that limit expiratory airflow including asthma, emphysema and chronic bronchitis (Rennard, 1998). It is strongly associated with cigarette smoking.

Prevalence

COPD was named as the underlying cause of 27,218 deaths in England and Wales in 1997 (ONS, 1998). It has been associated with around 28 million lost working days each year in the UK (Turner-Warwick et al., 1990).

Aetiology

Asthma was discussed earlier in this chapter so will not be mentioned here. It should, however, be clarified that airflow obstruction in asthma is reversible. In emphysema and chronic bronchitis it is irreversible.

The Medical Research Council defined chronic bronchitis as 'excessive cough, productive of sputum on most days, for at least three months a year during at least two consecutive years' (MRC, 1965).

The walls of the bronchi become hyperresponsive to irritants such as infection, cigarette smoke and air pollution, resulting in inflammation and bronchoconstriction. The bronchial mucous glands also become hyperresponsive, secreting copious amounts of sputum and further restricting airflow. Additional mucus-secreting goblet cells are produced as the disease progresses.

Emphysema results from the destruction of alveoli. The elasticity of the alveolar wall is damaged initially, and the weakened airways subsequently collapse during expiration. The cause is debatable but is thought to be related to an imbalance of the lungs' enzyme maintenance system (Kryger, 1995).

It is not particularly helpful for the nurse to distinguish between emphysema and chronic bronchitis in patients with COPD as most have a combination of airways and alveolar disease. The strong link to cigarette smoking relates to both diseases, and both are characterized by a relatively rapid decline in lung function. Patients are often well managed at home with a shared care plan involving the patient and relatives, the GP, respiratory specialist nurse and respiratory consultant. This is, at least anecdotally, the most successful model. Knowledgeable patients, confident and competent in the use of inhalers, peak flow meters, home oxygen and nebulizers, are likely to achieve optimum quality of life (Herbert and Gregor, 1997). A&E nurses may be able to initiate and reinforce patients' knowledge and technique but should also be aware of relevant specialist teams and support groups within the community.

Respiratory Drive

The rate and depth of breathing are involuntarily controlled by the respiratory centre in the medulla and by chemoreceptors in the aorta and carotid arteries. In a healthy individual the respiratory centre has dominant control, setting a moderate rate and depth. It is sensitive to acidosis, e.g. reduced pH and raised pCO_2 (hypercapnia). Once acidosis is detected, the respiratory rate and depth are increased and excess CO_2 is eliminated.

Patients with COPD are unable to efficiently eliminate excess CO_2. They gradually become accustomed to increased CO_2 tensions as their lung function deteriorates. Chemoreceptors in the aorta and carotid arteries that are sensitive to lowered oxygen tensions take over the dominant control of respiration. When the oxygen tension drops below 8 kPa the respiratory effort is increased to compensate. This is described as hypoxic drive. Conversely, if the oxygen tension rose the stimulus to breathe would be removed, reducing respiratory effort with potential for apnoea.

The implication for nurses is to cautiously administer oxygen to patients with COPD. It is unusual for a hypoxic patient with COPD to require more than 35% oxygen. Greater concentrations can be given but the patient's respiratory effort should be closely monitored: he/she may require encouragement and/or assistance to maintain adequate ventilation.

Oxygen should be administered using a ventimask with the appropriate percentage valve (if tolerated) until the patient is stabilized. Nasal cannulae are a less accurate mode of oxygen administration.

Acute on Chronic Respiratory Failure

Patients with COPD periodically experience acute exacerbations of their symptoms. These often require A&E intervention. The causes are wide ranging and include:

- infection (viral or bacterial);
- heart failure (cor pulmonale);
- respiratory depressants (alcohol, sedatives);
- lung cancer;
- pneumothorax;

- incorrect home oxygen administration;
- incorrect medication administration/abstention;
- general inability to cope at home.

Signs and Symptoms

The patient with acute exacerbation of COPD will present with increasing breathlessness leading to an inability to talk and intercostal recession. Hypoxia with associated confusion and cyanosis, may follow. The patient will be tachycardic and may have raised jugular venous pressure (JVP). The patient may complain of a productive cough with greater volume and sputum of a different colour than normal.

Nursing Assessment and Intervention

Whilst talking to the patient an assessment should be made of his/her colour and ability to talk. The initial ABC assessment will identify a patient experiencing a severe exacerbation requiring nursing in the resuscitation room. Vital signs to be recorded are respiratory rate, heart rate, blood pressure, PEFR and oxygen saturation using pulse oximetry, followed by regular observations. If spirometry is available record FEV1. Respiratory rate >25/min and FEV1 <1 litre are markers of severity (Spiro, 1998).

Oxygen should be administered at 24% via a ventimask intially, progressing to 28-35% to achieve oxygen saturations of at least 90%. Arterial blood gases should be measured, ideally but not essentially on air, to assess hypoxia, hypercapnia and pH. The latter is the better indicator of CO_2 retention in COPD.

Nebulized bronchodilators such as 5 mg salbutamol may be given to ease presenting symptoms and enable further assessment. If the patient's pCO_2 < 7kPa the nebulizer can be driven by 6 l/min oxygen over no more than 10 min. If the pCO_2 > 7kPa, the nebulizer should be driven by air with 1–2 l/min oxygen simultaneously administered via nasal cannulae, over no more than 10 min.

The history and context of this attack should be investigated. Details of the patient's usual performance including PEFR and activities of daily living and of his/her home management need to be obtained. The key to treatment will be the cause of the exacerbation. It will be influenced by the patient's existing treatment, e.g. theophylline as discussed in the asthma section. Old notes and/or A&E records should be obtained where possible.

A chest X-ray should be organized. This will help identify/eliminate pneumothorax, lung cancer, pneumonia and cardiomegaly. An ECG should be recorded to assess right heart strain and also to help identify/eliminate other diagnoses.

Venous blood should be taken for full blood count, urea and electrolytes, and blood cultures. Arterial blood gases should be rechecked 30–60 minutes after intervention. A sputum specimen should be obtained for culture and sensitivity. This may require suction or assistance from the physiotherapist.

Treatment

Oxygen and nebulized bronchodilators are the initial treatment. Any reversible cause should be treated appropriately, e.g. needle aspiration/chest drain for pneumothorax, antibiotics for pneumonia. Intravenous bronchodilators such as aminophylline should be considered in severe hypercapnia and in patients failing to respond to nebulized salbutamol. Ventilation may be required.

The usefulness of antibiotics in the treatment of acute exacerbations of COPD is subject to debate (Grossman, 1998). Sputum cultures take more than a week to develop. Antibiotics will be prescribed according to local protocol but should be used only if there is strong evidence of a bacterial infection. The value of steroids is also debatable. Hydrocortisone or prednisolone may be prescribed when there is thought to be an asthmatic component.

Ongoing Treatment and Discharge

Patients with acute exacerbation of COPD will be admitted for oxygen and bronchodilator therapy plus any additional treatments indicated. They may require chest physiotherapy and referral to a respiratory specialist nurse. The RCN Respiratory Specialist Nurses Forum has standards advocating patient self-management plans and education (RCN, 1995). Referrals to social services, physiotherapists and occupational therapists will most likely be required to facilitate safe discharge. The patient may require home oxygen and smoking-cessation counselling. It would usually be appropriate to involve family/friends in home management planning.

Anaphylaxis

There are four types of allergy/hypersensitivity:

(1) anaphylactic;
(2) cytotoxic;
(3) immune complex;
(4) cell mediated.

Anaphylaxis is an immune response to certain allergens. It can be localized, as in hay fever, or systemic. Systemic reactions occur within seconds or minutes of exposure and can lead to hypovolaemic shock and asphyxia. Six people died of anaphylactic shock in England and Wales in 1997 (ONS, 1998). The incidence is estimated to be in the region of 1 in 2300 in the UK (Henderson, 1998).

Aetiology

Antigens that cause allergic reactions are called allergens. Allergens can gain entry to the body by injection (including stings), by ingestion and by inhalation. Once the allergen has gained entry the immune system may produce IgE antibodies. These subsequently attach themselves to basophils and mast cells. Mast cells are located in the bronchi, gut mucosa, around blood vessels and in connective tissue in the skin. They contain histamine, spasmogens, inflammatory activators and anaphylactic bronchoconstrictors (Betts and Langelaan, 1996). Basophils are a type of white blood cell that contain histamine and heparin; they become mast cells when they enter tissue. The attachment of IgE causes the release of all these chemicals, which are known collectively as mediators of anaphylaxis. Their effects include increased capillary permeability, increased smooth muscle contraction and increased mucous secretion.

Signs and Symptoms

Increased permeability, smooth muscle contraction and mucous secretion present varying degrees of danger depending on where they occur. Airway obstruction due to laryngeal oedema is possible. The patient may complain of feeling as though his/her throat is closing. Airflow resistance will occur if there is bronchoconstriction and hypersecretion of mucus. The patient will complain of severe

difficulty in breathing with associated wheezin;
and chest tightness. Vasodilation will reduce the
increased permeability will decrease the blood
rate will increase to compensate and may lead
dizzy and faint. Syncope or even cardiac arrest m
swelling may occur. Histamine release will cause ;
urticaria. Nausea, vomiting, abdominal cramps a ....noea will
occur if the mast cells in the gut mucosa are involved. Anaphylaxis
should be considered in any A&E patient presenting with sudden
onset of breathlessness or collapse.

Nursing Assessment and Intervention

The initial ABC assessment will identify patients who should be
nursed in the resuscitation room. The airway should be secured by
intubation or by surgical means if necessary, e.g. cricothyrotomy. The
patient should be given high-flow oxygen and his/her vital signs
recorded – heart rate, respiratory rate, PEFR, blood pressure and
oxygen saturations – with subsequent regular observations. They
should also receive cardiac monitoring. Death usually occurs by asystole secondary to hypotension and hypoxia (International Liaison
Committee on Resuscitation [ILCOR], 1997).

The patient's history of allergies and context of this attack should
be obtained. It is often possible to identify the allergen. Any treatment self-administered or given *en route* by ambulance personnel
should be recorded. As in all emergency situations, a calm,
controlled environment should be promoted with an emphasis on
informing and reassuring the patient and his/her relatives.

Treatment

Epinephrine (adrenaline) is the front-line treatment for anaphylaxis.
Although ILCOR (1997) stated that there is no standard treatment
algorithm, Department of Health (DoH, 1996) guidelines advise that
0.5mg–1mg epinephrine be administered to an adult by intramuscular (IM) injection using 1 mg/1 ml solution (1:1000). Epinephrine
causes vasoconstriction, relaxation of smooth muscle and inhibition
of the mediators of anaphylaxis (Henderson, 1998).

Nebulized epinephrine or salbutamol and possibly ipratropium
bromide may be administered, driven by oxygen, instead of or in

on to IM epinephrine for bronchodilation. An antihistamine
ll be given, usually chlorpheniramine 20mg by IV injection. The
value of steroids is debated as they have no effect for at least four
hours; administration is by local policy. IV fluids are administered to
support the blood pressure. Epinephrine can be repeated IM after
10 minutes or by IV infusion in life-threatening cases. These patients
will most probably be transferred to intensive care.

Health Education and Discharge

Many patients will be discharged from A&E after successful treatment of anaphylaxis and a period of monitoring. Local policies and
clinical judgement, in the absence of national guidelines, will
determine the length of stay. Patients should be assisted to identify
the allergen and its mode of gaining entry. They should be given
clear information regarding the initial symptoms to recognize and
action they should take if they experience another attack. The
author advocates the use of patient information leaflets to support
this.

A patient may be advised to carry an 'Epi-pen' or similar self-
administration epinephrine device. They will require instruction,
practice and reassurance for this to be effective. Patients may benefit
from contact with the Anaphylaxis Campaign and from wearing a
Medic-Alert bracelet.

Conclusion

This chapter has covered several situations where an A&E nurse
may be presented with an acutely breathless patient. It has not,
however, aimed to cover all conditions. The nurse is responsible for
rapid ABC assessment and for taking appropriate intervention.
Oxygen should always be administered, monitoring the respiratory
effort of a patient with hypoxic drive. The importance of an accurate
history and the context of the event are stressed. Nurses are the
cornerstone of the A&E speciality. Their role is both interpersonal
and technical. They attend to all aspects of patient care, they coordinate the A&E team and act as a resource to patients, relatives and
colleagues in all disciplines. This chapter has reflected that role
within emergency respiratory care.

Suggested Further Reading

Cray JV, McMahon E, Ambrose M, Sloan G Wallace J (Eds) (1994) Life Threatening Disorders: A Guide to Priority Nursing Care. Pennsylvania: Springhouse.

Rutishauser S (1994) Physiology and Anatomy: A Basis for Nursing and Health Care. Edinburgh: Churchill Livingstone.

Walsh M (Ed) (1997) Watson's Clinical Nursing and Related Sciences, 5th edn. London: Baillière Tindall in association with RCN.

References

Amyes SGB (1998) Strategies and options for minimizing resistance emergence in pulmonary infections. Chest 113 (Suppl.): 228–32.

Anderson S (1990) ABGs: Six easy steps to interpreting blood gases. American Journal of Nursing August: 42–44.

Betts A, Langelaan DG (1996) Acquired defences. In Hinchliff SM, Montague SE, Watson R (Eds) Physiology for Nursing Practice, 2nd edn. London: Ballière Tindall.

British Thoracic Society (BTS) (1987) Community acquired pneumonia in adults in British hospitals in 1982–1983: a survey of aetiology, mortality, prognostic factors and outcomes. Quarterly Journal of Medicine 62: 195–220.

British Thoracic Society (BTS) (1993) Guidelines on the management of asthma. Thorax 48(2, Suppl.): S1–S24.

British Association for Accident and Emergency Medicine (BAAEM) (1993) Guidelines for the Treatment of Acute Asthma in A&E (Adults). London: Royal College of Surgeons Academic Committee.

British National Formulary (BNF) (1998) Number 36. London: British Medical Association and Royal Pharmaceutical Society of Great Britain.

Department of Health (1996) Immunisation against Infectious Diseases. London: HMSO.

European Community Respiratory Health Survey (ECRHS) (1996) Variations in the prevalence of respiratory symptoms, self-reported asthma attacks and the issue of asthma medication in the ECRHS. European Respiratory Journal 9: 687–95.

Grossman RF (1998) The value of antibiotics and the outcomes of antibiotic therapy in exacerbations of COPD. Chest 113 (Suppl.): 249–55.

Henderson N (1998) Anaphylaxis. In Thomas L (Ed) Maintaining an Airway, RCN Continuing Education Reader. London: RCN Publishing.

Herbert R, Gregor F (1997) Quality of life and coping strategies of clients with COPD. Rehabilitation Nursing 22(4): 182–7.

International Liaison Committee on Resuscitation (ILCOR) (1997) Special resuscitation situations. Resuscitation 34(2): 140–1.

Kryger MH (Ed) (1995) Introduction to Respiratory Medicine, 2nd edn. London: Churchill Livingstone.

Macfarlane JT, Finch RG, Ward MJ (1982) Hospital study of adult community acquired pneumonia. Lancet 2: 255–8.

Medical Research Council (1965) In Grossman RF (1998) The value of antibiotics and the outcomes of antibiotic therapy in exacerbations of COPD. Chest 113 (Suppl.): 249–55.

National Asthma Campaign (NAC) (1998) The National Asthma Campaign Asthma
    Audit 1998/1999. London: National Asthma Campaign.
Office of National Statistics (ONS) (1997) Monitor: Population & Health MB97/3.
    London: Government Statistical Service.
Office for National Statistics (ONS) (1998) Mortality Statistics 1997: Cause, England &
    Wales Series DH2 No.24. London: Government Statistical Service.
RCN Respiratory Nurses Forum (1995) Standards of Care for Respiratory Nursing.
    London: Royal College of Nursing.
Rennard SI (1998) COPD: overview of definitions, epidemiology and factors influenc-
    ing its development. Chest 113 (Suppl.): 235–41.
Sawicka EH, Braithwaite MA (1987) Respiratory Emergencies. London: Butterworth.
Spiro SG (Ed) (1998) Guidelines for the Management of Common Medical
    Emergencies and for the Use of Antimicrobial Drugs. London: UCL Hospitals.
Sprigings D, Chambers J, Jeffrey A (1995) Acute Medicine, 2nd edn. Oxford: Blackwell
    Science.
Turner-Warwick M, Hodson ME, Corrin B (1990) Clinical Atlas of Respiratory
    Diseases. London: Gower Medical.

Chapter 4
Surgical Conditions

Melanie Gunstone

Introduction

This chapter will address the surgical conditions that may present within the accident and emergency (A&E) department. The conditions that have been included cover the most common major presenting conditions. Those covered are as follows:

(1) leaking aortic aneurysm;
(2) intestinal obstruction;
(3) gastrointestinal bleeds;
(4) appendicitis;
(5) other causes of acute abdomen;
(6) peripheral vascular disease;
(7) testicular pain;
(8) acute urinary retention.

It is hoped that the material will provide the reader with sufficient insight to care for patients presenting to A&E with such surgical conditions, though with the proviso that what has been included is not exhaustive.

Leaking Aortic Aneurysm

Incidence

Aneurysms of the abdominal aorta occur as a complication of atherosclerosis. They are relatively uncommon and are found mainly in elderly patients, often over the age of 70, who may be unaware of the condition until they suddenly become very unwell. Aneurysms are

most prominent and significant in the aorta but can occur in peripheral vessels as well, especially in the popliteal arteries of the elderly.
However, this section will relate only to aortic aneurysms. If an aortic
aneurysm ruptures, mortality rates are between 20% and 70%. Post-
operatively, morbidity is high as a result of multi-organ failure,
myocardial infarction, strokes or haemorrhage (Hope et al., 1998).

Basic Anatomy and Physiology

Damage to arterial walls caused by factors such as atherosclerosis or
hypertension may lead to the formation of an aneurysm. This is
where a section of the artery wall becomes excessively dilated due to
a weakening within the wall. Sometimes aneurysms form a sac-like
extension of the arterial wall or are fusiform in shape, slowly
expanding in diameter. Aneurysms may also have a longitudinal
dissection between the outer and inner layers of the vessel wall. The
majority of abdominal aortic aneurysms only involve the infrarenal
aorta, although some extend to involve one or both of the iliac
arteries. Syphilitic aneurysms almost always occur in the thoracic
aorta involving the aortic arch, while atherosclerotic aneurysms
occur in the abdominal section below the renal arteries and above
the bifurcation of the aorta (Mosby, 1990). An enlarged abdominal
aneurysm may press on the vertebrae or other structures causing
associated pain.

The reasons for concern regarding aneurysms include possible
plaque formation as a result of atherosclerosis, which may cause a
blockage in vital tissue and, more importantly, the fact that they have
a tendency to burst causing severe haemorrhage or even death.
Aneurysms greater than 5cm in diameter must be considered for
surgery owing to the risk of rupture.

Presenting Signs and Symptoms/Complications

When a patient presents with chest, abdominal or back pain, or a
combination of the three, the nurse should always be aware of the
possibility of an aneurysm. Aortic aneurysms are often found incidentally, either on a routine abdominal examination where a
pulsatile mass may be felt or on a plain abdominal/chest X-ray film.
Rarely, patients may be able to feel a pulsating area within their
abdomen. However, the symptoms a patient may experience are

often as a result of the aneurysm leaking and it is these symptoms that cause the patient to seek medical attention.

Classic symptoms associated with leaking aortic aneurysms include chest, abdominal or back pain which may be unrelenting or described as tearing, and the patient may be cardiovascularly compromised. The patient is often very restless or even semi-conscious, is invariably tachycardic and tachypnoeic and is often found to have differing blood pressures in each arm. The patient will also look 'shut down' or cyanosed.

Complications include back pain due to erosion of the lumbar vertebrae, thrombosis with distal ischaemia and intraperitoneal haemorrhage, which is rapidly fatal. This is often an unrecognized cause of death in the elderly (Raftery, 1996).

Nursing Assessment and Intervention

Such patients should always have a triage rating of urgent to emergent. Any patient showing the signs and symptoms described should have one large-bore cannula inserted into either antecubital fossa and blood should be taken for routine investigation as well as typing and cross-matching. An ECG should be performed as it may identify the size and location of the aneurysm and oxygen therapy should always be commenced. The patient should remain under constant nursing observation as his/her condition can change very rapidly. Regular observations should be recorded including pulse rate and rhythm, blood pressure in both arms, pulse oximetry and respiration rate and depth. Time allowing, the patient should also be catheterized with urine output measurements recorded.

Analgesia must be administered, with intravenous morphine and diamorphine being the first drugs of choice because of their strength and action. Intravenous fluids may also be commenced, but owing to the risk of fluid overload and increased pressure they may be withheld.

Many relatives do not understand the nature of the condition or indeed the possible seriousness and it is vital to remember not to build up false hopes.

Potential Surgical Interventions

If time allows, an ultrasound scan will confirm the diagnosis and subsequent treatment may depend on this. Asymptomatic aneurysms under 5 cm in diameter may be treated conservatively, particularly if the patient is a poor surgical risk. In such cases routine ultrasound scans should be performed to observe the development of the aneurysm.

Aneurysms greater than 5 cm should be considered for surgery because of the risk of rupture if left untreated. In these cases of elective surgery, mortality rates are generally less than 5% (Berridge et al., 1995). With aneurysms that are leaking the patient is invariably taken to theatre straight from the A&E department. A leaking abdominal aortic aneurysm is a surgical emergency with fewer than half the patients actually reaching hospital alive and of those only about half survive (Burkitt et al., 1990).

Intestinal Obstruction

Basic Anatomy and Physiology

The small intestine is the longest portion of the alimentary canal, being approximately 18–20 feet in length and divided into the duodenum, the jejunum and the ileum. The small intestine is covered with villi and is where most digestion and absorption takes place.

The large intestine is much greater in diameter than the small intestine and is divided into the caecum, colon, rectum and anal canal. The large intestine does not have villi but has goblet cells to secrete mucus along with an arrangement of muscular tissues.

The most acute presentation is upper small bowel obstruction, whereas large bowel obstruction is often more chronic. Obstruction primarily results in proximal dilatation of the bowel, which disrupts peristalsis.

Causes of Intestinal Obstruction

The most common cause is a mechanical blockage within the intestine as a result of faecal matter, tumours, adhesions, hernia, intussusception (usually in children aged under two years), inflammatory bowel disease, strangulation or strictures (Mosby, 1990).

Presenting Signs and Symptoms

Patients may present with differing signs and symptoms depending on the degree and level of obstruction (e.g. whether large or small bowel).

The most common symptoms include abdominal pain, constipation or diarrhoea and vomiting, which may persist even when the patient has eaten nothing because of the amount of gastric juices which continue to be produced. The material vomited often gives doctors a good indication of where the obstruction has occurred (e.g. large amounts of bile indicates upper small bowel obstruction; faecal matter indicates more distal obstruction and semi-digested food indicates obstruction nearer the stomach outlet (Burkitt et al., 1990).

Signs include abdominal distension, tachycardia, dehydration, hypotension, hypo/hyperactive bowel sounds and rebound tenderness and guarding on examination of the abdomen. The patient's condition may deteriorate rapidly leading to shock if the bowel is not decompressed or essential fluids replaced. Patients with small bowel obstruction often experience greater pain than those with large bowel obstruction (Mosby, 1990).

Nursing Assessment and Intervention

Such patients should receive a triage category of urgent to emergent (Selfridge-Thomas, 1997). Baseline observations should be recorded with regular monitoring of blood pressure and pulse as these can alter with the patient's condition.

A nasogastric tube should be inserted and either attached to suction or regularly aspirated in order to relieve the patient's nausea and vomiting, remove any swallowed air, reduce the risk of inhaling gastric contents and measure the amount of gastric output. The patient should also be given adequate pain relief, preferably opiate based, with the effectiveness measured.

Mouth care is important for patients with obstruction as they are usually nil by mouth, have not eaten for some time and may well have vomited faecal fluid.

Potential Surgical Interventions

Patients with probable bowel obstruction will be admitted to a ward and kept under observation prior to any possible surgery. If the obstruction is uncomplicated, it may well be treated conservatively (e.g. if due to constipation) but in the presence of any possible complications surgery is usually the management. This can be delayed for one to two days if there is no risk of strangulation, allowing for any further investigations and patient stabilization (Burkitt et al., 1990).

If surgery is performed the section of bowel which has become obstructed is resected, anastomosing the remaining bowel. If the resection has been extensive the patient may require either a temporary or permanent stoma and will require considerable nursing care and support post-operatively. The two most common stomas are a colostomy or ileostomy, again depending on which part of the bowel is removed.

Gastrointestinal Bleeds

Causes

Gastrointestinal (GI) bleeding can occur at any part of the GI tract and may be manifested by haematemesis or melaena. There are various causes for GI bleeds, the most common being those summarized below:

(1) Mallory-Weiss tear;
(2) peptic ulceration;
(3) oesophageal varices;
(4) diverticulitis;
(5) ulcerative colitis;
(6) carcinoma;
(7) erosion of mucosa;
(8) laceration following foreign body ingestion;
(9) gastritis (Mosby, 1990; Raftery, 1996).

Non-steroidal anti-inflammatory analgesic drugs (NSAIDS) are often a cause of erosion if used over a prolonged period of time.

Basic Anatomy and Physiology

The gastrointestinal tract includes all the organs from mouth to anus. The alimentary canal, as it is commonly known, includes the oral cavity, pharynx, oesophagus, stomach, small intestine, large intestine and rectum. There are also accessory organs, which include the liver, gall bladder, pancreas and bile ducts (Kapit and Elson, 1993).

Presenting Signs and Symptoms/Complications

These will depend upon the severity and location of the bleeding although patients generally complain of vomiting blood or passing blood rectally.

Haematemesis usually indicates upper GI bleeding, e.g. from the oesophagus, stomach or even duodenum. This may be bright red with fresh blood or darker with the appearance of 'coffee grounds' within it, often occurring when the blood has been partially digested.

Any blood originating beyond the duodenum is usually passed rectally forming a classic black, tarry stool due to the effect of digestive juices on the blood.

Any fresh blood passed rectally is often due to bleeding from the colon, rectum or anus from erosion of mucosa, ulcerative colitis or haemorrhoids (Watson and Royle, 1987).

The patient may experience dizziness, weakness, syncope or may collapse as a result of the blood loss, especially if the bleeding has occurred for some time. He/she is often found to be restless or semi-conscious, to look pale with clammy skin, to be hypotensive, tachycardic and to have possible tenderness on examination of the abdomen. Again these are all dependent upon the extent of the blood loss (Selfridge-Thomas, 1997).

Complications generally relate to massive haemorrhage, which can result from ruptured oesophageal varices. If this happens there is an 80% mortality rate (Hope et al., 1998).

Nursing Assessment and Intervention

A nursing assessment identifying a patient who is pale, clammy, possibly hypotensive and tachycardic must always alert the nurse to the possibility of blood loss and associated hypovolaemia. Baseline observations should be recorded with regular monitoring of the patient's level of consciousness, blood pressure, pulse rate and rhythm, respiratory rate and pulse oximetry. These can all alter with the patient's condition and an increase in respiratory rate is often the first sign of increasing blood loss. By the time the patient's blood pressure has dropped he/she can have lost considerable amounts of blood volume owing to the body's compensatory mechanisms. An ECG should also be recorded, as arrhythmias can occur with blood loss.

A nasogastric tube may be passed if the patient is vomiting blood as it provides a record of output as well as alleviating patient discomfort.

Supplementary oxygen should always be administered as blood loss reduces oxygen-carrying capacity. If the bleeding is severe or fresh then one large-bore cannula should be inserted into each ante-cubital fossa and IV fluids commenced. Depending upon severity a blood transfusion may be required. These may be given as a bolus if the estimated blood loss is great or may be given slowly so as not to increase any pressure upon bleeding points.

If any active bleeding is evident, an estimated record of output should be maintained. If the patient is cardiovascularly compromised or collapsed an indwelling urinary catheter should also be inserted to measure urine production and output as renal failure can occur as a result of extensive blood loss. This will also give an indication of effective fluid replacement.

It is vital for the nurse to examine any blood passed through the mouth to determine whether it is actually haematemesis or haemoptysis. This is frequently found in patients who present to A&E with a history of vomiting blood, yet who look well on arrival and do not have any episodes for considerable periods of time.

Potential Surgical Intervention

Intervention is indicated if there is massive haemorrhage or continual re-bleeding with treatment being either operative or non-operative. Surgery is usually performed for oversewing of peptic ulcers, transection of varices or removal of tumours. Non-operative procedures are generally in the form of adrenaline injections or laser treatment. Tubes such as Sengstaken tubes may be passed to treat oesophageal varices if there is active bleeding within the A&E setting.

Minor bleeds, such as with a Mallory-Weiss tear or erosion from the use of NSAIDS, can be treated conservatively with the use of ulcer-healing drugs such as cimetidine or ranitidine. Mallory-Weiss tears often occur when a patient has forcibly vomited or even coughed and should resolve spontaneously. Diagnosis is usually confirmed via an endoscopy and treated according to the findings.

There is an overall 10% mortality rate for patients with upper GI bleeds (Raftery, 1996).

Appendicitis

Incidence

An inflamed appendix can occur at almost any age and in either sex but most commonly occurs in teenagers and young adults, being rare in the elderly and in infants under two years. Appendicitis is the most common cause of an acute abdomen, with an average of one in every six or seven people undergoing surgery for an inflamed appendix. However, the incidence of appendicitis has fallen by approximately 50% over the last ten years (Burkitt et al., 1990) and Barber et al. (1997) revealed that of patients studied, at least a third who underwent surgery had a 'normal' appendix removed.

Appendicitis is generally acute in onset, although some controversy remains as to whether recurrent or chronic appendicitis exists.

Basic Anatomy and Physiology

The appendix is a narrow, blind-ending tube containing a large amount of lymphoid tissue. It projects from the end of the caecum and is approximately the size of an adult's little finger. Its position can vary between individuals but is commonly mobile within the peritoneal cavity, suspended by mesentery, only becoming fixed in one place when it becomes inflamed. The appendix lies within the right iliac fossa and has no function in humans (Hinchliff et al., 1996).

The appendix can become enlarged if infection or inflammation is present, which may occur if the opening of the appendix becomes blocked. This may be due to a mass of faeces or swollen lymphoid tissue. If the inflammation becomes severe enough to cause the appendix to rupture then peritonitis is likely to occur as a result of faecal material and bacteria entering the abdominal cavity.

Presenting Signs and Symptoms/Complications

Acute appendicitis is typically associated with abdominal pain, yet it is often difficult to make a positive diagnosis. It classically begins with poorly localized, colicky type central abdominal pain. This may be as a result of muscular spasm in reaction to any obstruction or because embryologically the appendix develops in the midgut, lying in the periumbilical area, and its nerve supply reflects this. As inflammation develops the pain becomes localized in the right iliac fossa region. Depending on the exact location of the appendix, specific pain and symptoms may differ. For example, if the appendix lies near the bladder then the patient may experience symptoms that could be mistaken for a urinary tract infection.

Appendicitis is characterized by the early phase of poorly localized pain generally lasting for a few hours until inflammation produces localizing signs. There may also be nausea and/or vomiting and a low-grade fever. On examination the patient is often found to have rebound tenderness, a rigid abdomen and decreased or absent bowel sounds. The classic features of acute appendicitis are summarized below:

- abdominal pain for less than 72 hours;
- nausea/vomiting;
- tenderness over right iliac fossa;
- rebound tenderness in the right iliac fossa;
- tenderness anteriorly on rectal examination;
- low-grade pyrexia (often between 37.2° and 38.5°C);
- no evidence of urine infection;
- raised white cell count.

If left untreated the inflamed appendix often becomes gangrenous after 12–48 hours and then perforates causing peritonitis. Once this happens there is a rise in any fever and the whole abdomen becomes rigid and tender. Other indications of peritonitis include abdominal distension, tachycardia, restlessness and rapid, shallow breathing. Such signs should be apparent on nursing assessment.

The nurse should also have some insight into other possible causes of signs and symptoms which may mimic appendicitis. Briefly these include the following:

(1) constipation – may cause iliac fossa tenderness and colicky pain but fever is absent;
(2) urinary tract infection – this should reveal leucocytes or bacteria on microscopy;
(3) mesenteric adenitis – inflammation of the abdominal lymph nodes. This is often associated with respiratory tract infections or

sore throat. Fever is typically higher than with an appendicitis and there is no tenderness;

(4) gynaecological disorders – menstruation pain, salpingitis and ovarian cysts can cause abdominal or right iliac fossa pain, but vaginal examination often confirms diagnosis;

(5) pancreatitis – although abdominal pain is present, it is predominantly central and epigastric.

Nursing Assessment and Intervention

On assessing the patient in A&E the nurse should obtain an accurate history. This should include onset of pain, whether there is associated nausea and vomiting, other relevant medical history and whether anything has helped relieve the symptoms. Severity of pain should be noted along with the effectiveness of any home analgesia. Appendicitis should have a triage rating of urgent. The patient's baseline blood pressure, pulse, respirations and temperature should be recorded as these may change in the presence of appendicitis or peritonitis. A urine sample should be obtained and tested for any infection. A pregnancy test should also be performed on all females of child-bearing age since it is not uncommon for complications of pregnancy to mimic signs of appendicitis (e.g. an ectopic pregnancy).

Pain relief and an anti-emetic should be offered and administered to any patient in pain. Some doctors believe that if patients with abdominal pain receive analgesia prior to examination then certain signs will be masked. However, by administering analgesia the patient becomes more settled and the doctor is more able to examine the patient successfully. Analgesia does not mask diagnosis: it merely alleviates the symptoms, which is a prime nursing goal. Commonly administered analgesics are generally opiate based as they relieve moderate to severe pain, particularly those of visceral origin.

Drugs commonly prescribed include:

(1) analgesics:
  • pethidine: prompt, but short-lasting;
  • morphine: commonly causes nausea and vomiting;
  • papaveretum: often used after surgery;

(2) anti-emetics:
- metoclopramide: particularly useful in gastrointestinal disorders;
- prochlorperazine (although not licensed for IV use);

(3) other:
- antibiotics (e.g. metronidazole), may be given pre-operatively to reduce the risk of wound infection.

A nasogastric tube may also be passed if the patient experiences considerable nausea or vomiting.

It is important for the A&E nurse to ensure that both patient and relatives are kept informed of all procedures. A&E is a frightening place for patients who have become unwell suddenly and therefore feel out of control of their situation. It is vital to remember that dignity must be maintained at all times and patient embarrassment kept to a minimum where possible.

Potential Surgical Interventions

Diagnosis of acute appendicitis poses little difficulty if the patient exhibits signs and symptoms classically associated with it. The most common treatment is surgical removal of the appendix, preferably performed within 48 hours of the onset of symptoms so as to reduce the risk of perforation. Difficulties arise when signs and symptoms are atypical. If the evidence for acute appendicitis is insufficient the patient should be admitted and kept under observation with periodic review.

Other Causes of Acute Abdomen

The term 'acute abdomen' is one that describes many patients attending A&E with abdominal symptoms but is difficult to define. It covers a vast array of conditions including those which require urgent surgery, those which do not require surgery and those which do not need urgent investigation or treatment. Burkitt et al. (1990) stated that of all surgical admissions nearly 50% relate to an acute abdomen.

Causes

There are many causes for an acute abdomen and because of the amount of organs possibly involved the initial diagnosis can prove difficult. Typically the symptoms are acute in onset and reflect an abdominal cause. The common causes for an acute abdomen are summarized below:

(1) acute appendicitis;
(2) peptic ulceration;
(3) pancreatitis;
(4) gallstones;
(5) aneurysm (especially leaking);
(6) diverticulitis;
(7) hernias;
(8) tumours;
(9) constipation;
(10) acute urinary retention;
(11) gynaecological conditions;
(12) abdominal trauma;
(13) sickle-cell crisis.

The major causes of an acute abdomen have already been covered earlier in the chapter.

Basic Anatomy and Physiology

An acute abdomen relates to conditions that affect any part of the abdominal cavity. This may involve any of the following organs:

(1) stomach;
(2) liver;
(3) intestines;
(4) pancreas;
(5) gall bladder;
(6) bladder;
(7) kidneys
(8) biliary tract;
(9) reproductive organs.

Presenting Signs and Symptoms

These will vary greatly depending upon the exact cause, but the most common symptoms include pain and possibly nausea and vomiting. Pain may be due to muscular spasm of the smooth muscle, mucosal or peritoneal irritation, swelling, strangulation, obstruction or infection. Patients will often look pale and possibly dehydrated depending on how long they have been unwell. They may also be tachycardic and tachypnoeic, be restless, possibly pyrexic and may present with abdominal distension. Other common symptoms include dyspepsia, anorexia, pale stools, flatulence, rectal bleeding, jaundice and dark urine (McGrath, 1998). If the cause is truly abdominal there will often be pain, rigidity and guarding on palpation of the abdomen.

Nursing Assessment and Intervention

A nurse can gain a great deal of information about abdominal conditions following an accurate assessment of the patient. First, it is vital to determine the time of onset of pain and/or symptoms (e.g. whether sudden or gradual), the severity, type of pain (e.g. sharp, stabbing), location and associated radiation, including any associated nausea, vomiting, constipation or diarrhoea. The patient should also be asked if the symptoms have affected any normal activities such as movement, eating or breathing and if he/she has had any fever. If he/she has used first-aid measures at home, for example analgesia, the effects of these should be noted. It is often these details in a history that give doctors and nurses a clearer indication about possible causes.

Vital signs should be recorded as well as a urine sample being tested as it is very common for patients to present with abdominal pain when they have a urinary tract infection. This should also include a pregnancy test on all females of child-bearing age.

If the patient is vomiting continuously, a nasogastric tube should be passed with any output recorded and an anti-emetic administered. Analgesia should be administered depending upon the severity, remembering that it will not mask any signs during medical assessment. Non-steroidal drugs such as diclofenac should be avoided in case of exacerbation of irritation or pain. If a full bladder can be palpated, a urinary catheter may be inserted to exclude urinary retention as the underlying cause.

Patients will usually be kept nil by mouth and under observation either until signs and symptoms become clearer and treatment is obvious or until the condition resolves.

If there is any suspicion of infection then broad-spectrum antibiotics may be administered either orally or IV. Blood tests should also be performed to identify any abnormalities such as a raise in white cell count in infection or raised amylase indicating pancreatitis.

Potential Surgical Intervention

Approximately half of those patients who are admitted with an acute abdomen do not require surgical intervention. Diagnoses commonly include pancreatitis, diverticulitis, acute urinary retention, ulceration and constipation.

Surgery is indicated for patients where there is a spreading of abdominal tenderness, shock, free gas on X-ray, peritonitis and localized guarding (Raftery, 1996). These conditions may result from strangulation, obstruction, acute appendicitis, ruptured ulcers, varices, ovarian cysts or aneurysms. If a patient's condition deteriorates but a cause has not been found then a laparotomy may be performed to aid diagnosis.

Peripheral Vascular Disease

Vascular disease can originate in either the arterial or venous system. If the arterial system is affected there is a reduction of blood volume into the affected vessel through partial or complete occlusion, causing a lack of oxygen and nutrients to the tissues. If the venous system is involved the outflow of venous blood is affected causing oedema and congestion within the tissues (Watson and Royle, 1987). Vascular disease can be acute or chronic.

Peripheral vascular disease usually affects the lower limbs but can also affect the GI tract, the renal and cerebral vessels and the upper limbs. This section will address only lower limb disease as that is the most frequent presentation to A&E departments, but will examine both acute and chronic arterial and venous conditions.

Arterial

The majority of arterial complications are the result of ischaemia due to atherosclerosis; risk factors include smoking, diabetes, hyperlipidaemia, obesity and hypotension. Almost any vessel can be involved.

Causes

These complications result from thrombosis, embolism or external compression such as trauma. Thrombosis usually occurs where there has been a narrowing in the lumen of vessels, often associated with plaque formation. An embolus can be the result of complications within the heart, e.g. following an MI, disease of the valves or aneurysms (Raftery, 1996). Trauma may result from direct penetration following catheterization or angioplasty, damage following fractures or even misplaced injections into the artery instead of the vein.

Chronic occlusion is more of a gradual process where there is progressive narrowing within the walls of the vessels but carries the same risk factors.

Presenting Signs and Symptoms

There are classic signs and symptoms found in acute arterial occlusion known as the 'Ps'. These are as follows:

(1) pale;
(2) pain;
(3) pulseless;
(4) paraesthesia;
(5) paralysed;
(6) 'perishing cold' (Hope et al., 1998).

The patient may also have had intermittent claudication (pain induced by exercise due to ischaemia in the muscles), pain at rest which indicates more severe ischaemia or even gangrene. Claudication may prevent the patient from walking any great distance. Previous medical history should be sought identifying any contributory factors.

Patients with chronic ischaemia often experience more rest pain and may have more necrotic areas evident, especially where pressure occurs such as at the ends of toes and in bunion areas.

Nursing Assessment and Intervention

It is difficult to miss an ischaemic limb but A&E nurses must remember that they invariably see the patient long before the doctor does and so an accurate nursing assessment is vital. The triage rating should be urgent to emergent.

The patient's limb should be checked for colour and appearance. The skin may have a fixed mottled effect which indicates irreversible damage, may be white or marbled (indicating acute ischaemia), or may be shades of blue or red. There may also be a collapsed look in the veins known as 'guttering'. If the skin is shiny this is often an indication of chronic ischaemia.

Pulses within the limb should also be recorded and, if absent, a doctor should be informed immediately, especially if associated with the above signs. The nurse should also ask the patient to raise his/her leg to assess whether there is any loss of colour distally; the quicker pallor begins, the more severe the ischaemia. Pressure areas should also be assessed as ischaemic limbs break down much more quickly. The nurse may find the patient is more comfortable if his/her foot is able to hang down, as raising an already ischaemic limb only causes more pain with a further reduction in blood flow.

Baseline observations should be noted along with the temperature of the skin. The capillary refill time should be recorded and monitored regularly if the response is slow. A Doppler is the best measurement of pulses and should be available in every A&E department.

Pain relief should be offered to the patient and should be of an opiate base. The patient should also be commenced on anticoagulant therapy (usually intravenous heparin) and should be kept on strict bed rest.

Potential Surgical Intervention

Treatment very much depends on the vessel obstructed and the size of obstruction. If an end artery is occluded, any tissue beyond it will become necrotic. Any embolus originating from the right side of the heart could potentially lead to a pulmonary embolism, which has a high mortality rate. Any embolism originating from the left side of the heart could potentially cause a cerebral infarct (Watson and Royle, 1987).

If the symptoms are mild to moderate in chronic occlusion then surgery is not usually required. Minimizing risk factors could certainly assist in treatment and patients will require regular follow-ups.

If the cause is thought to be an embolus, surgery is usually performed to remove the blockage. More chronic ischaemia may require grafting. Limbs that are irreversibly ischaemic or gangrenous invariably require amputation. Surgery to correct any acute occlusion should ideally be undertaken within the first 8-10 hours of onset if blood flow is to be returned. Any delay beyond this time increases the likelihood of amputation or even death (Raftery, 1996).

Venous

Interference with blood flow through the veins causes oedema and congestion. The most common types of venous disease include deep vein thrombosis (DVT) and varicose veins. This section will discuss only DVTs as they are the most common presentation for venous conditions within the emergency setting. Other types also include leg ulcers, which are generally dealt with in the community. DVTs are a major cause of morbidity following surgery and trauma and are often associated with high levels of oestrogen found in the contraceptive pill.

Causes

Several factors are found to influence the incidence of DVT formation and are summarized below:

(1) prolonged bed rest;
(2) obesity;
(3) oral contraceptive pill;
(4) trauma and surgery;
(5) previous DVT;
(6) certain blood disorders;
(7) pregnancy.

Basic Anatomy and Physiology

There are two drainage systems for venous blood of the lower limb: the deep venous system draining the tissues of the foot and muscles of the lower leg and thigh (the posterior tibial, anterior tibial, popliteal, femoral and iliac veins) and the superficial venous system draining skin and tissues superficial to the deep fascial layer and comprising mainly the saphenous veins.

Presenting Signs and Symptoms

These generally include pain and swelling in the calf region, often associated with an increase in temperature. Depending on the site of occlusion the whole leg may become swollen. The limb is often found to be discoloured – either red or cyanosed.

Raftery (1996) stated that only 25% of patients with DVTs actually have any signs or symptoms. Many patients express a development of 'pulled muscle' feeling in the calf which they do not investigate until other symptoms occur. Tenderness on walking may be the only symptom a patient complains of. If the occlusion has been present for some time, the patient may have areas of ulceration or necrosis although most patients presenting to A&E have usually had concerns for a few days only and therefore not long enough for necrosis to set in without other complications being present.

Nursing Assessment and Intervention

Baseline observations should be recorded as patients with cellulitis may have symptoms which mimic a DVT and DVTs do not generally cause pyrexia or systemic illness. The nurse should take careful measurement of the patient's calves, normally measured at a point of 10 cm below the tibial plateau, noting any difference in diameter. In addition the skin should be felt for heat and tenseness.

The patient should be discouraged from walking about because of the risk of dislodging any clot present. This can involve effective communication skills as patients may report that they have been fully mobile until arriving at A&E.

Treatment is usually in the form of anticoagulation with either intravenous subcutaneous heparin or low molecular weight heparin (e.g. clexane) with regular monitoring of blood clotting times. The patient may be advised to rest or mobolize as able. Following a period of anticoagulation he/she may change to oral medication. Depending on local hospital policies, most patients are now discharged on clexane programmes.

Some doctors will endeavour to arrange a venogram if a DVT is not clearly indicated prior to commencing anticoagulation. Doppler ultrasound is another effective method of diagnosis and is now being used more readily owing to the time factor and ease of use. Doctors may also stipulate the use of thrombo-embolic (TED) stockings, either during treatment or as a preventive measure following thrombosis.

Potential Surgical Intervention

Surgery is rarely indicated for the treatment of DVTs unless there are underlying complications which cannot be treated conservatively. Surgery is generally used to treat arterial conditions only.

Testicular Pain

There are various causes and problems associated with the testes including undescended testes, hydrocele, cysts, varicocele, intussusception, epididymitis and torsion. However, the two most common conditions presenting to A&E departments are epididymitis and torsion of the testes, which will be discussed here.

Epididymitis

Male patients can present with inflammation of the epididymis at any age and is the most common disorder of the scrotal area. The inflammation can be acute or chronic with causes including urinary tract infections, venereal disease, following prostate or urethral surgery or infections such as mumps or TB.

Basic Anatomy and Physiology

The male genital system consists of two testes and their ducts, accessory glands and the penis. The testes are located within the scrotum with the ducts and tubules from each testis forming the epididymis. The vas deferens runs from the tail of the epididymis to the ureter.

Presenting Signs and Symptoms

Signs and symptoms commonly associated with epididymitis include pain in the testes or groin, pyrexia, scrotal swelling and redness (Mosby, 1990). Patients are often seen to walk with a waddle owing to tenderness when the legs are close together. Rarely, the testis itself becomes infected (orchitis) although generalized surrounding inflammation can cause tenderness in the testis. A good indication of epididymitis is relief of pain when the scrotum is elevated.

Nursing Assessment and Intervention

This condition should be triaged as urgent because of the associated pain. Baseline observation should be recorded, especially temperature, and a urine sample sent for microscopy. The patient should be encouraged to rest and if the infection is acute bed rest with scrotal elevation should be commenced. Ice packs may be offered to ease the swelling of the scrotal area but should be intermittent.

Analgesics should be given to the patient with any effects monitored, along with a broad-spectrum antibiotic until culture results are known. The patient should also be issued with a scrotal support to wear when mobile. Recurrent or chronic epididymitis is usually the result of inadequate antibiotic therapy, either due to non-compliance by the patient or through doctors not perceiving the need for an extended course of treatment.

Potential Surgical Intervention

This is unlikely for this condition as antibiotic therapy is the treatment of choice. There are rarely any long-term complications if appropriate treatment is given at the time of infection.

Torsion of the Testes

This is most common in young males between the ages of 10 and 30 (Hope et al., 1998). As the result of inadequate connective tissue some testes are more prone to torsion than others, or the condition may occur as a result of trauma.

Basic Anatomy and Physiology

The testis is usually suspended in the scrotum and held in place by the spermatic cord. Torsion of the testes occurs when there is rotation within the tunica vaginalis affecting the blood supply to the testicle or epididymis. Ischaemia occurs if untwisting is not carried out within six hours of symptoms and gangrene may possibly result.

Presenting Signs and Symptoms/Complications

There is usually sudden onset of pain in the scrotum, radiating to the groin and/or abdomen, often associated with nausea and vomiting. Abdominal pain occurs because the nerve supply for the testes is in the abdomen. The testis may be felt higher up in the neck of the scrotum due to the twisting effect. After a short time the scrotum becomes red and tender, often making it difficult to distinguish between torsion and epididymitis.

The patient is often tachycardic owing to the pain and the scrotal skin is tight over the testes. He may also have difficulty in walking. The main complication is necrosis if the torsion is not reversed.

Nursing Assessment and Intervention

Patients with suspected torsion should always be seen as an emergency because of the short time frame before necrosis of the testis forms. Baseline observations should be recorded and an opiate-based analgesic should be administered. The patient should be referred to a surgeon as soon as possible to prevent further delay in treatment.

Potential Surgical Intervention

Surgery is nearly always required to correct torsion of the testes, although occasionally the doctor may be able to manually untwist the testis with the use of local anaesthetic (Selfridge-Thomas, 1997). Regardless of this, patients are often operated on to explore the testis and to ensure there is no irreversible damage. At this point the testis is generally fixed in place within the scrotum.

It is possible that the other testis is also in an abnormal position and may require fixing at the same time. If the testis is found to be necrotic it will be removed as it may affect the antibodies of the sperm in the remaining testis (Raftery, 1996).

If surgery is performed within the first six hours of onset, the testis can normally be saved.

Acute Urinary Retention

Urinary retention may be acute, chronic or acute-on-chronic. Patients with acute retention present as surgical emergencies and should have a triage rating of urgent as the kidneys continue to produce urine, which is unable to be expelled. Urinary retention is most commonly seen in men.

Causes

There are various causes for urinary retention with the most common cause in the male population being benign prostatic enlargement. The causes of urinary retention are summarized below:

(a) blockage at the urethral lumen or bladder neck:
- urethral valves;
- calculi;
- tumours;
- blood clots;
- ulceration at meatus;

(b) blockage in the urethra or bladder wall:
- trauma;
- stricture;
- tumour;

(c) outside the bladder wall:
- prostatic enlargement;
- faecal impaction;
- pregnant uterus;
- tumours;

(d) others:
- spinal cord injury or disease;
- drugs, e.g. anti-cholinergics;
- antidepressants, alcohol;
- diabetes (Raftery, 1996).

Presenting Signs and Symptoms

Patients will often give a history of poor urinary stream, which may be sudden in onset or something which has worsened progressively. There may also be a history of frequency, haematuria or urinary tract infection.

On assessment the nurse will invariably find the patient in pain with a palpable distended bladder. On bladder percussion, dull sounds will be heard. The patient may also be tachycardic if the retention has been present for some time.

Nursing Assessment and Intervention

The first line of treatment for urinary retention is insertion of an indwelling catheter allowing the bladder to empty. This should be controlled so as not to shock the patient if a vast amount of urine is drained immediately following insertion. The nurse/doctor should aim to drain the bladder in 500–800 ml increments (Selfridge-Thomas, 1997). Depending on the severity of the pain, an analgesic may be administered prior to catheterization although emptying the bladder via a catheter will result in an immediate relief.

The procedure of catheterization should be performed under strict aseptic technique to avoid further risk of urinary tract infection.

If urine flow is obstructed following the insertion of a urethral catheter, irrigation of the bladder with normal saline may be required. This is particularly true if retention has occurred after bladder surgery, as blood clots tend to form readily.

The patient should have his/her baseline vital signs recorded, including measurement of subsequent urine output. Urinalysis should be performed to determine whether the retention has been caused by bacteria from an infection. If it is a nurse who performs the urethral catheterization it is vital that the patient receives a full medical assessment, particularly if the retention is a new symptom as causes for retention must be excluded. The nurse must provide supportive care, especially if the patient is enduring a catheter for the first time, as there are a variety of social implications.

Potential Surgical Interventions

If urethral catheterization proves difficult or impossible, the patient may require supra-pubic catheter insertion. This most commonly occurs if patients have impassable strictures or significant urethral trauma. This type of catheter is often seen as more permanent by the fact that it is surgically placed through the abdominal wall into the bladder. However, these catheters can also be temporary depending upon the reason for insertion.

If there are no complications from urethral catheterization, patients may be sent home with an indwelling catheter *in situ*. However, they must receive close follow up at home to determine the cause of urinary obstruction and may need to undergo further investigation including urodynamic assessment.

Conclusion

The A&E department encounters patients with surgical conditions on a regular basis, either through GP referrals for specialist opinions or because the patient self-presents. It is vital for all A&E nurses to have a general understanding about surgical conditions that they might encounter, and how best to assess and treat them.

This chapter has addressed the most common surgical conditions seen within the acute setting, usually as a result of their sudden onset/severity, and has highlighted the management required. It is not exhaustive, owing to the vast scope that surgery covers, but it is hoped that those conditions discussed have given A&E nurses sufficient information to relate to a variety of patients and their conditions, encouraging further reading where appropriate.

Suggested Further Reading

Anon (1989) Nursing Revision Notes: Surgical Nursing. London: Penguin Books.
Bates B (1995) Physical Examination and History Taking, 6th edn. Philadelphia: JB Lippincott.
Thibodeau GA, Patton KT (1992) The Human Body in Health and Disease. St Louis: Mosby Year Book.

References

Barber MD, McLaren J, Rainey JB (1997) Recurrent appendicitis. British Journal of Surgery 84: 110–12.
Berridge DC, Chamberlain J, Guy AJ, Lambert D (1995) Prospective Audit of Abdominal Aortic Aneurysm Surgery in the Northern Region from 1988 to 1992. British Journal of Surgery 82: 906–10.
Burkitt HG, Quick CRG, Gatt D (1990) Essential Surgery. Problems, Diagnosis And Management. Edinburgh: Churchill Livingstone.
Hinchliff SM, Montague SE, Watson R (1996) Physiology for Nursing Practice, 2nd edn. London: Baillière Tindall.
Hope RA, Longmore JM, Mcmanus SK, Wood-Allum CA (1998) Oxford Handbook of Clinical Medicine, 4th edn. Oxford: Oxford University Press.
Kapit W, Elson LM (1993) The Anatomy Colouring Book, 2nd edn. New York: HarperCollins.
McGrath A (1998) Abdominal Examination and Assessment in A&E. Emergency Nurse 6(4): 15–18.
Mosby (1990) Mosby's Medical, Nursing and Allied Health Dictionary, 3rd edn. St Louis: CV Mosby.
Raftery AT (1996) Churchill's Pocket Book of Surgery, 2nd edn. Edinburgh: Churchill Livingstone.
Selfridge-Thomas J (1997) Emergency Nursing. Philadelphia: WB Saunders.
Watson JE, Royle JA (1987) Watson's Medical-Surgical Nursing and Related Physiology, 3rd edn. London: Baillière Tindall.

Chapter 5
Gynaecological Conditions

KATHERINE POWER

Introduction

This chapter will address four gynaecological conditions that commonly present within the accident and emergency (A&E) setting. These are: ectopic pregnancy, toxic shock syndrome, pelvic inflammatory disease and miscarriage. Some present more often than others and some are more emergent. The incidence, possible causes and the subsequent nursing care required will be discussed.

Ectopic Pregnancy (Ruptured and Unruptured)

This is defined as a pregnancy in which the fertilized ovum implants on any tissue other than the endometrial lining of the uterus.

Incidence

Between 0.5 % and 1.4% of all pregnancies are believed to be ectopic (Gould, 1997) and there is an apparent rise in the incidence of the condition. The UK also appears to have the highest incidence rate at one in 60 reported pregnancies. Abound (1997) also concluded a 0.59 % rise in the incidence of ectopic pregnancy and a study between 1990 and 1994 demonstrated that 98 % of them were found to be tubal.

Pathology of Ectopic Pregnancy

The expected course of the ovum at ovulation is via the fallopian tube aided by the fimbriae. It is then transferred to the uterus by a combination of ciliary beating and muscular contractions. Essentially, an ectopic pregnancy occurs when there is a delay in this passage of the ovum to the uterus.

Main Risk Factors of Ectopic Pregnancy

Risk factors are present in 25–50% of patients (Ling and Stovall, 1994).

Age

Most ectopic pregnancies occur in females aged between 25 and 34 years of age, with women aged 35–39 having a 2.6 fold higher risk of death than women aged 25–29 years. This risk is increased to 5.9 fold for women aged >40.

Pelvic Inflammatory Disease (PID)

The rate of ectopic pregnancies in women with previously diagnosed PID is 6–10 times higher than in women with no previous history of the disease. Pelvic inflammatory disease is usually caused by invasion of either gonorrhoea or Chlamydia, from the cervix up to the uterus and fallopian tubes. The infection in these tissues causes an intense inflammatory response. Bacteria, white blood cells and other fluids fill the tubes as the body combats the infection. During the healing process the endosalpinx (lining of the inner tubal lumen) suffers agglutination (sticking together) of the mucosal folds in the tube and peritubal adhesions (scar tissue). The end of the tube by the ovaries may become partially or completely blocked and scar tissue often forms on the outside of the tubes and ovaries. All these factors can impact on ovarian and tubal function and the chances for future conception.

Chronic salpingitis has been attributed to sexually transmitted diseases, especially to Chlamydia trachomatis, a known major cause of tubal damage. However, Stabile (1996) claimed that only 50% of tubal specimens removed following ectopic pregnancy had evidence of chronic salpingitis by H and E staining. The risk of an ectopic pregnancy is greater when women with the infection are younger (possibly related to avoiding or delaying appropriate medical care). Furthermore, most women with Chlamydia infection have no symptoms and it has been suggested that routine screening should be considered if the prevalence of Chlamydia infection is high, otherwise screening should be offered to women with high risk factors.

Previous Surgery

When a bilateral tubal ligation is followed either by an unexpected pregnancy (failed tubal ligation) or is reversed with a tubal reanastomosis (tubal reconstruction), there is an increased risk of tubal ectopic pregnancy as a result of adhesion formation or scar tissue development within the fallopian tube. Other forms of previous pelvic surgery have also been identified as increasing the risk of ectopic pregnancies. Dimitry (1987), for example, reported that previous appendicectomy was one such underlying cause, again as a result of the formation of associated adhesions. Abound (1997) further concluded that 11% of women who underwent surgery for an ectopic pregnancy had a history of previous ectopic pregnancies.

Intrauterine Device (IUD)

The link between IUD and ectopic pregnancy is well documented. The World Health Organisation (1985) concluded that those women who used an IUD were six times more likely to have an ectopic pregnancy than non-users.

Assisted Reproductive Technology (IVF)

When multiple embryos or gametes are replaced into the uterus or the fallopian tubes, the risk of multiple pregnancy rises significantly. The development of assisted reproduction techniques has resulted in more women with previous tubal damage conceiving. Heterotrophic pregnancy is the combined occurrence of intrauterine and extrauterine gestations. It is significantly high after *in vitro* fertilization and embryo transfer, the reported rate ranging from 1% to 3 % of all clinical pregnancies and 10–15 % of all IVF-ET ectopic gestations (Rizk et al., 1991). This rate is probably related to the transference of large numbers of embryos (Tummon et al., 1994). The seriousness of the outcome depends upon the site of implantation and the degree of the development of the conceptus (Stabile, 1996).

The most common sites for an ectopic pregnancy are:

•   the ampullary (mid) portion of the fallopian tube (80–90%). This is the most common site for an ectopic pregnancy. In the tubal ampulla, the muscular area between the outer tubal serosa and the inner tubal lumen is relatively thick. Frequently ectopic pregnancies in the ampullary portion of the tube grow in this muscular area outside the tubal lumen, so even when the ectopic site has attained a large size the tubal lumen can escape any damage;

- the isthmic (area closer to the uterus) portion of the fallopian tube (5–50%). The isthmic portion of the fallopian tube is the second most common site for ectopic pregnancy. In the tubal isthmus the muscular area between the outer tubal serosa and the inner tubal lumen is very thin. Often, isthmic ectopic pregnancies grow within the lumen itself and therefore the lumen is destroyed as the pregnancy becomes larger in size;

- the fimbrial (distal end away from the uterus) portion of the fallopian tube (about 5%). This is the third most common site for ectopic pregnancy and many of these represent 'tubal abortions' in which the products of conception are already being excluded from the tube into the abdomen;

- the cornual (within the uterine muscle) portion of the fallopian tube (1-2%). A very uncommon site for ectopic pregnancy where the pregnancy is growing within the muscular wall of the uterus as the tube enters the uterine cavity. The potential for increased blood supply to this area will occasionally allow the pregnancy to grow to a very large size, making the removal of the pregnancy difficult;

- the abdomen (1–2%). Here the pregnancy has been expelled from the fallopian tube and implants into a highly vascular region of the abdomen. Most of the blood supply to these pregnancies may again result in the ectopic pregnancy growing to term;

- the ovary (less than 1%). This is very rare and may also be vascular;

- the cervix (less than 1%). This is again very rare and can be difficult to distinguish from an incomplete abortion since both can be located within the cervix. The uterine artery and vein approach the uterus at the level of the cervix so that these ectopic pregnancies often have a profuse blood supply.

Most embryos implanted in the fallopian wall die within six weeks of implantation owing to defective placentation and the embryo may be reabsorbed, become infected or mummify. When an ectopic pregnancy outgrows the limits of the space in which it is enclosed then life-threatening bleeding can result.

The clinical presentation of an ectopic pregnancy may vary from general vaginal spotting to vasomotor shock with haemoperitoneum, making the accuracy of diagnoses about 50%. Abbot et al. (1990) subsequently reported an alarming rate of missed and/or delayed diagnoses within the A&E setting.

Early Symptoms of an Ectopic Pregnancy

- Abdominal pain. This may be irregular and colicky, sometimes localized to one side. Pain is caused by distension of the gravid tube due to the associated effort in attempting to contract and expel the ovum.
- Late or missed period. However, women may start to experience the symptoms of the ectopic pregnancy prior to missing a period.
- Vaginal bleeding. This usually occurs after the death of the ovum and is an effect of oestrogen withdrawal. It is dark brown and scanty (vaginal spotting) and its irregularity may lead the patient to confuse it with menstrual flow.
- Tissue passage from the vagina. Women should subsequently try to save any tissue produced for later examination.
- Pregnancy symptoms.

An early diagnosis of an ectopic pregnancy is critical to a successful outcome. When an ectopic pregnancy is detected early in development, especially prior to tubal rupture or damage to surrounding tissue, major morbidity is decreased and the treatment options are enhanced. A diagnosis is generally made on the basis of a positive pregnancy test combined with ultrasonography.

The measurement of human chorionic gonadotrophin (hCG) is used as an indicator of both intra- and extra-uterine trophoblastic tissue as patients with suspected ectopic pregnancy have lower hCG levels. A negative quantitative serum measurement almost always excludes the presence of an ectopic pregnancy. Ultrasound can be either done abdominally or vaginally, the latter being more comfortable and less time consuming than an abdominal ultraound since there is no need to fill the bladder.

If a woman has a non-ruptured ectopic pregnancy, the pregnancy can be removed surgically by either laparoscopy or laparotomy dependent upon the site and/or progress of the pregnancy. Ectopic pregnancies may also be managed medically with the use of methotrexate management that results in the destruction of the growing pregnancy. This may take from four to six weeks and therefore there is a risk of the pregnancy rupturing within this time.

Late Symptoms

When the ectopic pregnancy continues to develop into a larger embryo and causes bleeding or rupture the acute presentation comprises brief amenorrhoea, severe pain in the illiac fossa or hypogastrium, syncope, shock, guarding, tenderness and rebound throughout the abdomen. Women with ruptured tubal pregnancies have a higher incidence of abdominal pain lasting less than 24 hours and associated adnexal tenderness. Where the ovum separates from the tubal wall by chorio-decidual haemorrhage, forming a haematosalpinx, blood may collect around the tube or run down into the rectovaginal pouch. Free intrapertineal blood may cause epigastric pain or shoulder-tip pain caused by blood irritating the phrenic nerve. A pelvic haematocele may cause tenesmus, dysuria and retention. If these symptoms present then no time should be lost with regard to instituting appropriate haemorrhagic shock management.

Signs and Symptoms of Hypovolaemic Shock

Classes of haemorrhage have been defined based on the percentage of blood volume loss. The difference between these classes in the hypovolaemic patient is often less apparent. Treatment should be aggressive and be directed more by response to therapy than by initial classification.

- Class 1 haemorrhage (loss of 0–15%):
  In the absence of complications, only minimal tachycardia will be seen. There are usually no changes in blood pressure, or respiratory or pulse rate. A delay in capillary refill of greater than three seconds corresponds to approximately a 10% volume loss.
- Class 2 haemorrhage (loss of 15–30%):
  Clinical symptoms include tachycardia > 100 bpm, tachypnoea, decrease in pulse pressure, cool clammy skin, delayed capillary refill and slight anxiety.

- Class 3 haemorrhage (loss of 30–40%):
  The patient will have marked tachycardia and tachypnoea and falling systolic blood pressure, oliguria and significant changes in mental state including confusion and agitation. Most of these patients will require blood transfusions, but this decision should be based on initial response to fluids.
- Class 4 haemorrhage (loss of > 40%)
  Symptoms include marked tachycardia, decreased systolic pressure, narrowed pulse pressure (or an unrecordable diastolic pressure), markedly decreased (or absent) urinary output, depressed mental status (or loss of consciousness) and cold, clammy and pale skin. This amount of haemorrhage is immediately life-threatening.

The human body responds to acute haemorrhage by activating four physiological systems:

- the haematological system responds to acute, severe blood loss by activating the coagulation cascade and contracting the bleeding vessels. Platelets are activated which form a clot on the bleeding source. The damaged vessel exposes collagen that subsequently causes fibrin deposition and clot stabilization;
- the renal system response to haemorrhagic shock is by stimulating an increase in renin secretion from the juxtaglomerular apparatus. Renin converts angiotensin 1, which is then converted to angiotensin 2 by the liver and lungs. This results in vasoconstriction of the arteriolar smooth muscle and stimulation of aldosterone secretion by the adrenal cortex that is responsible for active sodium reabsorption and subsequent water conservation;
- the cardiovascular system initially responds to hypovolaemic shock by increasing heart rate, increasing myocardial contractility and the constriction of peripheral blood vessels. This is a secondary response to an increase in release of norepinephrine and a decrease in baseline vagal tone. This is regulated by the baroreceptors in the carotid arch, aortic arch, left atrium and pulmonary vessels. The cardiovascular system also responds by redistributing blood to the brain, heart and kidneys and away from the skin, muscle and gastrointestinal tract;
- the neuroendocrine system responds by causing an increase in circulating antidiuretic hormone (ADH). ADH is released from

the posterior pituitary gland in response to a decrease in blood pressure (as detected by the baroreceptors) and a decrease in sodium concentration (as detected by the osmoreceptors). ADH indirectly leads to an increase in the reabsorbsion of water and salt.

Nursing Intervention

On arrival at the A&E department the nurse should record a baseline set of vital signs and continued recordings as deemed appropriate from the presenting symptoms and response to treatment. High-flow supplemental oxygen is advocated to optimize perfusion to vital organs.

Two large-bore IVs should be inserted and initial fluid resuscitation should involve a bolus of 1–2 litres of an isotonic crystalloid such as Ringer's lactate solution or normal saline. If vital signs return to normal then the patient should be monitored whilst blood samples are sent for type and cross-match. Treatment for all ruptured ectopic pregnancies is surgery and patients in shock should be taken to the operating theatre straight from the A&E department. The patient will require surgical intervention involving a laparotomy and, for women with irreparable damage to tubes, radical surgery involving resection of the fallopian tube will be necessary.

The nurse should remember that patients presenting with an ectopic pregnancy might not be aware that they were pregnant and may have a mixture of emotions to deal with. There may also be concerns regarding future fertility, the ability to conceive and the possibility of repeated ectopic pregnancies.

On average 30% of patients are infertile after an ectopic pregnancy (Toth and Jothivijayarani, 1999). Early diagnoses of women with a previous history of ectopic pregnancies, or those with high risk factors, may reduce the possibility of future tubal rupture and the associated complications. This can occur very early on in the pregnancy, before six weeks, by measuring hCG levels and endovaginal ultrasound (Cacciatore et al., 1990). However, early diagnoses may invite enthusiastic over-treatment of ectopic pregnancies that may later resolve spontaneously without complications (Ylostalo et al., 1992; Stabile, 1996).

Toxic Shock Syndrome

Definition

Toxic shock syndrome (TSS) is a bacterial infection that can cause acute multi-system failure through septic shock. The main source is Staphylococcus aureus, although TSS has also been identified with group A streptococci and group B streptococcus. Toxic shock syndrome is a potentially fatal illness.

Incidence

TSS was first recognized in 1978 and there are approximately 40 cases of TSS per year in the UK. Of these, two to three people will die each year. Although tampon-related toxic shock syndrome is rare, the number of menstrual-related cases having declined during the last 10 years, nurses still need to be aware of its causes and presenting symptoms and to become involved in making tampon users aware of the subsequent risk factors.

TSS occurs predominantly in 15- to 34-year-olds, with one-third of cases in the 15-19 age range and 65% of all cases in the under 25s. About 70% of TSS cases have been related to the use of certain brands of highly absorbent tampons and although these brands are no longer available on the market many tampons contain highly absorbent fibres. Menstrual-related cases of TSS account for around 50–70% of all cases of TSS in women of reproductive age, and women with a history of menstrual-related TSS have a 30% chance of reoccurrence (Bryner, 1989).

There are two theories about how tampons may promote TSS:

(1) Tampons may keep the bacteria blocked in the vagina where they breed abnormally and produce toxins.
(2) Tampons may cause very small lacerations in the vagina through which the bacteria or their toxins may enter the bloodstream.

Signs, Symptoms and Presentation

The symptoms of TSS may include:

• fever above 102°F;
• muscle pains;

- sore throat;
- vomiting;
- diarrhoea;
- dizziness and fainting;
- headache with a stiff and tender neck;
- a sunburn-like rash, which may be diffuse or localized to the trunk or extremities;
- shortness of breath.

For most women the condition does not progress beyond this stage. Fever is the most common early sign, although hypothermia may present in patients already in shock (Stevens, 1992). With early diagnosis TSS can be treated successfully.

For patients whose symptoms worsen, presentation may include:

- fever – temperature > 38.9 C (102°F);
- rash – diffuse macular erythroderma;
- desquamation – 1–2 weeks after onset of illness, particularly palms and soles;
- hypotension:
- systolic blood pressure < 90 mmHg for adults;
- systolic blood pressure less than one-fifth percentile by age for children (aged less than 16 years);
- orthostatic drop in diastolic blood pressure >15 mmHg from lying to sitting;
- orthostatic syncope or orthostatic dizziness;
- multisystem involvement (three or four of the following):
  - gastrointestinal (vomiting or diarrhoea at onset of illness);
  - muscular (severe myalgia or creatinine phosphokinase level at least twice the upper limit of normal for laboratory);
  - mucous membrane (vaginal, oropharyngeal or conjuctival hyperaemia);
  - renal (blood urea nitrogen or creatinine at least twice the upper limit of normal for laboratory or urinary sediment with pyuria (>5 leukocytes per high power field) in the absence of urinary tract infection);
  - hepatic (total bilirubin, serum glutamic oxaloacetic transaminase (SGOT) and serum glutamic pyruvic transaminase (SGPT) at least twice the upper limit of normal;

- haematologic (platelets < 100 000/3ul);
- central nervous system (disorientation or alterations in consciousness without focal neurological signs when fever and hypotension are present).

Septic shock occurs in about 20% of patients with Staphylococcus aureus bacteraemia and may be apparent at the time of admission or within 4–8 hours. The most consistent clinical feature in sepsis is an alteration in mental function. This may be non-specific such as fatigue or malaise or present with more severe signs including anxiety, agitation and apprehension. Neurological status may show early symptoms of shock or indicate the patient's condition is worsening. The symptoms include confusion, lethargy and irritability leading to unresponsiveness as cerebral perfusion decreases, and the nurse is responsible for observing response to verbal and tactile stimuli and monitoring the level of consciousness. Confusion is present in 55% of patients (Stevens, 1992).

Fever is another common feature of sepsis and fever from infectious aetiology results from a resetting of the hypothalamus so that heat production and loss are balanced to maintain a higher body temperature. Circulating pyrogens produced by stimulated circulating monocytes and tissue macrophages reset the hypothalamus. An abrupt onset of fever is usually associated with a large infectious load. Chills are a secondary symptom associated with fever that results from the need for muscular activity to increase heat production to raise body temperature to the level desired by the reset hypothalamus. Chills are seen at the onset of fever when body temperature is rising. Sweating occurs when the hypothalamus returns to its normal set point and senses that the body temperature is above the desired level. Perspiration is stimulated to evaporate away excess body heat. Sweats are commonly seen as the fever is breaking and the body temperature is falling. The hypothalamus can be reset to normal by the use of antipyretics.

Nursing Intervention

The airway should be assessed immediately upon arrival of the patient, noting depth, rate and breath sounds. Because of the changes occurring at cellular level in the lung tissue, the oxygen concentration decreases and carbon dioxide increases causing hypoxaemia. Acute respiratory distress syndrome occurs in 55% of patients and generally develops after the onset of hypotension, and supplemental oxygen, intubation and mechanical ventilation are necessary in 90% of the patients in whom this syndrome develops (Stevens, 1992).

All patients with sepsis will require supplemental IV fluids due to the risk of hypovolaemia resulting from leaky capillaries and fluid loss into the interstitial space. Regular vital signs should be recorded and the most important factor is how the blood pressure changes from any baseline recording, a fall of 30 mmHg or more from a person's baseline being considered a low blood pressure.

It must be remembered that the nurse should not rely on the systolic blood pressure reading as the main indicator for shock as this will result in a delayed diagnoses. Compensatory mechanisms will prevent a significant fall in systolic blood pressure until the patient has lost 30% of his/her blood volume. The nurse should therefore be attentive to heart rate, respiratory rate, skin perfusion and mental changes.

Because of the risk of hypovolaemic shock, rapid infusion of fluids should be started immediately and two large-bore IVs should be started. Poiseuille's Law states that flow is inversely related to the length of the IV catheter and directly related to its radius, hence the use of size 14–16 cannulae. Subsequent IV access should be obtained via percutaneous access to antecubital veins, cut down of saphenous or arm veins or access to central veins via a central line.

The amount and rate of IV fluid resuscitation is guided by an assessment of the patient's volume and cardiovascular status. For hypotensive patients, an isotonic crystalloid should be administered in boluses of 500 ml (in adults). Repeat boluses should be administered until signs of adequate perfusion are restored; a total of 4–6 litres may be required. Patients should be monitored for signs of volume overload such as dyspnoea and pulmonary oedema. Stabilization in the patient's mental status, heart rate, blood pressure, capillary refill and urine output will subsequently indicate sufficient volume replacement. CVP monitoring should also be considered.

If the patient does not respond to isotonic crystalloid (usually 4 litres or more) or there is evidence of volume overload, the depressed cardiovascular system can be stimulated by administration of IV dopamine. If the patient remains hypotensive despite volume infusion and dopamine then a vasoconstrictor such as norepinephrine may be commenced.

On admission, renal involvement is indicated by the presence of haemoglobinuria and by serum creatinine values that are >2.5 times normal. Renal dysfunction precedes shock/hypotension in 40–50 % of patients and is apparent early in the course of shock in all others. Renal dysfunction may progress or persists for 48–72 hours post-treatment. Urinary catheterization and the use of a urometer for accurate measurement of urine output is required. Urine output should be maintained at a minimum of 30 ml per hour since anything below this may indicate reduced kidney function.

An ECG should be recorded to observe for ventricular arrhythmias, bundle branch blocks, first-degree heart block and ST-T wave changes indicative of ischaemia. If appropriate the source of the infection should be removed. Therefore, with TSS caused by an indwelling tampon, this should be removed and irrigation with normal saline or povidone-iodine solution performed. IV antibiotics should be commenced: a combination of an aminoglycoside such as gentamicin and a broad-spectrum penicillin or cephalosporin. The patient should ultimately be transferred to an intensive care unit for further haemodynamic monitoring and/or ventilatory support. Parental antibiotic therapy should be continued for seven days, followed by seven days of oral therapy. Some patients may also require dialysis.

Pelvic Inflammatory Disease (PID)

Definition

PID can be defined as a clinical syndrome consisting of a complex combination of signs and symptoms that refer to an ascending inflammatory reaction which involves, to a variable extent, the entire female genital tract (Stacey, 1992). This includes the uterus, fallopian tubes and associated structures such as the ovaries, pelvic peritoneum and tubal-ovarian juncture (Westrom and Mardh, 1990). PID is actually a spectrum of disease, beginning with cervicitis and progressing to endometriosis and eventually salpingitis. It can be classified as primary, secondary or recurrent. PID is also known as salpingo-peritonitis, salpingo-oophoritis or salpingitis.

Incidence and Causes

Exposure to Sexually Transmitted Diseases

The same organisms responsible for bacterial sexually transmitted diseases such as Chlamydia and gonorrhoea are mostly responsible in cases of PID (Rice and Schachter, 1991) and at least 60% of cases of PID can be attributed to infection with a sexually transmitted organism (Munday, 1997).

Chlamydia

Chlamydia is the most common curable sexually transmitted disease. Up to 80% of women with uncomplicated Chlamydia have no symptoms at all ('silent PID') and, if they do, these occur within one week to one month after exposure. The condition is therefore often overlooked, yet, left untreated, these infections can lead to serious damage to the female reproductive organs.

Symptoms include:

- irregular vaginal bleeding;
- burning with urination;
- itching and burning in the genital area;
- vaginal discharge;
- lower abdominal pain, often accompanied by nausea and fever.

The subsequent cure rate is greater than 95%.

Gonorrhoea

The gonorrhoea bacteria can be transmitted by sexual penetration and in women it usually first infects the cervix. Often an infected person will have no detectable symptoms. When symptoms do appear they usually develop within two to five days after exposure, although may develop any time between one and 30 days.

Symptoms include:

- cloudy, yellow vaginal discharge;
- bleeding between menstrual periods;
- chronic abdominal pain;
- pain or burning when urinating;

- frequency of urination;
- sore throat (from oral sex).

Neisseria gonorrhoeae was the first organism found to be associated with PID and often produces the classical clinical features of PID: acute abdominal pain, purulent vaginal discharge and pyrexia. Gonorrhoea is detected through culture or antigen detection and treatment during the early stages is usually 100% effective.

History of PID

It is estimated that up to one-third of women with PID will suffer repeat episodes (Westrom and Mardh, 1990). This is due to re-exposure to untreated male sexual partners, inadequate initial treatment and post-infection damage to the fallopian tubes leaving them vulnerable to subsequent infection. Failure to educate women who are at risk to take adequate precautions to avoid re-infection with sexually transmitted diseases is also a causative factor.

Patients with recurrent disease may need repeated courses of antibiotics. Mitchell (1993) further advocated that any woman with a previous history of PID who is having a procedure involving instrumentation of the cervix should receive prophylactic antibiotic cover.

Age

The average age for women presenting with PID appears to be getting younger (Marchbanks et al., 1990). In industrialized countries the incidence of PID is 10–13 per 1000 of reproductive-age women, with the peak incidence of 20 per 1000 occurring in those aged 15–24 years.

Contraception

Oral Contraceptives

Studies have suggested that oral contraception may have protective qualities against PID (Aral et al., 1987; Wolner-Hanssen et al., 1990).

Intrauterine device (IUD)

Evidence in the past has seen a correlation between IUD use and elevated incidence of implicated STD infections (Aral and Holmes, 1990). Farley et al. (1992) concluded that PID among IUD users was most strongly related to the insertion process and that PID is an infrequent event beyond the first 20 days after insertion. It also has been reported that there is a practice of replacing an IUD irrespective of need (Edelman et al., 1990). The reported incidence of an 84% infection rate after coil insertion (Farley et al., 1992) could subsequently be reduced by prophylactic antibiotics given at the time of insertion (Sinei et al., 1990).

Barrier Method

Condoms or a diaphragm with spermicide have an obvious protective effect against STDs and therefore against possible related PID (Aral and Holmes,1990).

Iatrogenic PID

Procedures such as dilatation and curettage of the endometrium, insertion of an IUD or hysterosalpingogram may traumatize the genital tissues, compromising protective mechanisms and introducing bacteria (Spence, 1989).

Signs and Symptoms

- vaginal discharge (with abnormal colour, consistency or odour);
- irregular menstrual bleeding or spotting;
- increased menstrual cramping;
- absent menstruation;
- increased pain during ovulation;
- painful sexual intercourse;
- bleeding after intercourse;
- fever (may range from occasional to constant and be low to high grade);
- chills;
- abdominal pain;
- lower back pain;
- fatigue;
- lack of appetite;
- nausea, with or without vomiting;
- frequent urination;
- painful urination;
- point tenderness.

Chronic PID

One in six women will experience chronic pelvic pain after one proven episode of PID (Landers, 1994). The exact mechanism of persistent or recurrent pelvic pain is unknown, although empirical data suggest that adhesion formation resulting from inflammatory insult to the peritoneum may play a role (Kottman, 1995).

Jacobson and Westrom (1984) reported that diagnosis by experienced gynaecologists was incorrect 35% of the time when all cases were later checked by laparoscopy. Pearce (1990) subsequently stated that all too often the diagnosis of PID tended to be a 'dustbin' for all the varying presentations of non-specific lower abdominal pain in young women. However, not all women with PID will present with abdominal pain and associated atypical symptoms such as meteorrhagia and dyspareunia should therefore suggest diagnosis.

The patient presenting to A&E should receive a general examination which may reveal enlarged lymph nodes in the groin area (inguinal). Subsequent pelvic examination may reveal cervical discharge, cervical tenderness, a friable cervix (one that bleeds easily), uterine or adnexal (ovarian) tenderness.

Treatment/Nursing Intervention

Blood samples should be obtained for WBC, ESR and serum hCG levels. An endocervical culture for gonorrhoea, Chlamydia and other organisms will be required. A laparoscopy can prove invaluable in confirming the diagnosis and to exclude other disorders. It also allows fluid samples to be taken for bacterial analysis. However, most gynaecologists will do this only if the PID fails to respond to a trial treatment of antibiotics (Pearce, 1990).

If the patient presents with abdominal pain and mild PID it may be appropriate to treat with oral tetracycline, co-trimoxazole and metronidazole, which should cover more than 90% of organisms. More severe infections will require IV antibiotic administration (e.g. penicillin and gentamicin) in conjunction with PR metronidazole for the first three days. This may subsequently be followed by a 14-day course of oral tetracycline and metronidazole.

The implications of PID for the patient include infertility and ectopic pregnancy (due to scarring or blockage of the fallopian tubes) and long-term disabling effects, such as recurrent infection and chronic pelvic pain absent evidence of infection. The proportion of women who acquire tubal infertility is dependent upon the number and severity of attacks of PID and many gynaecologists no longer attempt to reverse tubal adhesions as the success rate is less than 10% (Mitchell, 1993). The emphasis should be on patient education and prevention of PID, including regular screening for Chlamydia and gonorrhoea and subsequent treatment of lower genital tract infections. Nurses therefore have a key role to play in subsequent PID prevention by ensuring early intervention, accurate patient assessment and comprehensive treatment, even within the acute A&E setting.

Miscarriage (spontaneous abortion)

Definition

Miscarriage is defined as the loss of a fetus during pregnancy as a result of natural causes (usually fetal death). Early pregnancy loss refers to spontaneous pregnancy loss up to 24 weeks (SDOH, 1997).

Incidence

Spontaneous abortion is the outcome of 14–19% of registered pregnancies (Hammerslough, 1992). Estimating the probability of spontaneous abortion in the presence of induced abortion, and vice versa, suggests that if very early miscarriages are included (before the woman knows that she is pregnant) the incidence may be as high as one in two conceptions ending in miscarriage (Hammerslough, 1992; Hey et al., 1996).

Pregnancy is divided into three trimesters:

- The first trimester is up to 14 weeks when the various body organs are being formed.
- The second trimester is between 14 and 24 weeks. If the baby was born now it would be too immature to survive.
- The third trimester is from 24 weeks to delivery date (40 weeks).

Causes

Genetic

Of first trimester miscarriages, 50–60% are genetic in origin(Hey et al., 1996). The contribution of the inappropriate number of chromosomes usually comes from the egg and most of the chromo-somally abnormal eggs are never identified as pregnancies; either they do not divide to produce an embryo or fetus, or the conception is lost very soon after implantation.

Eggs and sperm, collectively known as gametes, form differently than other cells in the body. With the exception of gametes, all normal cells in the human contain 46 chromosomes. There are 22 paired chromosomes called autosomes. These direct the overall formation of the body. There is also a twenty-third pair of chromo-somes, often referred to as sex chromosomes. In women and girls, there is a matched pair of 'X' chromosomes that are responsible for, among other things, the formation of ovaries. In men and boys, one of the 'X' chromosomes is replaced with a much shorter 'Y' chromo-some. The 'Y' chromosome carries the determinants of maleness. Formation of gametes (sperm and eggs) requires the separation of pairs of chromosomes into singletons which, on egg fertilization, recombine to form the 23 pairs of a new individual. Occasionally, in the formation of the gamete, some genetic material gets lost resulting in the loss of part of a chromosome or even an entire chromosome. The missing genetic material may become attached to another chro-mosome and be surplus genetic material in another gamete.

When a chromosome is lost during fertilization (hence producing only 45) this results in monosomy. An example of a monosomy is Turner's syndrome. Among chromosomally abnormal babies, 25% are identified as having the syndrome, with two-thirds miscarrying at around six weeks (Hey et al., 1996).

If a chromosome is gained (making 47) this is termed trisomy. A prime example of this is Down's syndrome. Trisomies are common in babies that are miscarried, accounting for 50% of babies that are lost because of chromosomal abnormalities. The incidence of trisomy increases with age (see Table 5.1).

Blighted Ovum

A blighted ovum or anembryonic pregnancy also occurs following chromosomal abnormalities. A blighted ovum is a fertilized egg that implants in the uterus, begins to develop a gestational sac (this sac eventually forming the membranes) but does not develop into a fetus. The condition does not increase the risk of future miscarriage. Without a fetus the placenta begins to die and so the pregnancy miscarries, usually six to ten weeks after the last normal period.

Table 5.1 Incidence of trisomy

Maternal age (years)	Risk of miscarriage (%)
15–19	9.9
20–24	9.5
25–29	10.0
30–34	11.7
35–39	17.7
40–44	33.8
44 and older	53.2

Hydatidiform Mole

In the UK, hydatidiform mole occurs in approximately one in 1000 registered births (SDOH, 1997). In the case of a hydatidiform mole the chorionic villi of the placenta grow into a grape-like bunch of cysts within the uterus. It can either be a 'complete mole' in which there is no fetus at any stage or a 'partial mole' where there is evidence of a fetus although it cannot survive. Most women with a molar pregnancy have vaginal bleeding, excessive nausea and vomiting, the latter being due to the swollen villi of the placenta producing a markedly elevated level of the pregnancy hormone beta-human chorionic gonadotrophin (B-hCG). Ultrasound confirms diagnoses. A molar pregnancy may also be diagnosed following a dilation and curettage (D and C) for a miscarriage or missed abortion. When the diagnosis of molar pregnancy is made, the abnormal pregnancy tissue is removed by D and C and serial blood tests are performed to document falling hormone levels. The B-hCG hormone level is monitored every one to two weeks until a normal level is reached. The hormone level is then checked every few months, for up to a year, to be certain that the disease is in remission and that no malignant changes have occurred. The chance of a mole occurring in a subsequent pregnancy is one in 75 (SDOH, 1997).

Infections

German Measles

German measles (rubella) is a mild but highly contagious virus that affects mainly children and young adults. It is one infection that can affect a pregnancy quite severely. If the infection occurs during the first four months of pregnancy there is a risk of either a spontaneous miscarriage or of the baby developing abnormally if the pregnancy continues. Babies born with congenital rubella often have serious birth defects including glaucoma, deafness, mental retardation and heart problems.

Measles, Mumps, Influenza and Chicken Pox

These are viral infections that may also cause miscarriage when contracted within the first three months. The high temperature and severity of the infection are the important factors.

Listeriosis

Although listeriosis is uncommon, anyone may become contaminated with the *Listeria monocytogene* bacteria. *L. monocytogenes* is found in soil and water and vegetables can become contaminated from the soil or from manure used as fertilizer. Animals can carry the bacteria without appearing ill and can contaminate foods of animal origin, such as meats and dairy products. Listeria has been found in processed foods that have become contaminated after processing, and unpasteurized milk or foods made from unpasteurized milk may also contain the bacteria. Although healthy people may consume contaminated food without becoming ill, pregnant women are at high risk from the infection and about one-third of listeriosis cases happen during pregnancy causing miscarriage, especially in the second trimester. Newborns are very likely to suffer the serious effects of the infection during their mother's pregnancy. Infants may be stillborn, born with septicaemia or develop meningitis very early in life, even if the mother is asymptomatic.

Toxoplasmosis

Toxoplasmosis is a parasitic disease caused by the protozoan *Toxoplasma gondii*. Infection in humans is common, although may result in no symptoms. Congenital toxoplasmosis is caused by infection with *Toxoplasma gondii* in pregnant women, with up to 50% of such infections transmitted to the fetus.

Once infection has occurred, the seriousness is dependent upon the trimester of fetal infection. If early on, the parasite causes a spontaneous abortion. If the miscarriage has not occurred and infection is present in the first trimester, then developmental effects are severe because this is when the majority of the significant systems are being developed; between weeks three and twelve important developments are occurring in the central and peripheral nervous systems, the heart, gastrointestinal and urogenital systems, limbs, eyes and ears. The protozoa form cysts and can impede neural migration, blocking the flow of cerebrospinal fluid and inhibiting organ development. Infections in the second trimester are not so severe, but there are still problems, with third trimester infections having the least severe effects. At birth a number of abnormalities can be identified: 94% of infants born with toxoplasmosis will have some level of chorioretinitis; 55% show abnormal spinal fluids; 51% will show signs of anaemia; 50% will have intercranial calcifications and convulsions. Only a very small percentage are normal by four years of age (Boyer et al., 1996).

Pregnant women should have their blood examined for Toxoplasma antibody and those with negative results should take measures to prevent infection by avoiding contact with cats, cooking meat thoroughly and washing hands after handling raw meat.

Cytomegalovirus (CMV)

CMV is a virus that gives an influenza-like illness and is an illness that most women have immunity to following childhood exposure. Healthy pregnant women are not at special risk for disease from CMV infection. When infected with CMV, most women are without symptoms and only a few have a disease resembling mononucleosis. It is their developing unborn babies that may be at risk of developing congenital CMV disease. For infants who are infected by their mothers before birth, generalized infection may occur with symptoms ranging from moderate enlargement of the liver and spleen (with jaundice) to fatal illness. With supportive treatment, most infants with CMV disease usually survive, although 80–90% will have complications within the first few years of life including hearing loss, visual and mental disturbances or coordination problems. Some 5–10% of infants infected are without symptoms at birth, but will then develop varying degrees of hearing, visual and mental problems.

The virus may also be transmitted to the infant at delivery from contact with genital secretions or later in infancy through breast milk. However, these infections result in little or no clinical illnesses in the infant. Women who develop a mononucleosis-like illness during pregnancy should be evaluated for CMV infection and counselled about the possible risks to the unborn child. The demonstrated benefits of breast-feeding outweigh the risk of acquiring CMV from the breast-feeding mother.

Uterine Abnormalities

In female embryos two separate tubes fusing together form the uterus, but this fusion may be incomplete. The incidence of miscarriage in women with anatomical abnormalities of the uterus is difficult to quantify because diagnoses will never be made in many women who have successful pregnancies (SDOH, 1997). Many women with congenital abnormalities do not have any reproductive problems (Simon et al., 1991). Hey et al. (1996) further suggested that the different shapes of the uterus are associated with miscarriages that occur in the second trimester. Sometimes there is a duplication of the uterine body and cavity, described as a 'bicornuate' or two-horned uterus. The risk of pregnancy loss in this condition is approximately 30–35%. More common is a less severe incomplete fusion. The septum, which either partially or completely divides the uterine cavity, has a very poor blood supply and this may be responsible for the two-thirds probability of losing a pregnancy. A partial septum increases the risk to 60–75%; a total septum carries a risk of pregnancy loss up to 90%.

The shape of the uterus can be altered by the presence of fibroids. If the fibroid is large and alters the shape of the uterine cavity it may subsequently affect the ability of the uterus to carry the pregnancy to full term.

Incompetent Cervix

Cervical incompetence is a recognized cause of second-trimester miscarriage and occurs when the cervix opens prematurely and the pregnancy is expelled (SDOH, 1997). This may be a natural weakness or it can be caused by surgery, for example a cone biopsy or forcible dilation of the cervix. In subsequent pregnancies a Shriodkar suture is inserted until removal around the thirty-eighth week of pregnancy. Inserting a cervical suture does not guarantee that premature labour will not occur and the suture may have some adverse effects for the women including leaving scar tissue around the cervix or infection and inflammation that can lead to premature labour.

Immune Factors

Approximately 10% of couples with recurrent pregnancy loss have immune problems. Systemic lupus erythematosus (SLE) is a disease of the immune system that may affect many organ systems including the skin, joints and internal organs. Normally the immune system controls the body's defences against infection, but in SLE these defences are turned against the body when antibodies are produced against its own cells. These antibodies fight against the body's blood cells, organs and tissues causing chronic disease. SLE may improve, exacerbate or be unchanged during pregnancy and the activity of SLE at the time of conception has a major effect upon pregnancy outcome. Those women who are found to have certain antibodies have a fetal loss rate of 50–70% (Perez et al., 1991). Other antibodies confer a risk of neonatal lupus that includes lupus dermatitis, congenital complete heart block, thrombocytopenia and cholestatic jaundice, in order of their relative frequencies (Reichlin, 1998).

Pregnancy with an IUD in the Womb

Many pregnancies occurring when there is a IUD *in situ* continue without problems although risks include bleeding through the pregnancy with an increased tendency to miscarriage, premature rupture of the membranes and premature labour.

Hormone Deficiency

The hormone progesterone is very important in the maintenance of a pregnancy by preparing the endometrium for implantation of the fetus and low progesterone levels in early pregnancy have been associated with miscarriage. The levels of progesterone in the early part of the menstrual cycle are increased with a drug called clomiphene.

This causes the ovary to produce more progesterone after ovulation. Progesterone pessaries or suppositories can also be used.

Recurrent Miscarriages

Recurrent (habitual) miscarriage is defined as two or more consecutive abortions and the cause is not always clear and may not be the same each time. Most couples who have had fewer than three consecutive miscarriages are not offered routine tests or treatment, unless there is a definitive reason such as an incompetent cervix. Where no cause is found after investigation, the chance of a successful pregnancy is still between 50% and 70% (Hey et al., 1996). Even after four or more miscarriages the chance of a successful pregnancy is still greater than 40% (Lachelin, 1996).

Symptoms

The following may all be symptoms of impending miscarriage in a currently pregnant woman:

- vaginal bleeding, with or without abdominal cramps;
- low back pain or abdominal pain; pain can be dull, sharp or cramping, persistent, constant or intermittent;
- tissue or clot-like material that passes from the vagina.

Approximately 20% of pregnant women experience some vaginal bleeding during the first trimester and less than half of these women will experience a spontaneous abortion.

Investigations

The following investigations should be undertaken:

- Pelvic examination may reveal moderate thinning of the cervix (effacement), increased cervical dilation and evidence of ruptured membranes.
- Blood sampling should include hCG, FBC and WCC.
- Ultrasound examination is often used to determine whether there is a live fetus inside the uterus.

Complications

Complications of miscarriage are listed below:

- Retained products of conception are referred to as an incomplete abortion. This may cause infection and the retained uterine tissue must be removed surgically (D and C).
- An infection may occur after either a complete or incomplete abortion.
- In a missed abortion the pregnancy has continued for four weeks or longer following the death of the fetus. This usually occurs in the second trimester. Sometimes (if early enough in the pregnancy) D and C can be performed to remove the dead tissue.
- Dead fetus syndrome is the term used to describe a condition that affects the mother. If the fetus has died but the dead tissue has not been discarded by the uterus, an abnormal activation of the blood clotting systems can develop in response to the release of anti-clotting chemicals from the retained dead fetus (missed abortion).

If a woman has a spontaneous abortion, the odds of her successfully completing her next pregnancy are greater than 85%. After two or more spontaneous abortions, if uterine anomaly, genetic abnormality and luteal phase defect have been ruled out, the odds of completing the next pregnancy are 70% and remain so for each successive pregnancy.

Emotional Support Following Miscarriage:

The attachment bond between mother and fetus is one of the closest with regard to physical, emotional and psychological intimacy and therefore has the capacity to cause a substantial degree of grief when the fetus is lost (Leick and Davidson-Neilson, 1991).

Grief

It has been stated that women who suffer an early loss, that is a spontaneous abortion before 20 weeks, show a significantly lower degree of grief than those who sustain a late perinatal loss, whether stillborn or neonatal death (Theut et al., 1989). However, each woman's experience of miscarriage is unique and individual and therefore should be treated as such. The duration and intensity of grief can be influenced by many factors including the degree of attachment and previous pregnancy loss. Normal grief reactions include both somatic and psychological symptoms. These usually happen in a recognizable pattern: the initial somatic symptoms such as sighing, lack of strength and shortness of breath are followed by a stage characterized by mental images of the deceased and feelings of grief, and are often followed by feelings of hostility towards hospital staff.

Guilt

Feelings of guilt and anger are also common and normal reactions to a miscarriage as some women feel responsible for the miscarriage and start to search for something they may have done wrong. Such losses have often been referred to as 'quiet tragedies' because of the silence that surrounds the event, and it is very important that the parents are encouraged to grieve for their loss. Grief should not be left unacknowledged and unresolved as it can lead to future psychological problems, with one-quarter to one-third of women suffering some degree of depression (Moscarello, 1989).

Terminology

The appropriate use of medical terminology is an essential component in developing a trusting and caring relationship with the patient. However, often the terminology is alien and can sound harsh in describing the process involved in miscarriage. Use of the term abortion can be particularly insensitive and terms such as failed pregnancy, incompetent cervix and abnormal chromosomal material are frequently used (Chambers, 1992). Care should therefore be taken because the parents will tend to focus on the words 'failed', 'incompetent' and 'abnormal'.

Subsequent Patient Advice

- Physically the recovery will take 4–6 weeks.
- There may be some spotting and discomfort for a few days.
- If the pregnancy was lost at more than 13 weeks the patient may still look pregnant and the breasts may still leak milk.
- There will be follow-up appointment with the GP after a couple of weeks to check on recovery.

The best time to start trying for another baby will vary, but generally it is advisable to wait about three months to get over the physical and perhaps more importantly the emotional effects of miscarriage as replacing the loss so quickly can impede the resolution of the primary loss and cause psychological problems with subsequent attachments. In summary, A&E nurses must appreciate that each woman is an individual and must explore the history she brings to the current event, the meaning she attributes to the miscarriage and its subsequent impact on her life (Stead, 1996).

Conclusion

It is hoped that this chapter has given nurses a greater insight into, and background and knowledge of the four main gynaecological conditions that present within the acute A&E setting as, with a greater understanding, they will be better equipped to care for these women in a more complete and holistic way.

Suggested Further Reading

Lachelin G (1996) Miscarriage: The Facts. Oxford: Oxford University Press.
Hey V, Hzin C, Saunders L, Speakman MA (1996) Hidden Loss, Miscarriage and Ectopic Pregnancy, 2nd edn. London: Women's Press.

References

Abbott J, Emmans LS, Lowenstein SR (1990) Ectopic Pregnancy: Ten Common Pitfalls in Diagnoses. American Journal of Emergency Medicine 8: 515–22.
Abound E (1997) A five year review of ectopic pregnancy, Clinical and Experimental Obstetrics and Gynecology 24(3): 127–9.
Aral S, Holmes KK (1990) Epidemiology of sex behaviour and sexually transmitted diseases. In Holmes KK et al. (Eds).Sexually transmitted diseases, 2nd edn. New York: McGraw-Hill.
Aral SO, Mosher WD, Cates W (1987) Contraceptive use, pelvic inflammatory disease and fertility problems among American women. American Journal of Obstetrics and Gynecology No. 157: 59–64.
Boyer K et al. (1996) Resolution of intercranial calcifications in infants with treated congenital toxoplasmosis. Radiology 199(2): 433–40.
Bryner L (1989) Recurrent toxic shock syndrome. American Family Physician 39(3): 157–64.
Cacciatore B, Tiitinen A, Astenman DH, Ylostalo P (1990) Normal early pregnancy: serum hCG levels and vaginal ultrasonography findings. British Journal of Obstetrics and Gynaecology 9: 899–903.

Chambers B (1992) Terminology used in early pregnancy loss. British Journal of Obstetrics and Gynaecology No. 99: 357–58.

Dimitry ES (1987) Does previous appendicectomy predispose to ectopic pregnancy? A retrospective case-controlled study. British Journal of Obstetrics and Gynaecology 7: 221–24.

Edelman DA, Porter CW, Van Os WA (1990) When should intrauterine devices be removed and replaced? British Journal of Family Planning No.16: 132–8.

Farley TM, Rosenberg M, Rowe P, Chen J, Meirik O (1992) Intrauterine devices and pelvic inflammatory disease: an international perspective. Lancet No. 339: 785–8.

Gould D (1997) Ectopic pregnancies: causes and outcomes. Nursing Times 93(14): 53–5.

Hammerslough CL (1992) Estimating the probability of spontaneous abortion in the presence of induced abortion and vice versa. Public Health Report No. 107: 269–77.

Hey V, Hzin C, Saunders L, Speakman MA (1996) Hidden Loss, Miscarriage and Ectopic Pregnancy, 2nd edn. London: Women's Press.

Jacobson L, Westrom L (1984) Objectivised diagnoses of acute pelvic inflammatory disease. American Journal of Obstetrics and Gynecology No. 105: 1088–98.

Kottman LM (1995) Pelvic inflammatory disease; clinical overview. Journal of Obstetric, Gynecologic and Neonatal Nursing 24(8): 759–67.

Lachelin G (1996) Miscarriage: The Facts, 2nd edn. Oxford: Oxford University Press.

Landers D (1994) Pelvic Inflammatory Disease in STD Update '93: STDs in the 90s. The Association of Reproductive Health Professionals Clinical Proceedings. Washington, DC: ARHP.

Leick N, Davidson-Neilson M (1991) Healing pain; attachment, loss and grief therapy. Genetic, Social, and General Psychology Monographs No.95: 55–96.

Ling FW, Stovall TG (1994) Update on the diagnoses and management of ectopic pregnancy. In Advances in Obstetrics and Gynaecology. Chicago: Mosby Year Book.

Marchbanks PA, Lee C, Peterson B (1990) Cigarette smoking as a risk factor for pelvic inflammatory disease. American Journal of Obstetrics and Gynecology No. 162: 639–44.

Mitchell S (1993) Recurrent pelvic inflammatory disease. The Practitioner 237: 218–19.

Moscarello R (1989) Perinatal bereavement support services: three-year review. Journal of Palliative Care 5(4): 2–8.

Munday PE (1997) Clinical aspects of pelvic inflammatory disease. Human Reproduction 12 November: 121–6.

Pearce JM (1990) Pelvic inflammatory disease (diagnoses and treatment). British Medical Journal 300: 1090–1.

Perez MC, Wilson WA, Brown HL, Scopelitis E (1991) Anticariolipin antibodies in unselected pregnant women: relationship to foetal outcome. Journal of Perinatology 11(1): 33–6.

Reichlin M (1998) Systemic lupus erythematosus and pregnancy. Journal of Reproductive Medicine No. 43: 355–60.

Rice PA, Schachter J (1991) Pathogenesis of pelvic inflammatory disease. What are the questions? Journal of the American Medical Association No. 288: 2587–93.

Rizk B et al. (1991) Heterotopic pregnancies after IVF and ET. American Journal of Obstetrics and Gynecology 164(1), Part 1: 161–4.

Scottish Department of Health (1997) The Management of Early Pregnancy Loss: A Statement of Good Practice. Edinburgh: Stationery Office.

Simon C, Martinez L, Pardo F, Tortajad M, Pellicer A, Mulerian A (1991) Defects in women with normal reproductive outcome. Fertility & Sterility No. 56: 1192–3.

Sinei SKA et al. (1990) Preventing IUD related pelvic infection; the efficacy of prophylactic doxycycline at insertion. British Journal of Obstetrics and Gynaecology No. 97: 412–19.

Spence MR (1989) Pelvic inflammatory disease. Journal of Reproductive Medicine No. 34(8s): 605–9.

Stabile I (1996) Ectopic Pregnancy: Diagnoses and Management. Cambridge: Cambridge University Press.

Stacey C (1992) Pelvic inflammatory disease. Maternal and Child Health January: 11–14.

Stead CE (1996) Nursing management in the accident and emergency department of women undergoing a miscarriage. Accident & Emergency Nursing 4(4): 182–6.

Stevens DL (1992) Invasive group A streptococcus infections. Clinical Infectious Diseases No. 14: 2–13.

Theut S, Henderson F, Zaslow M, Cain R, Rabinovich B, Morihsa J (1989) Perinatal loss and perinatal bereavement. Journal of Psychiatry 147(5): 635–9.

Toth PP, Jothivijayarani A (1999) Family Practice Handbook, 3rd edn. Ames: University of Iowa, Department of Family Medicine.

Tummon IS, Whitmore NA, Daniel SA, Nisker JA, Yuzpe AA (1994). Transferring embryos increases risk of heterotopic pregnancy. Fertility and Sterility 61(6): 1065–67.

Westrom L, Mardh PA (1990) Acute pelvic inflammatory disease (PID). In Holmes KK, Mardh PA, Sparling PJ, Wiesner W, Cates SM (Eds) Sexually Transmitted Diseases, 2nd edn. New York: McGraw-Hill.

Wolner-Hassen P et al. (1990) Association between vaginal douching and acute pelvic inflammatory disease. Journal of the American Medical Association 263: 1936–41.

World Health Organisation (1985) Task Force on Inter Uterine Devices for Fertility Regulation: a multinational case control study of ectopic pregnancy. Clinical Reproduction and Fertility No. 3: 131–9.

Ylostalo P, Cacciatore B, Bsjoberg J, Kaarainen M, Tenhumen A, Astenman UH (1992) Expectant management of ectopic pregnancy. Obstetrics and Gynaecology No. 80: 345–8.

Chapter 6
The Unconscious Patient

Andrew Rideout

Principles of Unconsciousness

Unconsciousness follows an interruption of the normal activity within the cerebral cortex or reticular activating system of the brainstem. This can be due to trauma or as a result of central or systemic metabolic disturbances or disease processes. Neurones are dependent on the metabolism of oxygen and glucose and do not have reserves of energy stores or the ability to survive under anaerobic conditions. Any disruption to the supply of these two nutrients, or any changes within the body's chemistry that prevent their utilization, will quickly result in unconsciousness. This chapter will discuss the common causes of unconsciousness, the nursing interventions required and the rationale behind them.

Initial Assessment

Initial assessment of the unconscious patient should follow the recognized ABC system adopted by the Advanced Life Support/Advanced Trauma Life Support courses (Alexander and Procter, 1993).

Airway (with Stabilization/Control of the Cervical Spine)

For the unconscious patient, the most immediately life-threatening concern is the inability to keep his/her airway open. The airway can be obstructed by anatomical structures such as the tongue, epiglottis, soft tissues of the oropharynx, or by foreign objects such as dentures, vomitus or food boluses. Correct airway position will prevent obstruction by anatomical structures. In the adult this position is the head-tilt/chin-lift position or the jaw-thrust position. If an underlying neck injury is suspected then the head-tilt/chin-lift procedure is inappropriate and a jaw thrust must be used instead. The airway can then be inspected and solid matter removed with the gloved hand or Magill's forceps. Fluids such as saliva, blood and vomitus can be removed by suction using a wide-bore Yankeur sucker. If suction is not available then the head (and possibly the whole body) needs to be turned to one side and the trolley tilted to a 'head down' position to allow fluids to flow out away from the airway.

Adjuncts may be used to help maintain a patent airway. These include the oropharyngeal (Guedal) airway, the nasopharyngeal airway and the laryngeal mask airway. The 'gold standard' for protecting a patient's airway is intubation with a cuffed tube. Often the anaesthetist will perform this procedure, although in practice any competent practitioner can carry it out. Patients may be brought to the accident and emergency (A&E) department already intubated and it is good nursing practice to check that the endotracheal tube is still in the correct place on patient arrival as movement on and off ambulance trolleys may dislodge the tube.

Breathing

The next stage of assessment is the patient's breathing. This is assessed by looking for movement associated with respiration (rib cage, abdomen, and accessory muscles), listening for sounds of breathing both by ear and with a stethoscope, and feeling for chest movement and flow of exhaled air from the mouth. The rate of breathing may be changed abnormally. Hypoxia or metabolic acidosis will cause an increase in rate whilst metabolic alkalosis, raised intercranial pressure or some toxic agents (particularly opiates) cause decreased respiratory rate or respiratory arrest. Uneven chest movement may occur secondary to a pneumothorax or the obstruction of one bronchus. An unconscious patient may also display rhythmical breathing, particularly Cheyne-Stokes respiration, where the breathing rate cycles through apnoea to hyperventilation. This may be a sign of raised intercranial pressure or overdose of opiates, but is often an end stage in the moribund patient.

As well as recording the respiratory rate it is often useful to estimate oxygen saturation using a pulse oximeter although this will give unreliable recordings in a patient who is peripherally vaso-constricted due to cold or hypovolaemia. Certain conditions will also affect the accuracy or usefulness of this recording, including carbon monoxide and cyanide poisoning. There are expired-breath carbon monoxide measuring devices that may give an indication of carboxyhaemoglobin, although the unconscious patient will be unable to use them. Therefore arterial blood gas sampling should be performed as early as possible in patients who are suspected of carbon monoxide poisoning.

Patients who are breathing spontaneously should have supplemental oxygen administered as hypoxia is a common causative or associated factor in unconsciousness. This should be delivered at a high flow rate, 10–15 l/min, through a mask and reservoir (non-rebreathing mask), giving 90–100% oxygen. Those patients whose respiratory rate is inadequate should be ventilated using a bag/valve/mask with reservoir and intubation considered.

Circulation

The circulation should be assessed by feeling for a major pulse (in adults the carotid or femoral pulse), assessing capillary refill, observing skin colour and measuring blood pressure. Two possible methods for assessing capillary refill are either to press the skin of the forehead firmly with a finger or to raise the patient's arm above the height of the heart and squeeze on the tip of the finger. In the patient with a good circulation, blood will return to the blanched area within about two seconds. However, a patient who is peripherally vaso-constricted because of the cold will also show a delayed capillary refill in the fingers, making this technique less useful. In the shocked patient there will be signs of increased autonomic activity including sweatiness associated with pallor and cool skin. In the absence of circulation, cardiopulmonary resuscitation should be started.

Both cardiac and cerebral disease processes may affect heart rate and blood pressure. Overdoses of a number of drugs can also affect cardiac rate and contractility. The patient who appears to have a heart rate that is irregular, is outside the normal parameters or who is known to have taken cardiotoxic drugs should have continuous cardiac monitoring performed.

An absence of peripheral pulses with prolonged capillary refill time indicates poor perfusion due to low blood pressure. Patients with low blood pressure should have at least one (and preferably two) large-bore cannulae inserted into large proximal veins, such as those in the ante-cubital fossae. If venous access cannot be obtained by this method then an alternative method should be tried: either central venous cannulation, peripheral venous cut-down or, as an extreme measure, use of an interosseous needle. IV fluids can then be administered to support the circulation. There is some debate comparing crystalloid and colloid fluids, but 1 litre of Hartmann's (Ringer's lactate solution) or normal saline is a suitable first-line treatment.

Disability

Initial observations should include a record of the Glasgow Coma Score (GCS). There is no current research to suggest an optimum interval for repeating GCS observations, although the nurse must be satisfied that he or she is able to detect changes in consciousness level early enough to allow appropriate intervention. Dependent upon the stage of patient care, observations may be made as frequently as every fifteen minutes or as seldom as every four hours.

The Glasgow Coma Score ranges from 3 to 15 and consists of three components:

- verbal response;
- eye opening;
- motor function.

A simple *aide-mémoire* for the different scores is:

Eyes – maximum score 4	'four eyes'
Vocal response – maximum 5	'V is the Latin symbol for 5'
Motor function – maximum 6	'M6 motorway'

An alternative measure of consciousness is the AVPU score (Alert, responds to Verbal, or Painful stimuli, Unresponsive) although this is more of a rapid assessment tool, suitable for exchange of information between professionals.

In the presence of raised intercranial pressure, changes in the pupillary reaction to light are a very late sign with poor prognosis. Pupils may be dilated due to hypoxia or as an effect of drugs such as barbiturates, ecstasy (**MDMA**) or anti-cholinergic drugs (atropine).

Pinpoint pupils may be a result of drugs (opiates) or a brain-stem infarction.

Necessary observations on the unconscious patient include pulse and respiratory rates, blood pressure, temperature, blood sugar concentration, pupil size and reactivity. Additionally, urinalysis, blood/breath alcohol and blood chemistry can be useful. The ABCs need to be constantly monitored to prevent or correct any deterioration in condition.

Physical Care of the Unconscious Patient

Safety is a major consideration in caring for the unconscious patient. The preferred position for the unconscious patient who is not thought to have any injuries is the recovery position. This allows the airway to remain clear in the event of passive regurgitation of stomach contents and also prevents the tongue from occluding the airway. Care must be taken whilst putting the patient into the recovery position as there is a risk of nerve damage in limbs caused by awkward positioning. However, the reality of positioning a patient on an A&E trolley means that the technique used is often less than perfect and staff need to be aware of their own safety in moving and handling of patients.

Some patients may remain unconscious for several hours and care needs to be taken of their pressure areas. It is tempting to place patients on a soft mattress and leave them, but for effective pressure area care the patient must be moved frequently to allow capillary blood flow to return to areas under high pressure. Tradition has dictated that patients should be turned every two hours, but pain and damage to tissues can occur in a much shorter period. For the supine patient, normally only those with a protected airway, 30° turns are sufficient to relieve pressure but the patient in the recovery position will probably have to be moved fully onto his/her other side.

No unconscious patient should be left on a trolley without the sides in place, and it may be safer to nurse some unconscious or semi-conscious patients on a mattress on the floor. Some of the conditions leading to unconsciousness (e.g. alcohol intoxication) can lead to increased susceptibility to hypothermia and for the semi-clothed patient the A&E environment can be a very cold place. The nurse should therefore ensure that the unconscious patient has sufficient blankets to cover him/her.

All patients will need ongoing nursing care including suctioning of the oropharynx, and mouth and eye care. There is also a risk of incontinence and so frequent condition checks should include checking for dampness and soiling. Frequent nursing review subsequently aims to prevent any deterioration in the patient's condition going unnoticed.

Psychological Care of the Unconscious Patient

Many unconscious patients are still aware of their surroundings and will benefit from physical contact and verbal reassurance. If painful procedures are being performed, analgesia or local anaesthetic should be administered first.

Unconsciousness is a very distressing condition for friends and family and they will need support from nurses. They may be unwilling to touch or speak to the patient and will need reassurance to do so. Conversely, they may make inappropriate comments in front of the patient assuming that he/she is unable to hear. When giving explanations about tests, equipment and likely outcomes for the patient it is wise to give one piece of information at a time and to repeat it as often as necessary. The relative who is showing signs of intense emotion is unlikely to remember much of what is said to him/her and may need information repeated or written down.

Legal Aspects of Care of the Unconscious Patient

The nurse is the advocate for the unconscious patient, representing him/her before relatives, police and other healthcare professionals.

A recurrent problem with unconscious patients in A&E is that of missing property. All departments will have a procedure for recording property and it is often in the form of a duplicate or triplicate book. It is often tempting not to record clothing and other belongings, but the frequency with which problems arise makes this unwise. Any damage to property, whether caused in the department (e.g. cutting off clothing) or before arrival should be noted. If clothing is cut in the department it is often worth recording the reason why this was thought to be necessary, even if this seems obvious. If it is known where any other property has gone, then this should also be noted (e.g. taken by police, family member or left with neighbour).

If the police remove property from the A&E department they will either give a receipt or should sign the case notes to acknowledge that they have done so. If the property is required as evidence then the police will have a procedure for removing it, involving separate bagging to minimize contamination. The nurse will normally have to sign police paper work and may have to give a statement, and may be asked to appear in court at a later date, to identify clothing or property that he or she has removed from an unconscious patient. If it seems that this is likely then it is worth making a separate record of property and clothing with full descriptions (including damage, stains etc.) for the nurse's own records.

Full and accurate record keeping is vital in the care of unconscious patients, both to mark any change in condition and also in case of later problems where the original notes need to be reviewed.

Some unconscious patients will be carrying illegal drugs, whether drug overdose is the primary cause of unconsciousness or not, and many departments will have their own procedures for dealing with these substances. Patients may have other illegal articles on their person such as offensive weapons, explosives or paedophilic literature and the UKCC (1992) makes it clear that, in such instances, the nurse has a responsibility to society as well as to the patient.

Further Assessment

The ambulance crew, friends or relatives may be able to give information about recent medical history, which will help in reaching a diagnosis and planning care. They should therefore be encouraged to stay until all possible information has been elicited. It may be possible to gain information from previous A&E or hospital attendances, and so the relevant computer systems should also be checked.

If there is no evidence of obvious injury or focal neurological signs (e.g. weakness in one side, or focal fitting) then the cause is more likely to be toxic, metabolic or shock related. The presence of focal signs suggests an intercranial cause (meningitis, haemorrhage, etc.) although such signs may also present following hypoglycaemia, or hepatic or renal failure.

Common signs

Below is a list of common signs and their possible significance:

- increased respiratory rate – airway compromise (e.g. physical obstruction, infection), acidosis (e.g. DKA, aspirin poisoning);
- reduced respiratory rate – CVA or poisoning (opiates, barbiturates);
- tachycardia – sepsis, hypovolaemia, poisoning (numerous drugs) or primary cardiac cause;
- bradycardia – hypoxia, CVA or other cause for raised intercranial pressure, poisoning (digoxin, beta-blockers) or primary cardiac cause;
- hypertension – raised intercranial pressure, particularly if associated with bradycardia, causative of CVA;
- hypotension – hypovolaemia, sepsis, anaphylaxis, cardiac cause;
- pyrexia – sepsis, heat stroke, intercranial lesion;
- hypothermia – environmental, myxoedema.

Specific Causes of Unconsciousness

One useful mnemonic to help remember possible causes of unconsciousness is the vowel sounds AEIOUH:

A Alcohol/Acidosis/Alkalosis/Anaphylaxis/'At it'
E Epilepsy/Electrolyte/Endocrine/Encephalopathy
I Insulin/Intercranial lesion/Infection
O Overdose
U Uraemia
H Hypoxia/Hypothermia/Hypovolaemia/Heart problems/Head injury

Some of the more common causes will now be discussed.

Alcohol Intoxication

It has been estimated that alcohol consumption is a contributory factor in 25% of hospital admissions and that acute alcohol intoxication is a factor in much of the routine work of A&E departments over weekends and in the evenings (Yates et al., 1987).

Alcohol is a central depressant, rapidly absorbed from the GI tract with peak blood levels occurring 30 to 90 minutes after drinking. Complete absorption may take six hours and excretion from the body normally takes about thirty minutes to an hour for every unit of alcohol (equivalent to 10 mg/100 ml blood) drunk. Chronic alcoholics clear alcohol from their systems much faster and may show fewer signs of impaired function and intoxication.

If the patient is unconscious he/she is likely to have a smell of alcohol on the breath and may have alcohol-containing vomitus on his/her clothing. Containers for alcohol may be found around their person. He/she may be flushed, have slow deep breathing, nystagmus and incontinence. Alcohol ingestion can also precipitate a hypoglycaemic episode and may contribute to other causes of unconsciousness including smoke inhalation, overdose and head injury.

If a breathalyser is available breath alcohol can be measured on the unconscious patient by passive expiration, otherwise blood alcohol levels may be measured if deemed necessary. Blood glucose, urea and electrolyte levels should be measured, and if the patient is thought to be a chronic alcoholic then liver function tests and full blood count may be performed. If the circumstances in which the alcohol has been taken are unknown then plasma paracetamol levels should be measured to exclude self-poisoning. The chronic alcoholic may show anaemia, thrombocytopaenia or leucocytosis.

In the occasional drinker, the effects of varying blood alcohol levels are listed below:

mg/100 ml	Effects
20–50	Decreased fine motor function
50–100	Impaired judgement/coordination
100–150	Difficulty with walking and balance, lethargy
250–300	Hallucinations
300	Coma
400	Respiratory depression
500	Death

If the patient is thought to be a chronic alcohol user then IV thiamine should be given to prevent Wernicke's encephalopathy. This is particularly important before any glucose is administered. Otherwise care of ABCs is the first priority. Additional complications such as poisoning, hypoglycaemic coma or head injury should always be excluded before a diagnosis of alcohol intoxication is accepted.

Acidosis/Alkalosis

Acid-base imbalance can be either metabolic or respiratory in origin and should be regarded as a symptom of some other pathology. Acidosis is defined as a pH < 7.35 and alkalosis as a pH > 7.45 on blood gas analysis. Blood gas analysis will also demonstrate whether the imbalance has a respiratory or metabolic cause. Treatment should always aim to address the underlying cause initially, with possible use of drugs to alter or stabilize the blood pH (such as sodium bicarbonate or methylene blue) if treatment of the underlying cause is initially slow or unsuccessful.

Causes include the following:

- *metabolic acidosis*: high blood lactic acid levels (e.g. following vigorous exercise, fitting, trauma or liver failure), high levels of other physiological acids (e.g. diabetic ketoacidosis), ingestion of acidic substances (e.g. aspirin) or renal failure;
- *metabolic alkalosis*: vomiting;
- *respiratory acidosis*: any cause of reduced respiration such as smothering or chest trauma;
- *respiratory alkalosis*: any cause of increased respiration such as anxiety-induced hyperventilation, hyperventilating before diving, pyrexia or CVA.

Anaphylaxis

Anaphylactic shock is caused by an antibody reaction to a specific antigen to which a person has previously been sensitized. Histamine and kinins are released causing a systemic effect. In an anaphylactoid reaction there needs to be no previous sensitization. The most common causative agents are IV antibiotics (one in 5000 patients may experience a reaction), bee and wasp stings, peanuts or shellfish.

When an antigen attaches to its specific IgE on a basophil or mast cell an inflammatory mediator (such as histamine, leukotriene or prostaglandin) is released. This causes the typical allergic reaction of bronchospasm, mucus secretion, vasodilatation, increased capillary permeability and skin erythema and wheals.

Signs of anaphylactic shock include:

- hypotension;
- tachycardia;
- tachypnoea;
- wheeze;
- respiratory distress;
- a sense of impending doom.

Treatment follows the pattern of ABC, oxygen, IM adrenaline and IV fluids (an initial 1 litre bolus of normal saline or Hartmann's solution). Any antigen should be removed where possible (e.g. drug infusions should be stopped). The mainstay of drug therapy is adrenaline: 0.5 ml of 1:1000 adrenaline (500 µg) IM repeated every five minutes as necessary. Other drugs that may prove useful include bronchodilators such as salbutamol, antihistamines and steroids. The latter two have a comparatively slow onset of action, with steroids taking up to six hours to work, but are useful in preventing recurrences of the reaction.

'At it'

This diagnosis should be made with caution, after all other possible causes for unconsciousness have been excluded.

There are two recurrent features in this group of patients. The first is a history of a stressful situation. Typically this may involve being taken into police custody, but can also include an argument with a friend or relation (often partner or parent) or a recent minor overdose. There is also a group of patients who are well known to their local A&E department with frequent attendances after collapsing in public places and becoming 'unconscious'.

The second feature of this group is the common finding of very low GCS (typically 3) with atypical features such as screwing up of the eyelids and resistance to having the eyelids opened by the nurse.

Epilepsy

If a patient is fitting within the A&E department he/she should be placed flat and protected from injury. High-flow oxygen should be administered through a mask and nasopharyngeal airway and if the seizure is not self-limiting then anti-epileptic medication should be considered (IV or rectal diazepam or rectal paraldehyde).

Many epileptic patients will be post-ictal with reduced consciousness for a period of time post-seizure. This may last for several hours and during this time the patient will require observation to maintain his/her safety. Nursing observations should include a coma score and blood sugar. Precipitating factors for a seizure may include alcohol consumption, electrolyte imbalance or non-therapeutic serum medication levels and it may be appropriate to test for these. However, a seizure is commonly caused by environmental factors such as flashing lights, weather changes or an underlying infection such as a common cold and no further investigation may be required.

Status epilepticus is a continued seizure, or recurrent seizures, with no time for recovery in between. Whilst it is commonly accepted that a seizure lasting more than 30 minutes counts as status epilepticus, cerebral damage has been shown to occur after only ten minutes of seizure activity. During a seizure there is a rise in body temperature, release of lactic acid and catecholamine secretion because of the intense physical effort required. This results in tachycardia, hypertension, cardiac dysrhythmias and an increased cerebral metabolic rate. In a normal epileptic seizure cerebral blood flow and oxygenation increase to meet this demand. In status epilepticus this mechanism fails, causing neuronal damage as well as the direct effects of abnormal neuronal activity and the damage that this causes. Subsequently there is a 20% mortality rate from status epilepticus, although this is due in part to underlying pathology.

Status epilepticus may have a different presentation from the initial seizure, with only a persistent focal twitching of perhaps an eyelid, hand or foot. If IV diazepam fails to stop the seizure then a phenytoin infusion may be needed and, in some cases, ventilation following drug-induced paralysis will be required. The patient should be closely monitored after cessation of the seizure as diazepam may cause respiratory depression and arrest, especially following administration via both IV and PR routes.

Endocrine disorders

The most common endocrine disorder resulting in unconsciousness and subsequent A&E attendance is diabetes mellitus. The patient can suffer from both low blood sugar (hypoglycaemia) and high blood sugar (hyperglycaemia, with two serious presentations: diabetic ketoacidosis or hyperosmolar non-ketotic hyperglycaemia).

Hypoglycaemia

Hypoglycaemia is the condition where serum glucose is low (< 2.8mmol/l). This will initially affect nervous tissue as the cells are dependent upon glucose for energy. There will be associated signs of central nervous system depression (primarily confusion and unconsciousness) and there may also be signs of increased sympathetic activity including grey skin, sweating, dilated pupils and cardiac dysrhythmias. Prolonged periods of hypoglycaemia can lead to permanent neurological deficit including focal neurological signs (e.g. hemiparesis) or poor cognitive skills.

Hypoglycaemia leading to unconsciousness is rare in those individuals who have not taken insulin or oral hypoglycaemic medication. Rarely there will be another cause such as alcohol ingestion, liver disease or an insulin-secreting tumour. In the diabetic patient, increasing the dose of insulin, failure to take adequate nutrition, excessive exercise, interaction with other drugs/alcohol or a systemic infection may cause hypoglycaemia.

Administration of IV glucose (50–100 ml 50% dextrose) or glucagon (1 mg by IM injection) rapidly reverses hypoglycaemia. However, a hypoglycaemic patient may become very agitated and violent as the hypoglycaemia resolves. Once conscious, patients should be given sugary food and drinks followed by complex carbohydrates (e.g. milk or biscuits) to maintain blood sugar levels.

Hyperglycaemia

Diabetic Ketoacidosis (DKA)

This condition most commonly occurs in young diabetics (< 20 years old) and may be the first indication that a patient has diabetes. Common features include high blood glucose, dehydration and hypokalaemia. The patient often has a history of vomiting, drowsiness and increased confusion over a two- to three-day period. There will be the smell of ketones (pear drops) on their breath and ketones will be found in their urine. Patients with DKA often have epigastric pain and DKA should always be ruled out as a cause for non-specific abdominal pain by performing a blood glucose check on such patients.

The precipitating factors for DKA are most commonly:

- infection – especially urinary infection (40%);
- poor management of diabetes (25%);
- undiagnosed diabetes (15%).

DKA can readily be treated and mortality rates are negligible.

Hyperosmolar non-ketotic hyperglycaemia (HONK)

This is generally a condition of the elderly with non-insulin dependent diabetes (type II diabetes) and may also be the first sign that a patient has diabetes. It has a long onset of about a week, typically following an infection, and unlike DKA has a high mortality rate (10–20%). Patients give a history of recent acute infection followed by gradual deterioration and may have dehydration and focal neurological signs. Unconsciousness is rare.

For both DKA and HONK treatment involves fluid replacement, treatment of electrolyte and acid-base imbalances and reduction of blood glucose to normal levels. Insulin should be given through a continuous IV infusion, with the amount of insulin titrated against the blood glucose levels. For this reason the patient needs frequent blood glucose testing. These patients are at risk as a result of the aggressive fluid replacement and should be monitored for signs of fluid overload.

Other Endocrine Causes of Unconsciousness

Addisonian Crisis

This occurs as a result of insufficient corticosteroids. This may be due to reduced secretion (such as adrenal gland disease including malignancy, infarction and tuberculosis, hypopituitarism or drug therapy) or secondary to stopping steroid therapy too rapidly. It may be precipitated by infection or trauma. Symptoms may have a gradual onset including apathy and depression, weakness and anorexia, increased thirst with a craving for salt, and postural hypotension.

Initial supportive treatment is with oxygen, fluids, antibiotics and IV steroids.

Myxoedema

This is caused by hypothyroidism, often with a gradual onset of symptoms. Coma may be precipitated by the elderly using benzodiazepine sedatives, causing the patient to become hypothermic. Patients may also be bradycardic, have respiratory depression and have seizures. Signs of hypothyroidism (goitre and periorbital oedema) may give a clue to the cause of the unconsciousness. Treatment in the first instance is supportive (particularly respiratory support), warming and IV fluids.

Thyrotoxic crisis

This may be confused with sepsis since patients will normally present with pyrexia and tachycardia. However, they may have a history of hyperthyroidism or signs consistent with being hyperthyroid (goitre and exophthalmos). Nursing measures include temperature control (paracetamol and cold sponging/ice packs), cardiac monitoring and regular recording of blood sugar levels.

Intercranial Lesions

Haemorrhagic Stroke

Worldwide, strokes are the second most frequent cause of death with 25% occurring in individuals aged below 65 years. Haemorrhagic strokes make up about 15% of all cerebrovascular accidents (CVAs) and have a higher mortality (up to 80% mortality after one month) than ischaemic strokes. Although the signs and symptoms are the same as an ischaemic stroke they tend to be more severe and patients may become progressively worse during their time in A&E, with about half of deaths occuring within the first 48 hours. There is more likely to be hypertension in these patients and a history of preceding headache. It is patients with haemorrhagic strokes who are more likely to present with fitting and coma.

Bleeding normally occurs as a result of damage to small vessels following chronic hypertension. The haematoma causes direct brain injury which is compounded by secondary oedema. Symptoms will depend upon the site of the bleed, but typically include hemiparesis, upgoing plantars and nystagmus. If the cerebellum or brainstem is involved there is a greater risk of respiratory involvement, including respiratory arrest.

An ECG should be recorded because CVAs predispose to cardiac dysrhythmias. Treatment involves maintenance of the ABCs, frequent blood pressure monitoring and care of mouth and skin. If the systolic blood pressure is greater than 200 mmHg, or the diastolic blood pressure is consistently greater than 100 mmHg (three readings over half an hour) then it may be appropriate to start anti-hypertensive therapy.

Ischaemic Stroke

Symptoms are similar to those found in haemorrhagic strokes although they tend to be less severe and have a lower incidence of unconsciousness. They are caused primarily by thrombosis of cerebral arteries but may also be caused by emboli or arterial spasm. The symptoms of a CVA can often (in about a fifth of cases of apparent ischaemic stroke) be caused by other diseases such as seizure, infection, brain tumour or hyponatraemia.

Within the UK treatment of CVAs tends to be palliative, although elsewhere thrombolysis, elective ventilation and Mannitol have all been used to try and improve tissue perfusion.

Subarachnoid Haemorrhage

Subarachnoid haemorrhage (SAH) is the term for blood within the subarachnoid space. It accounts for almost 10% of all strokes, occurs in younger patients (mean age 50 years) and affects women more than men. There is a high mortality rate, with 15% of patients dying before they reach A&E and 40% dying within the first week.

Although transient loss of consciousness is common when the bleed first occurs, persistent coma is a serious sign with a poor prognostic outcome. A CT scan should be performed and, if negative, a lumbar puncture may show the presence of blood and increased CSF protein, although this may take a couple of hours to develop. An ECG will often show widespread changes with ST elevation in all leads, prolonged QRS and QT intervals and U waves. Treatment is aimed at reducing intracranial pressure and hyperventilation;

Mannitol or hyperosmotic saline and frusemide may all be used. Nimodipine may further reduce secondary vasospasm.

Infection

This may be either localized to the central nervous system (meningitis or encephalitis) or systemic.

Meningitis

Meningitis may be viral or bacterial and often presents as flu-like symptoms with a generalized headache. Typically patients with meningitis demonstrate photophobia and neck stiffness. The petechial rash often associated with meningitis is a symptom of a systemic infection caused by the meningococcal bacteria. It is caused by tiny haemorrhages within the skin and so has a deep red or purple appearance similar to a bruise. Pressing the rash with a finger or a transparent object does not cause the colour of the rash to diminish (the blanche test). Meningitis is confirmed by analysis of cerebrospinal fluid collected by lumbar puncture and/or the isolation of meningococcus from scrapings of the rash. If meningitis is suspected, the patient should be given high-dose IV penicillin and cephalosporin antibiotics as soon as possible before waiting for a definitive diagnosis. Other treatment is supportive of symptoms.

Septic Shock

The symptoms of septic shock may vary according to the severity and the source of the infection. There will often be pyrexia and localized signs. Systemic signs of infection include hypotension, mottled skin, cool extremities and petechial rash. There may also be neurological signs such as fitting. Cultures should be taken from all areas that could be the source of infection. Blood tests may show raised white cell and neutrophil counts or c-reactive protein levels. Blood gas analysis may show metabolic acidosis due to lactate excretion from hypoxic tissues.

If the patient is hypotensive then rapid 500 ml boluses of crystalloid fluid should be given, with reassessment after 1 to 2 litres. It is common to transfuse up to 6 litres of fluid for patients in septic shock before the blood pressure is maintained. Signs of fluid overload (e.g. pulmonary oedema) or a failure of the blood pressure to stabilize may warrant commencement of an inotrope infusion.

Overdose

Management of overdose should be governed by advice from one of the regional poisons units. There is now little support for gastric lavage and the preferred treatment for oral ingestion of drugs or other poisons is with activated charcoal. In the unconscious patient this can be given via a nasogastric tube, although the airway may need protecting by intubation, and the patient should always be kept in the recovery position. If there is a suspicion of opioid poisoning, either through injection or ingestion (i.e. respiratory depression with pinpoint pupils or presence of needle marks), then naloxone should be given.

Common signs following overdose include:

- pinpoint pupils – opiates, organophosphate insecticide;
- dilated pupils – tricyclic antidepressants, alcohol;
- hyperventilation – salicylates, methanol (methylated spirits), ethylene glycol (antifreeze);
- increased muscle tone – tricyclic antidepressants;
- reduced tone – barbiturates;
- deeply asleep – benzodiazepines.

Assessment and treatment should follow the standard ABC guidelines. Cardiac monitoring is advocated since many poisons can cause cardiac dysrhythmias. All patients should be followed up postoverdose. Those who have had an accidental overdose may need health and safety education with possible social service or health visiting input and those who have had a non-accidental overdose will need review by a psychiatric team.

Opioid Overdose

Opioids (primarily heroin) are common drugs of abuse and a frequent cause of unconsciousness and death. Precipitating factors include a period of abstinence (such as during a prison sentence), a supply of unusually pure heroin or mixing opiates with benzodiazepines and/or alcohol. Serious side-effects most commonly arise following intravenous injection although the oral route may also cause unconsciousness. Smoking heroin infrequently causes coma.

Patients who have taken opiates typically show unconsciousness, depressed respiration, pinpoint pupils and often needle marks and signs of old abscesses. However, if respiratory depression is severe and cerebral hypoxia exists there may be pupillary dilation.

Maintenance of the airway and breathing are the first priorities, although the effects of opiates can quickly be reversed with naloxone. The half-life of naloxone is much shorter than that of heroin (about 2 to 3 hours) and so it is a wise precaution to establish an intramuscular depot before giving an intravenous dose to aid recovery. Administration often causes sneezing in the patient and possible agitation when he/she becomes sufficiently awake.

Hypoxia

Hypoxia exists as a problem secondary to a number of different conditions that can be subdivided into airway problems and breathing problems.

Airway

Airway Obstruction

Airway compromise may be upper or lower and may be pathophysiological or from a foreign body. Assessment of the airway should identify whether there is an obstruction that can be cleared. Other causes may be exacerbation of asthma, heart failure, pneumothorax or thermo-trauma.

Asthma

The prevalence of asthma within the community is about 3% and in urban A&E departments between 2.5% and 10% of all attendances may be for acute asthma. There has been an increase in asthma in recent years, particularly among children (50% of asthma cases are in children aged below ten years) and in the younger age group twice as many boys as girls have asthma. However, in adulthood greater numbers of women are asthma sufferers than men. The increase in asthma prevalence is thought to be related to environmental pollution although there is also a strong relationship with socioeconomic deprivation.

In acute asthma there is narrowing of the bronchial airways caused by smooth muscle contraction, inflammation and mucus secretion. It is characterized by an expiratory wheeze caused by airway restriction. Prostaglandins and leukotrienes are secreted as an end result of a pathway started by an antigen-antibody reaction. It is the action of NSAIDs on prostaglandin secretion that causes their dangerous side-effects for asthmatics.

Beta-agonists (specifically beta-2 agonists such as salbutamol) allow bronchodilation and are the main treatment for relief of an asthma attack. An acute attack of asthma may be exacerbated by a respiratory infection, anxiety, breathing cold air (especially whilst exercising), contact with an allergen or exposure to fumes or smoke. If the patient has reached the stage of being unconscious then he/she will require immediate intubation and ventilation. The patient may have a silent chest on auscultation, be cyanosed and bradycardic. Blood gases will show hypoxia and hypercapnia. Salbutamol may be given down the endotracheal tube, as a spray, via a nebulizer or intravenously (250 mg IV over 10 minutes). Steroids may be given to reduce the inflammatory response within the airways; their action is not immediate but they are beneficial in preventing recurrence of the attack.

Chest X-ray excludes pneumothorax and pneumonia as contributory or secondary problems from the acute asthma attack.

Breathing

Tension Pneumothorax

Tension pneumothoraces are a complication of a simple pneumothorax (air in the pleural space) which may be traumatic or spontaneous. Those at greatest risk of spontaneous pneumothoraces are young, thin men (at a rate six times greater than in women) but the condition may also be a secondary complication of asthma, emphysema or intrathoracic pathology.

The pleural cavity normally exists with a negative pressure and so any communication with the atmosphere (either through the chest wall or through the lungs) will cause air to flow into the pleural space. As the pneumothorax becomes larger the lung becomes smaller and, in a tension pneumothorax, a valve mechanism develops which prevents air leaving the pleural space once it has been drawn in. The lung space, and eventually the space occupied by the great vessels of the thorax, therefore become so compressed that function is severely restricted. The risk of death from a secondary pneumothorax (i.e. with some other underlying pathology) is 3.5 times higher than for a primary pneumothorax.

Tension pneumothorax presents as:

- reduced or absent air entry on the affected side;
- hyperresonance when the chest is percussed;
- deviation of the trachea away from the affected side, felt in the sternal notch.

Although pneumothoraces can be demonstrated on a chest X-ray, tension pneumothoraces should be identified clinically and treated before X-ray confirmation as this is a life-threatening condition leading to hypoxia and ultimately cardiac arrest due to pressure on the heart and great vessels. Immediate treatment involves needle decompression. A wide-bore IV cannula is inserted into the affected side of the chest at the level of the second intercostal space in the mid-clavicular line. Once *in situ* the needle can be removed and the cannula left. An escape of air may be heard and the patient should show a rapid improvement in condition. A chest drain should then be inserted, although this should not be attached to suction owing to the increased likelihood of pleural oedema.

Left Ventricular Failure

Acute left ventricular failure (LVF) will have a sudden onset, sometimes preceded by an episode of chest pain. It is the cause of death in 45% of patients with chronic congestive cardiac failure (CCF) and is caused by a failure of the heart to pump effectively. It results in altered pressures within the pulmonary circulation with a resultant fluid loss from the blood to the alveoli. The presence of fluid in the alveoli reduces gaseous exchange and increases respiratory effort that can quickly lead to hypoxia, exhaustion and unconsciousness. There may be evidence of frothy fluid at the mouth and nose that may be tinged pink. The patient may show systemic signs of heart failure including lower limb/trunk oedema, clammy grey skin, distended neck veins, pulsus alternans (alternating weak and strong pulse) and fluid in the lungs on X-ray or auscultation. Investigations should include ECG, chest X-ray, blood gases, pulse oximetry, cardiac enzymes and routine blood analysis.

The unconscious patient will require ventilation and drug therapy including IV opiates, a glyceryl trinitrate (GTN) infusion and a fast-acting loop diuretic to reduce the pre-load on the heart. Placing the trolley in a head-up position may also help to reduce venous return. Sublingual GTN spray or sustained-release tablets may be used until an infusion can be established. The patient should be given one spray every three minutes, with a maximum of three sprays or up to two 5 mg GTN tablets. The unconscious patient with LVF will need a urinary catheter and central venous monitoring.

Smoke/Fume Inhalation

Patients who have been exposed to a fire will be affected in two ways: they may have damage to their airways and they may have inhaled toxic fumes. This is particularly true when the fire is within an enclosed space. Children under 11 years, the elderly over the age of 70, and those living in socioeconomic deprivation suffer the effects of fire much more frequently than other groups (OPCS, 1988). Alcohol consumption is another common associated factor.

If a patient has been close to the source of heat damage to tissues will cause scarring, oedema and reduced function for gaseous exchange. If the heat source was dry (i.e. a fire) there may be scorching, charring of hairs in the nose and soot in the mouth. If the heat source was wet (e.g. steam) there may be blistering and tissue damage with no further signs of fire. Dry heat is quickly dissipated within the airways so that by the time the air reaches the lungs it is at body temperature. Steam, however, retains heat and is damaging much further down the respiratory tree. Patients who have suffered burns to their airways require immediate intubation and transfer to a specialist burns unit.

Priorities for these patients are:

- intubation with low inflation of the cuff of the endotracheal tube to prevent further tracheal damage;
- IV access and fluids;
- arterial blood gas analysis;
- possibly nebulized salbutamol via the endotracheal tube.

Steroids and antibiotics should not be given routinely as steroids have been shown to increase pulmonary oedema and bacterial infection can be cultured at a later stage.

Older furnishing materials release cyanide gas when burnt and any burning material, in the absence of adequate oxygen, releases carbon monoxide – a colourless, odourless gas. Patients may have been exposed to such fumes whilst at some distance from the heat source. If cyanide inhalation is suspected a closed circuit ventilator should be used with gas scavenging. If this is not possible the treatment area should be well ventilated with continuous fresh air to prevent harm to staff.

Carbon Monoxide Poisoning

Other sources of carbon monoxide include faulty heating appliances and car exhausts. Carbon monoxide binds to haemoglobin in the blood about 200 times more readily than oxygen. Oxygen is subsequently displaced, resulting in tissue hypoxia.

Symptoms of carbon monoxide poisoning may first be noticed at blood levels of 10% as a headache and lethargy. Levels of 50% can lead to unconsciousness, fitting and death. Carbon monoxide is excreted via the lungs with a half-life of 3 to 4 hours in atmospheric air. This is reduced to 30 to 90 minutes in 100% oxygen and down to 15 minutes in a hyperbaric chamber. Treatment in a hyperbaric chamber also causes oxygen to be dissolved directly into the blood serum at sufficient concentrations to maintain cerebral oxygenation.

In elderly patients with poor tissue perfusion there may be secondary myocardial or cerebral damage, with blood levels of 20% proving fatal. Although carbon monoxide poisoning is typically reported to cause a 'cherry red' appearance owing to an inability of oxygen to dissociate from haemoglobin, a patient may also show cyanosis or pallor. He/she may have an ischaemic ECG and exhibit cardiac arrhythmia. The definitive test for carbon monoxide poisoning is blood gas analysis, although expired breath analysers are available for conscious patients. Oxygen therapy (at atmospheric or hyperbaric pressures) must continue until carboxyhaemoglobin falls below 5%. A good history of likely exposure to carbon monoxide is helpful. Often more than one person will be affected and may be suffering from vague flu-like symptoms. There may also be evidence of palpitations, gastrointestinal disturbance, lethargy or poor concentration.

Because carboxyhaemoglobin has the same colour as oxyhaemoglobin, pulse oximetry will give no indication of oxygenation. Arterial blood gas analysis must therefore be performed. PCO_2 may be normal or slightly decreased, but there may be a metabolic acidosis due to the release of lactic acid from ischaemic tissue. This should not be treated as the shift of the oxygen dissociation curve to the right improves the release of oxygen to the tissues. Cardiac monitoring may show sinus tachycardia or a tachydisrhythmia.

Hypothermia

Hypothermia is termed primary hypothermia if its cause is environmental rather than pathological. Three principle causes exist for hypothermia:

- involvement in outdoor pursuits (such as hill-walking or boating);
- staying out in the cold (e.g. because of homelessness or as a result of intoxication);
- poorly heated homes.

Different mechanisms affect different groups, although it is primarily the elderly who suffer, with one study in Scotland showing a mean age of 76 years for those suffering from hypothermia in the home (Hislop et al., 1995), with similar ages in England and Wales (Chantler and Kelly, 1999).

Heat production is controlled by the hypothalamus in the healthy person. Metabolism produces heat, and the rate at which it is produced can be increased by exercise, or shivering (by a factor of 2 to 5). Heat is lost through the skin and from the lungs. More than half of the heat lost is through radiation, with conduction accounting for about 15% of heat loss. Immersion in cold water increases this loss by up to 25 times.

The adverse effects of hypothermia are primarily on the cardiovascular and central nervous systems. There is increasing confusion, drowsiness, poor judgement and eventually unconsciousness. The patient may also go through a stage of paradoxical undressing, when he/she starts removing clothes as a response to cold. As the core temperature falls, focal neurological signs such as hemiparesis may become apparent. The heart slows and becomes more susceptible to arrhythmias, with ventricular fibrillation (VF) and asystole frequently occurring below 25°C. The mortality rate of those whose body temperature falls below 32°C is 21%.

Primarily, assessment is by establishing a core temperature using a rectal thermometer or probe. Care must be taken to ensure that the thermometer is placed next to the mucosa of the rectum, since burying it in faeces will result in inaccuracies owing to the increased temperature latency. An ECG may also show diagnostic J waves and shivering artefact.

Care must be taken whilst examining the hypothermic patient as over-vigorous movement may precipitate cardiac dysrhythmia.

Physical symptoms develop as hypothermia intensifies, although the exact temperature at which they appear will vary between patients (Table 6.1).

Table 6.1 The physical symptoms of hypothermia

Mild hypothermia (32–35°C)	Moderate hypothermia (28–32°C)	Severe hypothermia (< 28°C)
Vigorous shivering	Absence of shivering	Increased muscular tone
Minor deterioration in mental state	Coma	Apnoea
Increased respiratory rate	Reduced respiration	Absent pulse (asystole or EMD)
No cardiovascular disturbance	Cardiac dysrhythmias	Absent reflexes
	Fixed dilated pupils	

Rapid hypothermia may cause hyperkalaemia and hyperglycaemia, whilst slow-onset hypothermia may cause hypokalaemia and hypoglycaemia. There may also be a failure of the blood-clotting mechanisms and a diuresis causing increased haematocrit. Blood gas analysis should be adjusted to the patient's temperature before being performed.

Cardiac arrhythmias develop at about 30°C and lignocaine is ineffective in controlling them. However, bretylium may be used prophylactically. Defibrillation of VF is generally unsuccessful until the core temperature has been raised and treatment should involve cardio-pulmonary resuscitation and active rewarming. All wet clothing should be removed and the patient warmed using warm blankets, warmed IV fluids, warmed humidified oxygen and warm-air machines. There is no place for using foil blankets within the A&E setting as they only prevent radiant heat loss and do not assist in rewarming.

Hartmann's solution should not be used to rewarm the hypothermic patient as the hypothermic liver can not metabolize lactate, resulting in a lactic acidosis. If a fluid-warming cupboard is not available then fluids can be warmed by immersion in hot water and normal saline can be heated in a microwave. Although fluids are normally warmed to 41-45°C, fluids at 65°C may be used.

It is often suggested that the rate of warming should mimic the rate of cooling. However, in all patients with severe hypothermia rapid rewarming should be considered.

- Slow rewarming (< 1.2°C rise per hour):
  - shivering;
  - warm IV fluids;
  - warm blankets;
  - warm humidified oxygen.
- Moderate rewarming (3°C rise per hour):
  - gastric lavage with warm fluids;
  - hot IV fluids (65°C);
  - warm water immersion.
- Rapid rewarming:
  - cardiopulmonary bypass (18°C rise per hour);
  - thoracic lavage with warm fluids (6° to 20°C rise per hour).

Hypovolaemic Shock

Shock is a state in which the body's tissues and organs are underperfused. This leads to tissue and organ death, the build-up of toxic metabolites and associated metabolic problems. Other causes of shock include sepsis, anaphylaxis and spinal cord damage.

Hypovolaemic shock is caused by fluid loss from the intravascular compartment. This may be due to haemorrhage (internal or external), vomiting, diarrhoea or excessive sweating. For a patient to become unconscious through hypovolaemic shock he/she will normally have to have lost > 40% of his/her circulating volume.

This level of blood loss can be external (including into the bowel) but can also be accommodated internally in the chest, abdomen or thighs. Blood loss may be caused by trauma, cardiovascular damage, gastrointestinal loss or in pregnancy. In the patient who has not received trauma most bleeding will be within the abdomen.

The symptoms of shock are part of the body's stress reaction, mediated by catecholamines and involving four body systems: the cardiovascular, renal, autonomic systems, and the blood.

These symptoms are:

- peripheral vasoconstriction;
- coldness;
- greyness;
- reduced capillary refill;
- sweating;
- tachycardia;
- tachypnoea;
- reduced urinary output.

Assessment should include identifying the source of fluid loss so that appropriate remedial action can be taken. This will involve history taking and examination of the patient from head to foot. In women of childbearing age this will include pregnancy testing to rule out a ruptured ectopic pregnancy. Initial laboratory studies should include a full blood count (FBC), electrolytes, coagulation studies, blood group and cross-match and arterial blood gases (ABGs). Ultrasound and X-rays can help to identify the source of bleeding.

Subsequent treatment is aimed at restoring oxygenation and perfusion of the tissues and organs by administering 100% oxygen, stopping further fluid loss and replacing fluids. External bleeding can be controlled by direct pressure and, in extreme circumstances, use of arterial clamps or a tourniquet. However, if an artery needs to be clamped or a tourniquet applied then the patient should be taken immediately to theatre for vascular repair and restoration of the blood supply. Internal bleeding needs an immediate operation to control it. The patient should have two large bore cannulae inserted into large veins (e.g. ante-cubital fossae) and IV fluids commenced. The aim is to restore circulating volume without increasing haemorrhage and a systolic BP of about 90–110 mmHg should be attained to prevent dislodging any clot that may be forming.

Cardiac Causes

There are two forms of cardiac arrhythmia that can lead to unconsciousness owing to decreased cerebral perfusion:

- bradycardia;
- tachycardia.

Bradycardia

Bradycardia is defined as a heart rate slower than 60 beats per minute, although many people will be asymptomatic until their rate slows to 40 or 50 beats per minute. Most commonly it will have one of three causes:

- a primary cardiac cause, often secondary to a myocardial infarction or myocardial ischaemia;
- secondary to hypoxia;
- following drug ingestion.

Any underlying causative factor should be corrected, with oxygen as a first-line treatment. Assessment should be clinical in conjunction with a twelve-lead ECG to determine the nature of any cardiac abnormalities. The most common cause of symptomatic sinus bradycardia is sick sinus syndrome, a condition where electrical impulses are not correctly formed in the SA node. Drugs that commonly cause bradycardia are digoxin, beta-blockers and calcium channel blockers, although a wide range of other drugs may also have this effect.

Secondary treatment will follow two routes, pharmacological and electrical. Pharmacological treatment involves blocking the effect of the vagus nerve on the heart with atropine, usually given as boluses of 500 μg up to a total dose of 3 mg. Electrical treatment involves external or internal pacing of the heart. As a temporary emergency treatment for bradycardia the heart can be forced into a faster rate by sharply tapping over the sternum at the desired rate (normally about 60 beats per minute) causing sufficient transfer of energy to cause a contraction.

Tachycardia

Tachycardias fall into two main categories: those that originate in the ventricles (ventricular tachycardia – VT), which are characterized by broad complexes, and those that originate above the ventricles (supra-ventricular tachycardia – SVT), which have narrow complexes. VT is a potentially unstable rhythm that can deteriorate into ventricular fibrillation and is likely to be associated with poorer cardiac function. The treatment for either VT or SVT with marked cardiovascular compromise is a synchronized DC electric shock (cardioversion), starting at a lower dose of 100 J with additional sedation if necessary. Other techniques that may cause reversion to a more stable rhythm include vagal manoeuvres (e.g. carotid massage), a sharp blow to the chest or stimulating coughing. Alternatively, pharmacological interventions may be used.

In the symptomatic patient with tachycardia, further examination should follow after treatment by synchronized or unsynchronized DC shock. When the patient is stable further tests should include an ECG and blood electrolytes, to additionally include calcium, magnesium and phosphate as discrepancies in serum levels of these electrolytes may be a predisposing factor. Cardiac enzymes should also be measured to exclude myocardial infarction as the underlying cause.

Initial drug treatment should involve correction of any electrolyte imbalance and cardiac ischaemia. A lignocaine (lidocaine) infusion may be started to prevent recurrence of VT, although this may increase the difficulty in reverting VT to a stable rhythm at a later stage. Drug treatment of SVT will depend upon its precise aetiology.

Conclusion

Although much of the investigation and treatment of the unconscious patient is medically directed, the nurse has an important responsibility in both the initial and ongoing assessment and care of the unconscious patient. The nurse also has a responsibility in supporting the family and friends of the patient. Health education is often vital in preventing a recurrence of the unconsciousness and this should be commenced at an early stage by the A&E nurse, prior to continuation by community and outpatient colleagues. It is beyond the scope of this chapter to cover all causes of unconsciousness in depth, and it is suggested that the reader use a clinical medicine or pathology textbook to understand more of the processes involved.

Practices in treatment also change with time, and vary between different settings, and so small variations may be found from the good practice laid out in this chapter. However, the principles of nursing care can be followed for all unconscious patients, to ensure that they receive the best care possible whatever their individual circumstances.

Suggested Further Reading

Benner P et al. (1999) Clinical Wisdom and Interventions in Critical Care. Philadelphia: WB Saunders.

Brown A (1992) Accident and Emergency Diagnosis and Management. Oxford: Butterworth Heinemann.

Colquhoun M et al. (1999) ABC of Resuscitation. London: BMJ Publishing.

Jamieson E et al. (1999) Clinical Nursing Practices, 4th edn. Edinburgh: Churchill Livingstone.

Wyatt J et al. (1998) Oxford Handbook of Accident and Emergency Medicine. Oxford: Oxford University Press.

References

Alexander R, Procter H (1993) Advanced Trauma Life Support. Chicago: American College of Surgeons.

Chantler C, Kelly S (Office for National Statistics) (1999) Deaths from hypothermia in England and Wales. Health Statistics Quarterly Summer (2): 50–2.

Hislop L et al. (1995) Urban hypothermia in the west of Scotland. British Medical Journal 311(7007): 725.

OPCS (1988) Occupational Mortality: Childhood Supplement. London: HMSO.

UKCC (1992) The Code of Professional Practice. London: UKCC.

Yates DW, Hadfield JM, Peters K (1987) Alcohol consumption of patients attending two accident and emergency departments in north-west England. Journal of the Royal Society of Medicine 80(8): 486–9.

Chapter 7
Neurological
Emergencies

Jacqueline Willan

Introduction

Accident and emergency (A&E) nurses are frequently faced with the challenge of caring for patients with life-threatening or potentially life-threatening neurological emergencies. These patients require a high standard of clinical competence, particularly if the patient is vulnerable due to an altered conscious level or unconsciousness. A&E nurses therefore need to be fully aware of the knowledge that underpins the practice of nursing patients with neurological conditions if favourable patient outcomes are to be achieved. This knowledge will subsequently enable nurses to create a significant impact in reducing the high incidence of morbidity and mortality associated with this patient group.

Overview of Neuroanatomy and Neurophysiology

The Central Nervous System

The central nervous system consists of the brain and the spinal cord. The forebrain, the cerebrum, includes two cerebral hemispheres: the right cerebral hemisphere controls voluntary muscle activity on the left side of the body and vice versa. The cerebral cortex is the peripheral part of the cerebrum and is formed from the nerve cells or grey matter. In each hemisphere there are deep fissures or sulci which artificially form four separate areas called lobes: the parietal, the frontal, the temporal and the occipital. The lobes are connected by masses of fibres, or tracts, which make up the white matter within the brain. The brainstem contains three areas: the midbrain, the pons and the medulla oblongata. The hindbrain, the cerebellum, is

172

situated behind the pons. All of these areas are contained within the skull. The brain continues with the spinal cord at the foramen magnum, the largest opening in the base of the skull.

Functions of the Cerebrum

These are:

- higher centre activities such as memory, thinking, reasoning, intelligence, judgement and personality;
- sensory perception such as pain, temperature and the special senses of sight, hearing, taste, touch and smell;
- muscle activity concerned with the initiation and control of voluntary muscle contraction.

Functions of the Brainstem

There include:

- decussation of the majority of the motor nerves;
- decussation of some sensory nerves;
- the reticular formation to control the state of activity and wakefulness;
- the nerve cells of some cranial nerves;
- the cardiac centre to control heart rate and force;
- the respiratory centre to control rate and depth of respiration;
- the vasomotor centre to control blood vessel tone;
- the reflex centre concerned with coughing, sneezing and vomiting.

Functions of the Cerebellum

These are:

- to control and coordinates groups of muscle movements such as in talking and walking;
- to ensure smooth, even and precise movement;
- to maintain balance.

The Meninges

Three coverings, the meninges, protect the brain and spinal cord with the outer membrane, the dura mater, lining the skull. It has two layers of dense fibrous tissue and has a potential space, the subdural space. Between its layers inside the skull lie the great venous sinuses. The web-like arachnoid mater, the middle membrane, loosely covers the brain. It is separated from the innermost layer, the pia mater, by the subarachnoid space containing the cerebrospinal fluid (CSF). The CSF is formed and secreted by the ventricles and flows throughout the brain and spinal cord.

Functions of the Meninges

These are:

- to support and protect the CNS by acting as a water cushion and shock absorber;
- to assist in the maintenance of a uniform intracranial pressure;
- to provide moisture and the interchange of some substances.

Intracranial Pressure (ICP)

Considerable emphasis needs to be placed on the nurse's knowledge of monitoring the ICP of patients presenting with neurological conditions, and its significance to patient outcomes. Knowledge of the pathophysiology involved will subsequently create meaningful understanding of the nurse's important role in undertaking both baseline and ongoing neurological observations.

Intracranial pressure is the pressure exerted by the CSF within the ventricles. ICP fluctuates in response to many factors: the individual's position, an increase in intra-abdominal pressure and activities such as nose blowing, sneezing and coughing. The ICP is therefore variable, although the accepted range is 0 to 10 mmHg.

The Modified Monro-Kellie Hypothesis states that the rigid skull compartment is filled to capacity with essentially non-compressible contents (this principle does not apply to infants or very young children where the skull has suture lines):

- the brain   80%;
- intravascular blood   10%;
- CSF   10%.

The volume of these components remains fairly constant in a state of dynamic equilibrium and reciprocal compensation occurs to accommodate any alteration. If any one component increases in volume another component must decrease for the volume and dynamic equilibrium to remain constant, otherwise the ICP will rise.

Intracranial hypertension will occur with a sustained elevated ICP of 15 mmHg or higher. In the A&E setting, intracranial hypertension often occurs as a result of the following:

- increased brain volume due to cerebral oedema, cerebrovascular accident and infection;
- increased blood volume due to haematoma, hypercarbia and hypoxia;
- increased CSF volume due to subarachnoid haemorrhage.

A point of decompensation will occur if ICP remains unrelieved, leaving the patient vulnerable to secondary brain injury. Robinson and Stott (1989) reported that a significant rise in ICP might be due to primary brain injury (e.g. the initial injury sustained) and that subsequent rises in ICP may be as a result of delayed secondary brain injury. These secondary events caused by hypoxia, hypercarbia, hypovolaemia, hypotension, seizures and infection are often preventable and reversible.

Monitoring Neurological Homeostasis: Neurological Assessment

All patients who present with life-threatening or potentially life-threatening neurological emergencies will require neurological observations and the knowledge base required will now be addressed.

It is of paramount importance that patients presenting to A&E with neurological conditions and trauma receive careful monitoring. Hickey (1992) stated that baseline and ongoing neurological assessment by knowledgeable practitioners is the most sensitive indicator of neurological change.

The three cardinal features of neurological assessment are:

- level of consciousness;
- pupil size and reaction;
- blood pressure, pulse and respiration.

The Glasgow Coma Scale (Table 7.1) is widely recognized and accepted as the tool to accurately measure the level of consciousness. The scale measures the best response of each of the three motor responses:

- eye-opening ability;
- motor response;
- verbal response.

The range is from 3 to 15 and a GCS score of 8 or less has become the generally accepted definition of coma.

Table 7.1 Glasgow Coma Scale

	Adult	Child	Infant	Score
Eye opening	Spontaneous	Spontaneous	Spontaneous	4
	To speech	To verbal stimuli	To verbal stimuli	3
	To pain	To pain	To pain	2
	None	None	None	1
Verbal response	Orientated	Orientated	Coos and babbles	5
	Confused	Confused	Irritable cries	4
	Inappropriate words	Inappropriate words	Cries to pain	3
	Incomprehensible sounds	Incomprehensible sounds	Moans to pain	2
	None	None	None	1
Motor response	Obeys commands	Obeys commands	Moves spontaneously and purposefully	6
	Localizes painful stimuli	Localizes painful stimuli	Withdraws to touch	5
	Withdraws in response to pain	Withdraws in response to pain	Withdraws in response to pain	4
	Abnormal flexion	Flexion in response to pain	Decorticate posturing (abnormal flexion)	3
	Extensor response	Extension in response to pain	Decerebrate posturing (abnormal extension)	2
	None	None	None	1
Total				3–15

Level of Consciousness

The area of the brain responsible for the individual's state of activity and wakefulness is a network of cells within the brain stem called the reticular formation. These cells are extremely sensitive to changes in neurological homeostasis caused by hypoxia and hypercarbia. There are many causes of brainstem dysfunction including infection, head injury, brain haemorrhage and metabolic disturbances. These causes can account for an alteration of the conscious level, from being simply dazed to a profound loss of consciousness lasting days and weeks.

Deterioration in the level of consciousness is the most sensitive, early and reliable indicator of neurological dysfunction in head trauma. The patient may display signs of lethargy, confusion, disorientation, agitation or restlessness. The patient often becomes progressively drowsy and finally comatose.

The utilization of the GCS therefore ensures uniformity of assessment and enables the nurse to assess consciousness level accurately.

Pupillary Size and Reaction

Pupil dysfunction causes changes in size and reaction to light and occurs in unrelieved increased ICP. The pupillary dysfunction is the result of pressure on the third cranial nerve (the occulo-motor nerve) resulting in an inability to constrict.

Tentorial Herniation

The tentorium is a tent-like dome of thickened meninges that separates the cerebral hemisphere from much of the brain stem and cerebellum. The upper brain stem passes through a large opening known as the tentorial hiatus. As the ICP rises, the hiatus represents an escape valve for relieving the supratentorial pressure. The nearest part of the cerebral hemispheres to the tentorial hiatus is the temporal lobe, the uncus. The temporal lobe will start to herniate through the tentorium if the ICP continues to increase, giving rise to the phenomenon of tentorial or uncal herniation.

The third cranial nerves are situated on either side of the tentorial hiatus. The displacement of the brain causes compression of the third cranial nerve and will produce pupillary dysfunction on the same side, initially causing mild dilation of the pupil and a sluggish response to light. With a worsening herniation the pupil may become fixed and dilated followed by ptosis and paresis. The eye is seen to be in a 'down and out' position as a result of third-nerve palsy. In addition, the unrelieved ICP will be transmitted to the opposite side of the brain and will result in bilateral pupillary dysfunction.

Blood Pressure and Pulse

In the early stages of raised ICP the blood pressure and pulse will remain stable. As a response to the continued rise in ICP an ischaemic reflex is activated – Cushing's response.

The signs and symptoms of this response are:

- rising systolic pressure;
- widening pulse pressure;
- bradycardia.

The arterial pressure is increased in an attempt to improve cerebral blood flow (CBF) and maintain cerebral perfusion pressure (CPP). This increase in blood pressure causes an increased force of cardiac contraction with a resultant widening pulse pressure. As the ICP continues to rise the pulse will decrease to 60 beats per minute or less. These signs indicate cerebral dysfunction caused by the raised ICP, which may still be reversible at this stage.

The following signs that indicate brain stem dysfunction are known as Cushing's triad:

- hypertension with a wide pulse pressure;
- bradycardia;
- abnormal respiratory patterns.

If the ICP continues to increase and remains unrelieved then a decompensatory phase will occur. The respiratory rate and depth becomes slow and laboured and the patient will often develop a Cheyne-Stokes breathing pattern. The pulse may become irregular, rapid, thready and finally cease. These late signs often indicate that it is too late for effective intervention to reverse cerebral dysfunction, tentorial herniation and impending death.

Motor Response

Tentorial herniation also causes compression of the corticospinal (pyramidal) tracts in the midbrain. These motor tracts decussate (cross over) in the brain stem to the opposite side at the level of the foramen magnum. Compression will result in a weakness (flaccidity) on the opposite side of the body. This accounts for the classic picture of ipsilateral pupillary dilation associated with contralateral hemiparesis seen in tentorial herniation. Motor posturing (Figure 7.1) can occur and can reveal the level and severity of neurological deficit, although does not distinguish between structural and metabolic dysfunction.

In decorticate posturing the arms are flexed at the elbow and the legs extended. There is cerebral dysfunction but generally the brainstem is unaffected. In decerebrate posturing the arms and legs are extended. Decerebrate posturing is more serious owing to associated brain stem dysfunction.

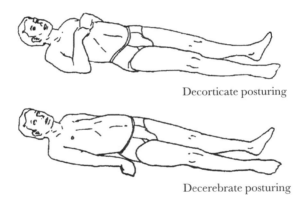

Decorticate posturing

Decerebrate posturing

Figure 7.1 Diagram to illustrate motor posturing

Temperature

The hypothalamus is part of a group of nerve cells known as ganglia that lie deep within the cerebral hemispheres. One of the functions of the hypothalamus is the control of body temperature and an extreme increase in temperature is usually associated with dysfunction within this area of the brain. It is this extreme level that differentiates the increase in temperature as being caused by an infection, albeit an uncommon occurrence.

A rise in ICP constitutes a real emergency and A&E nurses therefore perform a crucial role in monitoring neurological observations. Neurological diseases and trauma are frequently associated with a high incidence of morbidity and mortality and a significant reduction in this incidence can be achieved by the nurse's conscientious recording and understanding of neurological observations and the recognition for timely inventions.

Head Injuries

Incidence and Aetiology

Over 1,000,000 patients present with head injuries to A&E departments annually (Treadwell and Mendelow, 1994). A&E nurses therefore require considerable knowledge and skill in assessing the widely differing degrees of head trauma that may present, from the mild through to the severely head-injured patient who requires specialized neurosurgical intervention. It is estimated that head injuries account for nine deaths and over 300 hospital admissions per 100,000 population per year in the United Kingdom (Waldmann and Thyveetil, 1998).

The Department of Health (1993) outlined the recent progress that has been achieved in reducing death and disability through accidents, although there is still some way to go to reach the target reductions identified.

Government health policy has certainly reduced the incidence of head trauma due to road traffic accidents (RTAs). For example, the use of seat belts for front- and rear-seat passengers in motor vehicles has reduced serious RTA injuries by more than half and the compulsory wearing of motorcycle helmets has also created a significant decline in head trauma. Tough legislation and continued debate regarding the safe alcohol limit for driving also continues to create an impact on reducing the incidence of RTA trauma further.

In 1997, the Royal Society for the Prevention of Accidents (RoSPA) reported 255 deaths and 6197 serious injuries within Great Britain due to road accidents in children between the ages of 0 and 15 years. Work subsequently continues between government agencies and voluntary organizations to formulate measures to reduce these figures.

The motor industry appears to be acting more responsibly by designing more protective vehicle-cage frameworks and by the use of driver and passenger air bags.

Health and Safety at Work legislation for the use of safety helmets at work has also been effective in reducing the number of work-related head injuries.

Recommendations for protective headgear for sporting activities such as horseriding, cycling and rock-climbing assist further in preventing the occurrence of severe head injuries.

The elderly are especially at risk because of the associated pathology of old age as arteriosclerosis increases the risk of intracranial bleeds following seemingly minor head trauma. The elderly frequently present with head trauma following a collapse and can present a considerable challenge for clinical assessment and diagnosis.

Infants and young children are also more at risk of head trauma owing to the disproportionate size and weight of their heads in relation to their body weight and size. The developing young child will lack the stability of fluid mobility and gait, and blood vessel fragility in children makes them more vulnerable to intracranial injury.

A&E nurses must also be mindful of patients with an altered consciousness level or who are suspected to have taken alcohol or illicit drugs as both may increase the individual's vulnerability to significant head trauma.

Classification of Head Trauma

The American College of Surgeons (1997) classified head trauma as follows:

Mechanism:	Blunt or Penetrating Trauma		
Severity:			
	Mild	(GCS Score	14–15)
	Moderate	(GCS Score	9–13)
	Severe	(GCS Score	3–8)

Morphology:		
	Skull Fracture:	
Vault		Basilar
	Intracranial Lesions:	
Focal		Diffuse
Epidural (extradural)		Mild concussion
Subdural		Classic concussion
Intracerebral		Diffuse axonal injury

Common Clinical Signs and Symptoms of Head Trauma

The specific clinical presentation is discussed under the different types of brain injury, but the following are the common signs and symptoms that frequently occur following head trauma:

- altered level of consciousness;
- headache;
- nausea and vomiting;
- visual disturbances;
- dizziness;
- changes in behaviour;
- memory disturbances.

Blunt Trauma

Injury will occur when the direct force of the trauma exceeds the protection supplied by the skull. Blunt trauma is associated with falls, assaults and road traffic accidents. Acceleration-deceleration is the principle mechanism of head trauma owing to movement of the brain within the rigid skull. Different regions in the brain have different resistance movement. Following head trauma the individual's head comes to an abrupt stop but the contents of the skull continue to move, causing a direct impact between the brain and the skull. Further injury can arise as the brain reverses its forward movement backwards or laterally – the contracoup injury. Such injuries may produce an atypical clinical picture because of the transmitted force from the initial point of impact creating trauma to the opposite side.

Penetrating Trauma

The involvement and penetration of the dura determine the severity of penetrating head wounds. Penetrating head trauma is associated with impalement injuries, gunshot or stab wounds and is associated with high mortality rates.

Skull Fractures

It takes significant force to fracture the skull and therefore the risk of brain and cervical spine injury is increased considerably. Fractured skulls are classified into vault or basilar (base of skull). Vault fractures are linear or stellate, depressed or non-depressed, open or closed.

Basilar fractures are classified further as being with or without CSF leak and with or without seventh-nerve palsy. The presence of drainage of CSF from the nose (rhinorrhoea) and ears (otorrhoea) will indicate a fractured base of skull. Another feature is haemotympanum – bleeding behind the tympanic membrane. Commonly, haemorrhage from the nose or nasopharynx will also be apparent. In addition, periorbital ecchymosis (Racoon's eyes), conjunctival haemorrhage and mastoid ecchymosis (the late 'Battle's sign') should also alert the nurse to the probability of underlying bony injury.

Intracranial Lesions

Torn dural arteries in the temporal or temporo-parietal area most commonly cause an extradural (epidural) haematoma. They often result when a linear fracture crosses a vascular bed and are frequently seen when a temporo-parietal fracture tears the middle meningeal artery. Blood drains in the potential space between the skull and the dura, collecting and enlarging fairly rapidly. There is a common history presentation of loss of consciousness followed by a period of consciousness (the lucid interval) followed by a rapid progression to coma. The high incidence of mortality with this type of haematoma has coined the expression 'talk and die' (American College of Surgeons, 1997). Mortality and morbidity is directly related to neurological status before surgery, with a more favourable outcome being achieved if the haematoma is evacuated within two hours of neurological dysfunction (Treadwell and Mendelow, 1994).

Subdural haematomas most frequently arise as a result of torn bridging veins between the cerebral cortex and the venous sinuses. They can also occur if the fine arteries or veins that run between the arachnoid and the dura are damaged. Bleeding collects in the subdural space and enlarges much more slowly than the extradural bleed. This gives rise to a further classification related to the time of presentation: acute within 48 hours, subacute from two days to two weeks and chronic over two weeks. The clinical presentation differs from the acute lesion. Chronic subdural haematomas are associated with minor trauma in the elderly, the chronic alcohol user and infants of less than six months old owing to the increased fragility of blood vessels within these groups.

Presenting features often include persistent headaches and behavioural changes such as confusion, apathy, restlessness and agitation. The patient may present with a hemiparesis.

An intracerebral haematoma arises when bleeding occurs deep within the brain. Bleeding is commonly seen in the frontal and temporal lobes although may occur in any area of the cerebral hemispheres, the brain stem or the cerebellum. This type of bleed may evolve over a period of hours or days. The intracerebral bleed occurs commonly with penetrating head trauma. Intraventricular or intracerebellar bleeding is associated with high mortality rates. The specific signs associated with this type of bleed are directly related to the location and size of the bleed. If they occur in the brain stem, patients may show signs of impending death from respiratory and cardiac dysfunction.

A subarachnoid haemorrhage may result from head trauma if bleeding occurs between the arachnoid and pia – the subarachnoid space. The patient may show signs of meningeal irritation including severe headache, photophobia and neck stiffness.

Patients on anticoagulant therapy or those with diseases affecting clotting mechanisms have an increased risk of developing a cerebral bleed, even after a relatively minor head injury.

Diffuse axonal injury (DAI) is the term given to describe prolonged post-traumatic coma that is due not to a massive lesion or from ischaemic brain injury but as a result of diffuse shearing of nerve fibres within the brain. There are difficulties in distinguishing DAI from hypoxic brain injury as they frequently coexist. The patient often remains deeply comatose for long periods and survival is associated with severe neurological dysfunction. Cerebral deterioration may be due to the development of cerebral oedema – an abnormal accumulation of water or fluid in the intracellular or extracellular space, or both. The ICP will increase due to the associated increase in brain tissue volume and may result in herniation and brain stem compression if left untreated.

Nursing Care and Interventions for the Head-injured Patient

This section will discuss the care of a patient with life-threatening or potentially life-threatening head trauma, although many of the principles discussed will be common practice to all head-injured patients. This chapter does not address other concurrent injuries.

The majority of A&E departments now manage patients with head injuries using the standard Advanced Trauma Life Support (ATLS) guidelines (American College of Surgeons, 1997) as a structured, coordinated and multidisciplinary approach to trauma management is essential in reducing morbidity and mortality. McNamara (1999) highlighted the similarities of the systematic method of the ABC assessment within the primary survey to Roper, Logan and Tierney's (1996) Activities of Daily Living. These activities are commonly taught throughout nursing education and nurses will be able to recognize the commonality with the primary survey assessment when applied to the head-injured patient.

Aim: the identification and treatment of life-threatening injuries

Management of the patient with head trauma is often complicated by concurrent injuries and this group of patients should always be considered to have a cervical spine injury until proved otherwise.

The first priority is the ABC of the Primary Survey:

- airway (with C-spine control);
- breathing ;
- circulation.

Airway objective: To assess, protect and secure the patient's airway

Special Considerations

C-spine immobilization must be maintained until spinal clearance is obtained.

Endotracheal intubation is indicated when patients cannot protect their airway, to reduce the risk of aspiration due to an impaired level of consciousness where the GCS is generally less than 8. Hopkins (1993) documented that even a brief episode of airway obstruction will significantly increase intracranial pressure.

If significant facial trauma exists, making oral or nasotracheal intubation difficult, a surgical airway may be required. To reduce the risk of aspiration the stomach may need to be decompressed using a nasogastric tube. However, the tube may have to be placed orally if a fractured base of skull is suspected, to avoid migration of the tube to the brain through the fracture site. Suction should be kept to an absolute minimum because of the associated rise in ICP from this procedure.

If anaesthetic agents are used, those selected should not increase cerebral blood flow as this would increase ICP. Combined therapy of a hypnotic (Propofol) and an opioid (Alfentanil) is commonly used. These drugs may be required to enable a CT scan to be undertaken if the patient is restless or agitated, as both these conditions can increase the ICP further. Before the use of paralysing and sedating medication a rapid brief mini-neurological assessment should be made.

Breathing objective: To ensure adequate oxygenation and ventilation

Special considerations

The facilitation of early ventilation with 100% oxygen, intubation and prevention of hypercarbia is an extremely effective measure in reducing a raised ICP. Consequently these measures assist in the prevention of secondary brain injury.

Circulation objective: To achieve cardiovascular stability and control haemorrhage

Special Considerations

It is crucial that intravascular volume is effectively restored and control of haemorrhage is established. Hypotension will cause secondary brain injury and must be reversed as soon as possible. Hypotension does not occur from brain injury except as a terminal event because of brainstem dysfunction.

Disability objective: To perform a rapid mini-neurological evaluation

This can be performed easily by assessing pupil size and reaction and by using the AVPU method:

A *A*lert;
V responds to *V*erbal stimuli;
P responds to *P*ainful stimuli;
U *U*nresponsive.

Exposure/environment objective: To remove all clothing for a 'top to toe' secondary assessment, but with consideration of the prevention of hypothermia

Subjective Assessment

(1) Mechanism of injury.
(2) Loss of consciousness and, if so, for how long.
(3) Pre-hospital clinical signs and the care given.
(4) Use of illicit drugs or alcohol as these may impair assessment.
(5) Medical and drug history, including tetanus status.
(6) Allergies.

Objective Assessment

The GCS score is determined and the frequency of ongoing assessment established at the end of the primary survey. The scalp is assessed for lacerations, foreign bodies, and arterial or venous bleeding. Open wounds should be checked for the presence of brain tissue. The skull must be palpated gently for loss of continuity in the integrity of the skull. A depressed fracture can easily be palpated but palpation should be kept to an absolute minimum to prevent further depression. Depressed fractures of the skull may give rise to post-traumatic epilepsy, usually a tonic-clonic seizure type. Infants and very young children need to have their fontanelles examined as bulging or tenseness may indicate a significant raise in ICP.

An assessment for drainage of CSF must be performed as the presence of CSF will be suggestive of a basilar skull fracture. Any suspected CSF drainage should be evaluated; the presence of CSF can be differentiated from mucus by testing for glucose with BM stix, and a halo sign may be produced caused by the drainage of CSF onto gauze or bed linen.

The face and mouth will need to be examined for signs of bleeding and fractures.

It must be stressed that severe brain injury can occur without a fractured skull or any overt signs of injury, particularly in children and the elderly.

Specific Diagnostic Tests

The following tests may be required:

• a trauma series of X-rays: C-spine, chest and pelvis;

- full blood screen, blood group and cross-match, especially if haemorrhage is present;
- biochemical analysis of electrolytes and glucose;
- blood gas analysis (ABGs) to assist in the management of hyper-ventilation.

Skull X-rays are of little value with severe head trauma since a CT scan will be indicated.

Intervention and Management

The principles of caring for unconscious patients or patients with an altered consciousness level are very familiar to nurses and should be applied to this group of patients. In addition the patient will most probably be ventilated throughout their stay in A&E.

Reassessment of the ABCs and continued monitoring of neurological status are of paramount importance and nurses play a crucial role in the early recognition of deterioration by ensuring that timely interventions take place.

The patient will require rapid glucose estimation using BM stix. This is particularly important as hypoglycaemia will alter the consciousness level and, if the patient has been drinking, alcohol can also cause a serious fall in the blood sugar. Hypoglycaemia may be treated by IV administration of 50 ml of 50% glucose in adults and 0.5 to 1 g/kg in children, with boluses of 10 to 20 ml/kg 5% or 10% dextrose. Care must be exercised as hypertonic glucose can cause sclerosis of peripheral veins. Glucose levels may need to be monitored to ensure the glucose remains within normal limits.

Indications for Neurosurgical Consultation

Neurosurgical consultation is indicated in the following instances:

- skull fracture associated with:
- any impairment of consciousness;
- one or more seizure;
- neurological signs or symptoms;
- coma persisting after resuscitation;
- deterioration in the level of consciousness (using the GCS assessment);

- confusion or any neurological disturbance which persists after 8 hours;
- depressed skull fractures;
- basilar or suspected basilar skull fracture.

Early neurosurgical consultation is the most important factor in reducing the high morbidity and mortality associated with severe head trauma (American College of Surgeons, 1997) and the ability to transmit CT scans down a telephone line to Regional Neurosurgical Centres has made specialist review an accessible option.

Neurosurgical intervention may be required for elevation of the depressed skull fragment. Post-traumatic epilepsy may arise and seizures are often controlled with Diazemuls and the neurosurgical team will decide whether a particular focal lesion requires surgical intervention. In an absolute emergency, the patient with an extradural haematoma may require burrhole surgery in A&E to remove the clot and control the bleeding point.

Management of ICP

Hyperventilation is the most rapid and effective method of reducing a raised ICP (Hickey, 1992). Hyperventilation acts by reducing pCO_2 by causing vasoconstriction, although its aggressive and prolonged use can be associated with cerebral ischaemia. Waldmann and Thyveetil (1998) advocated that hyperventilation should therefore be used cautiously and as a temporary measure only. The recommended reduction in the pCO_2 level is from 35 mmHg to 25–30 mmHg (3.3 to 4 kPa). These levels can lower the ICP by 25–30%. Pulse oximetry will only evaluate oxygenation and not effectiveness of CO_2 elimination, whereas an end-tidal CO_2 detector will reflect the patient's CO_2 status. Blood gas analysis should also be obtained and appropriate adjustments made as indicated.

The administration of Mannitol, a hyperosmotic diuretic, is widely used to reduce ICP in comatose patients with pupillary dysfunction with or without hemiparesis. The use of Mannitol for patients without focal neurological signs remains controversial and it should not be used in hypotensive patients since it will aggravate hypovolaemia. The recommended Mannitol regime is a 20% solution of 1g/kg IV bolus rapidly. Frusemide, a loop diuretic, may also be prescribed in conjunction with Mannitol. A dose of 0.3 to 0.5 mg/kg is used in a combined diuretic approach, although it is recommended that diuretic agents should be used in consultation with the neurosurgeon. The patient will need an indwelling urinary catheter and strict monitoring/recording of all fluid input and output.

Intravenous access is obtained during the primary survey and fluid management will be required if there are signs of shock. If shock is not present it should be aimed to keep the patient in a normovolaemic state and to maintain systolic blood pressure appropriate for the patient's age. Fluid overload needs to be avoided. Basic measures like the use of continued sedation assist in controlling the ICP.

After spinal injury has been eliminated, the patient's head should be slightly elevated to 30° as this position will facilitate intracranial venous drainage and arterial blood flow.

Wound Management

Compound skull wounds need to be covered with a dressing or gauze, which may be soaked in saline. Brisk bleeding from scalp wounds may need to be controlled with a pressure bandage. Scalp lacerations may produce significant blood loss that requires fluid replacement, especially in a child or infant because of their small blood volume.

A gauze pad may be placed *in situ* to absorb CSF drainage. Suction or packing of CSF drainage must be avoided and the patient discouraged from blowing his/her nose as these actions will increase the drainage of CSF and will increase the patient's ICP.

The prophylactic use of penicillin for compound and basilar skull fractures is recommended as pneumococcus is the most likely organism to cause post-head-injury meningitis (Robinson and Stott, 1989). The patient's tetanus status should be established and appropriate measures taken to ensure protection. With severe head trauma, scalp lacerations will be managed by the neurosurgeons to prevent any delay in treatment.

In the case of penetrating head trauma, the object causing penetration is left *in situ* for removal by the neurosurgeons as indicated. The use of high-dose corticosteroids remains controversial and most research fails to demonstrate any benefit. Furthermore, experimental hypothermia studies and barbiturate therapy have not shown any reason to continue with these treatments in the management of severe head injuries.

Transfer to Neurosurgical Unit

It is of paramount importance that the condition of the patient is made stable, particularly if transfer to a Regional Neurosurgical Centre is required, and suitably trained nursing staff should accompany the patient.

Meningitis

Aetiology

Meningitis is the inflammation of the meninges that cover the brain and spinal cord, and is caused by different organisms: bacterial, viral and fungal. Meningococcus and pneumococcus are common bacteria that live in the nose and throat, but how they are passed from the nasopharynx is not clearly understood. Droplet or direct contact from individuals transmits the bacteria in the early stage of the disease. Some individuals are carriers of the disease. The incubation period is between 2 and 10 days and the onset of the disease varies from fulminant to insidious.

Incidence

Meningococcal disease is life-threatening but fortunately is relatively uncommon, although there has been a reported increase in the incidence of meningococcal disease in the last 10 years. Mortality from bacterial meningitis remains at 20–30% and is associated with such factors as type of organism, underlying illness, clinical presentation and age (Guberman, 1994). The disease is most common in infants over 6 months, children under five, teenagers and young adults. Most cases are isolated and outbreaks are uncommon although clusters of bacterial meningitis have been recorded at schools and colleges.

Causes and Types of Meningitis

Meningococcal meningitis

Meningococcal meningitis (caused by the bacterium *Neisseria meningitidis*) is the most common bacterial form in the UK, accounting for half of the cases. It is fatal in one in ten cases and one in seven is left with severe handicap. There are several different groups, with Group B accounting for approximately two-thirds of all cases. Meningococcal septicaemia will occur in approximately one-fifth of patients presenting with this form of meningitis.

Hib meningitis (caused by Haemophilus influenzae type b)

About two-fifths of bacterial meningitis were due to Hib before the introduction of the vaccine in 1992 and this form is now rare.

Pneumococcal Meningits (caused by Streptococcus pneumoniae)

This form accounts for approximately a tenth of meningitis cases and is associated with around a 20% mortality rate and a high incidence of morbidity. It is often associated with patients who have suffered a fractured skull or infection of the middle ear.

Other Forms

Viral meningitis is more common than bacterial, although much less serious, and very few cases will need to be admitted to hospital.

Neonatal meningitis caused by *Escherichia coli* (E coli) and *Streptococcus agalactiae* are rare, but when they occur are associated with high fatality rates.

TB and fungal meningitis are very rare within the UK.

Clinical Features

Meningitis is not easily recognized because of the similarity to influenza symptoms in the prodromal phase. The illness can take 2–3 days to develop but some individuals will become seriously ill within hours. Early recognition and treatment with antibiotics will significantly reduce the mortality and morbidity associated with meningococcal disease (Cartwright et al., 1992).

Symptoms include:

* fever;
* severe headache;
* pyrexia;
* neck stiffness with a positive Kernig's sign;

- photophobia;
- nausea and vomiting;
- petechial rash.

In the very young:

- irritability, poor feeding and drowsiness.

Febrile children with a petechial rash should be considered to have meningococcal disease and should be treated immediately with antibiotics if prognosis is to be improved. In addition, even if signs of shock are not present, almost all children with meningococcal disease will have evidence of underperfusion. The signs of septic shock are subtle, but recognition is crucial as septicaemia is particularly associated with meningococcal meningitis.

The characteristic features are:

- purpuric rash. If untreated, petechial lesions may develop into a purpuric rash. In some cases the bleeding can appear like fresh bruises that may form large areas of purple skin discoloration and damage;
- tachycardia;
- pale and cold periphery with a delayed capillary refill;
- tachypnoea;
- drowsiness or confusion;
- poor urine output;
- hypotension (which is often a late and sinister sign of cardiovascular decompensation).

Diagnosis

Diagnosis is mainly based on clinical findings although it may be difficult to differentiate between meningococcal disease and meningococcal septicaemia in the early stages. Lumbar puncture can be performed in patients with meningitis but should not be considered if the patient has septicaemia or if there is any evidence to suggest a raised ICP, because of the possibility of cerebral herniation. Full blood screen, clotting screen, blood cultures, blood gas analysis and grouping and cross-matching will be required.

Nursing Care and Interventions

Patients presenting with meningococcal septicaemia will require admission to the ITU or PICU and early involvement of these specialities is advised.

Cardiorespiratory failure is a common feature of septic shock, especially in infants and children, and it is essential that A&E nurses acquire knowledge of the principles of paediatric resuscitation because of the age groups most commonly affected. Most deaths from meningococcal septicaemia are as a consequence of shock, and initial interventions are aimed at assessing and supporting the airway, breathing and circulation.

> Aim: Resuscitation and management of life-threatening events as multi-organ dysfunction is common in this condition
> Airway objective: To assess, protect and secure the patient's airway

Special Considerations

Patients who cannot protect their airway because of impaired consciousness will require airway protection with intubation. Often a definitive airway is required because early elective ventilation is indicated. The stomach may need to be decompressed using a naso-gastric tube.

> Breathing objective: To ensure adequate oxygenation and ventilation

Special Considerations

The facilitation of 100% oxygen is urgently required. Early elective ventilation may be required because respiratory failure is common with meningococcal septicaemia.

Regular arterial blood gas analysis will be indicated as metabolic acidosis is often a consequence of septic shock. The patient's oxygen saturation should be monitored by pulse oximetry and loss of lung compliance may require the advance treatment strategy of extracorporeal membrane oxygenation (ECMO) at a specialist centre.

> Circulation objective: To achieve and maintain haemodynamic stability

Special Considerations

Septicaemia produces a distributive type of shock that results in hypovolaemia. This is caused by the systemic vasodilation and widespread increase in vascular permeability. Prompt vascular access is crucial to achieve fluid resuscitation and there should be no delay in establishing it. If peripheral venous access proves difficult in infants and children 6 years and under, it may be necessary to secure intraosseous access. In older age groups cannulation of central veins or venous cut-down may be required. The fluid of choice is 4.5% human albumin to replace protein-rich fluid, expand blood volume and restore peripheral circulation. In infants and children fluid replacement is based on their weight and given as a 20 ml/kg bolus stat with a further 20–40ml given over the next 10–30 minutes without risk of pulmonary oedema. Positive pressure ventilation reduces the risk of pulmonary oedema, thereby allowing more aggressive fluid resuscitation. However, strict monitoring of fluid balance must be undertaken to assess the effect of these measures.

Severe anaemia may be identified, which requires blood replacement following the initial fluid resuscitation. Coagulopathy may be evident from a rapidly progressive purpuric rash. A clotting screen is indicated and treatment will depend on the results obtained. Disseminated intravascular coagulopathy can occur and is life threatening.

Appropriate management of a number of complex electrolyte disturbances such as hypocalcaemia, hypokalaemia and hypomagnesaemia will also need to be considered. It may be difficult to achieve and maintain haemodynamic stability despite aggressive fluid resuscitation and inotropic support may be indicated, dopamine, dobutamine and epinephrine infusions being the agents of choice. These catecholamine agents are primarily associated with an increase in myocardial contractility, heart rate, pulse pressure and systolic blood pressure. The nurse needs to observe for the potential side-effects of these agents, especially cardiac arrhythmias and compromise of peripheral perfusion. Myocardial dysfunction is often present in septic shock and cardiac monitoring and frequent assessment of vital signs is required.

Disability objective: To monitor and achieve neurological stability

The principles of caring for patients with an altered consciousness level may need to be applied. The mini-neurological assessment of eye-opening ability, pupil reaction, and the use of the AVPU system are recommended to provide a rapid neurological assessment as patients may present with signs of a raised ICP. Initial management will involve ventilation with control of $PaCO_2$ and cardiovascular stability to improve CPP pressure. The use of Mannitol is to be considered very cautiously after treatment of shock.

Baseline and continued neurological observations are required to monitor for early signs of neurological dysfunction. Meningococcal disease can also cause the development of seizures that are commonly treated with the anti-convulsive agent Diazemuls.

Environment/exposure objective: To provide a cool environment and employ measures to reduce the patient's pyrexia

If the GP has seen the patient and suspects meningococcal disease it is recommended that benzylpenicillin is commenced: 300 mg in infants, 600 mg in children 1–9 years and 1.2 mg in patients over 10 years of age (Hodgetts et al., 1998). Early antibiotic treatment is of paramount importance; cefotaxime or ceftriaxone with its wide spectrum of action and the ability to penetrate the CSF is commonly prescribed (Guberman, 1994). The cephalosporins are also effective against all major childhood infections. Measures to reduce the patient's temperature should be employed and an antipyretic medication such as paracetamol prescribed. Frequent temperature monitoring is therefore required. Hypoglycaemia is commonly seen in seriously ill patients, particularly in infants and children owing to their limited glycogen stores. Low glucose levels may persist, therefore glucose monitoring must be maintained and hypoglycaemia corrected as necessary. The benefits of dexamethasone remain controversial and its use is often left to the preference of ITU or PICU medical staff.

Early transfer to ITU or PICU should occur as soon as cardiorespiratory stability is achieved and some A&E departments may need to request retrieval from a specialist paediatric facility for babies, infants and children.

Status Epilepticus

The majority of epileptic seizures are self-limiting, although occasionally the condition known as status epilepticus can occur. This condition can be defined as prolonged seizure activity or repeated seizures for 30 minutes, without the patient regaining consciousness. The seizure type giving the most concern is the convulsive tonic-clonic (grand mal) status epilepticus as long periods of hypoxia can occur. This is a life-threatening state and presents a medical/nursing emergency.

Aetiology and Incidence

Epilepsy is the most common serious neurological condition in the UK with tonic-clonic seizures being the most common (Russell, 1997). It is estimated that there are 15,000 cases of status epilepticus per year in the UK (Scholtes et al., 1994). Ryan et al. (1998) further reported that death or serious injury has been shown to occur in 15% of patients suffering a seizure as a result of airway obstruction, head injury or drowning.

The known causes of status epilepticus are:

- inadvertent or intentional withdrawal from anticonvulsant medication;
- intercurrent infection;
- metabolic disturbance;
- cerebrovascular disease;
- space-occupying lesions;
- poisoning and drug abuse;
- withdrawal from alcohol and/or drugs;
- traumatic head injury.

Status epilepticus is more common in symptomatic than in idiopathic epilepsy (Shorvon, 1993).

Diagnosis

Diagnosis is based on the clinical presentation although a number of investigations will be required, first to correct the systemic changes that occur as a result of seizure activity and second in an attempt to determine and treat the underlying cause. A CT scan may be required if neurological disease or trauma is suspected and the patient's condition needs to be stabilized before further investigations can take place.

Nursing Care and Interventions

Aim: To employ resuscitative measures, obtain cessation of seizure activity and treat the underlying cause
Airway objective: To assess, protect and maintain the patient's airway

Special Considerations

Initially, a simply manoeuvre such as a chin lift (in the absence of c-spine injury) is all that is required to prevent the tongue falling backwards and obstructing the airway and no attempt should be made to insert an oral airway during the tonic stage of the seizure. Oral and nasopharyngeal airways are well tolerated but if the gag reflex is absent and if the patient needs to be ventilated then a definitive airway is indicated.

Breathing objective: To maintain adequate oxygenation and ventilation

Special Considerations

The facilitation of early ventilation with 100% oxygen is required as neurological dysfunction may develop due to hypoxia from periods of apnoea. Pulse oximetry therefore needs to be undertaken and blood gases obtained. In some instances it may be necessary to ventilate the patient if cessation of seizure activity is difficult to achieve to ensure adequate cerebral oxygenation. A chest X-ray may be required to exclude aspiration once the patient has been stabilized.

Circulation objective: To achieve and maintain cardiovascular stability

Special Considerations

Urgent intravenous access to enable the administration of an anticonvulsant agent is paramount, and blood samples should be obtained to monitor electrolytes and a wide range of blood values that will aid in establishing the underlying cause.

Initially, in an attempt to meet CBF and metabolic demands, cardiac output and blood pressure may rise. However, in prolonged untreated status hypotension may develop and become severe. This needs to be considered as hypotension will lead to an inadequate CPP and many of the drugs that are used to control seizures have the side-effect of hypotension. The use of inotropes may be necessary, with the dose titrated to haemodynamic response. Cardiac monitoring is required and an ECG will be necessary if there is any suspicion of arrhythmia. Assessment of the patient's vital signs must be continued regularly including baseline and regular blood sugar evaluation as muscular activity may produce a hypoglycaemic state.

Disability objective: To perform a rapid neurological evaluation

Special Considerations

Hypoxia can cause an oedematous brain and raise the ICP, and the importance of the nurse's role in recording and reporting neurological observations cannot be overemphasized. The nature and duration of seizure activity also needs to be observed and recorded. A complete neurological medical assessment will be required when cessation of seizure activity is achieved.

Exposure/environment objective: To remove all clothing to allow further assessment and control pyrexia that may occur as a result of seizure activity

Special Considerations

Further assessment is required in an attempt to identify and control the underlying cause of the disorder. Increased muscular activity may produce excessive sweating and the patient may become pyrexial. The temperature will therefore need to be monitored as the underlying cause may be an infection.

Control of Seizure Activity

If termination of the seizure activity does not occur within 1 to 2 hours, unfavourable outcomes due to cerebral damage and systemic metabolic dysfunction have been reported (Petty, 1997). Ryan et al. (1998) studied the treatment of patients in A&E with epileptic seizures and showed wide variations in practice. These worrying results in the variable quality of care delivered led the authors to propose guidelines for a uniform approach to seizure management. Indeed, common care pathways may be the way forward to increase understanding, develop standards and achieve clinical excellence in many illnesses.

Early drug intervention is essential because once the condition becomes established it is more difficult to treat. Variations will exit in relation to the drug regime and management protocol and these decisions will be based largely on seizure duration and activity. A common approach to management principles is shown in Figure 7.2.

Although 80% of status epilepticus patients do respond to Diazemuls, the drug may produce hypotension and respiratory depression and if there is a high index of suspicion of pseudoseizures a prolactin level may be requested.

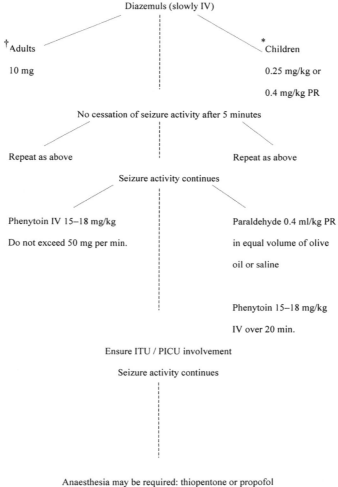

Figure 7.2 Management protocol for status epilepticus
† Adult – Based on management principles by Shorvon, 1994
* Children – Based on APLS Guidelines, 1997

Transfer to PICU or ITU should occur as soon as the patient's condition has been stabilized.

Cerebrovascular Disease/Strokes

In England, heart disease and strokes kill 550 people every day although the Department of Health (1993) reported that there appeared to be a move towards their target reduction of 40% in these figures. Evidence suggests that following initial presentation of a transient cerebral ischaemic attack (TIA), a number of people will go on to develop a stroke within 3 to 6 months (Guberman, 1994). There also appears to be a general consensus that cerebrovascular disease can be prevented or the incidence reduced. Consequently it is advised that A&E departments should be proactive in early referral of patients presenting with a TIA to medical or neuromedical outpatients. Modifiable risk factors can be identified and advice in adjusting lifestyle and the use of low-dose aspirin recommended as widely established measures to prevent strokes. Furthermore, the beneficial effects of carotid endarterectomy to certain people who have recently suffered from a TIA or mild stroke have been shown (Warlow, 1996).

Incidence

The Stroke Association reports that every year approximately 100,000 people suffer first strokes. It is the largest cause of severe disability with 350,000 people affected at any one time, and is the third commonest cause of death after heart disease and cancer (Hopkins, 1993). Subarachnoid haemorrhage further affects 1 in 10,000 of the population, commonly occurring in the middle years with a reported women to men ratio of 3:2 (Illingworth, 1995).

Aetiology

A stroke can be defined as a clinical syndrome characterized by rapidly developing neurological dysfunction lasting more than 24 hours or leading to death, with no apparent cause other than that of vascular origin. It may be of ischaemic or haemorrhagic origin.

Ischaemic strokes can be classified further as atherothrombotic (thrombosis of a cerebral vessel) or embolic (an embolism carried to the cerebral circulation, usually from the heart).

Haemorrhagic strokes can be classified further as intracerebral and subarachnoid haemorrhages. The cause of the bleeding is usually the result of a ruptured cerebral aneurysm or arteriovenous malformation.

Irrespective of the different causes the consequences are ischaemia and infarction of cerebral tissue.

Strokes can be considered in relation to the:

- clinical syndrome – the clinical presentation;
- anatomical area involved – the vessel and area it supplies;
- pathological basis – the cause.

Clinical Features and History

The clinical features will be dependent upon the anatomical area of the brain affected, the middle cerebral artery being the most commonly involved.

An array of neurological deficits can occur but common features include:

- impaired consciousness level or unconsciousness;*
- hemiplegia;*
- speech disturbances;
- visual disturbances;
- difficulty in swallowing;
- hypertension;*
- nausea and vomiting.

Specific signs of meningeal irritation occur with a subarachnoid haemorrhage:

- very sudden severe headache;
- neck stiffness;*
- photophobia.

The history of the stroke may help to determine whether the stroke is of ischaemic or haemorrhagic origin as difficulties may occur in differentiating on the basis of clinical presentation alone.

---

*Hopkins (1993) reported that these findings are unfavourable prognostic features of a stroke.

Ischaemic strokes tend to evolve over time, reaching a peak at 2 to 3 days and often with an accompanying history of TIAs. However, there is frequently an abrupt onset with embolic strokes and it is often established that the patient has a history of cardiovascular disease including valvular and/or ischaaemic heart disease. The single most common risk factor is the presence of atrial fibrillation.

Haemorrhagic strokes frequently present as a catastrophic event with a sudden onset of symptoms. A history of hypertension, especially with poor control, is strongly associated with this type of stroke.

Diagnosis

The diagnosis of stroke is often made on the medical history and clinical presentation of the patient and neurological examination aims to determine the cause of the stroke. CT scanning is recommended because treatment strategies vary and are based largely on causative factors. However, controversy exits as to the timing and reliability as the scan may appear quite normal in the early hours following ischaemic strokes. Intracerebral haemorrhages are also difficult to distinguish from ischaemic infarcts on a scan and with haemorrhagic strokes only large bleeds may be detected immediately (Hopkins, 1993).

Nursing Care and Interventions

Aims:
- To establish resuscitative measures and maintain vital functions
- To treat surgically or conservatively as appropriate when the patient has been stabilized

Airway objective: To assess, protect and maintain airway

Special Considerations

An assessment is made to determine the patency of the patient's airway. An altered consciousness level with loss of protective reflexes makes patients particularly vulnerable to aspiration and the patient may require endotracheal intubation to protect the airway. The patient may also require the insertion of a nasogastric tube to reduce the risk of aspiration and decompress the stomach. Suctioning of excess secretions may be necessary but should be kept to an absolute minimum to prevent a further raise in ICP. Simple manoeuvres may be all that is required, including inserting an oral or nasopharyngeal airway and placing the patient in a lateral position with a 30° head elevation.

If the patient needs a CT scan or to be ventilated then a definitive airway will be indicated.

Breathing objective: To ensure adequate oxygenation and ventilation

Special Considerations

The facilitation of early ventilation with 100% oxygen will be required to prevent further cerebral hypoxia. Pulse oximetry needs to be undertaken and blood gases may be required.

Circulation objective: To achieve and maintain cardiovascular stability

Special Considerations

Early intravenous access should be achieved in the resuscitative period and blood values monitored. Patients should be kept in a normovolaemic state and hypotension must be avoided for the maintenance of normal CBF and CPP to prevent a raise in ICP.

A frequent problem with both ischaemic and haemorrhagic strokes is the control of hypertension. Normally CBF and CPP are influenced by relatively minor fluctuations in systemic arterial blood pressure, but in patients with a longstanding history of hypertension, autoregulatory disturbances occur and a pressure shift in CBF results. Hopkins (1993) advised caution in rapidly reducing blood pressure as a normotensive blood pressure in these patients will barely maintain CBF and if CBF is not maintained then further cerebral ischaemia can ensue. Guberman (1994) recommended that pressures up to 190/110 mmHg should not ordinarily be treated owing to the risk of hypotension in patients with cerebral ischaemia. One of the major reasons for admission to ITU is associated with the difficulty in managing vital signs (Hickey, 1992).

Cardiac monitoring and an ECG will be required to establish whether any cardiac conditions are present that may have predisposed the stroke and cardiac arrhythmias must be treated if present.

An early estimation of the patient's blood sugar should be performed and measures taken to maintain blood sugar within the normal range. Hopkins (1993) reported hyperglycaemia to be an unfavourable prognostic feature following a stroke.

Disability objective: To monitor and achieve neurological homeostasis

The principles of caring for patients with an altered consciousness level or unconsciousness may need to be applied. Basic nursing interventions are incorporated early to achieve restoration of function and prevention of complications and so reduce the incidence of permanent disabilities.

Initially the mini-neurological assessment of eye-opening ability and pupil reaction with the AVPU system is undertaken. A full neurological assessment is completed when the patient's condition stabilizes, to establish the cause and anatomical area involved. Continued monitoring and early detection of neurological deterioration are vital to favourable patient outcomes.

Medical intervention may incorporate measures to reduce a raised ICP as cerebral oedema tends to develop and often progresses up to 48 hours after the stroke. If any form of diuretic therapy is used an indwelling catheter must be inserted and a strict input and output regime maintained.

The patient may present or develop a seizure or repeated seizures and this will worsen the cerebral ischaemia. Russell (1997) reported that the commonest cause of epilepsy in later life is cerebrovascular disease.

When the patient's condition is stabilized, the main aim of nursing interventions is focused on restoration of function with a strong emphasis on the prevention of complications.

Specific Treatments

The use of anticoagulants to reduce platelet stickiness is beneficial for those patients with ischaemic strokes and to prevent further development of thrombi, although a haemorrhagic cause must be excluded before treatment commences.

Hickey (1992) discussed the use of hypervolaemia-haemodilution therapy to increase CBF by reducing blood viscosity in the management of thrombotic strokes.

Although no definitive treatment of associated vasospasm seen in stroke pathology has been established, some patients have been treated successfully with the calcium-channel blocker nimodipine (Guberman, 1994).

Following CT scan, patients suffering from a haemorrhagic stroke who will benefit from surgical repair of an aneurysm may be identified although the timing of surgical intervention is controversial, being performed between 1 and 10 days after the initial bleed. The early evacuation of a cerebral haematoma may be a life-saving measure.

Indications for neurosurgery mainly depend upon the size, location and clinical condition of the patient. Often it presents too high a risk because many patients are elderly and other serious diseases frequently coexist, in which case conservative management is preferred.

The management strategy and condition of the patient will largely determine what speciality the patient is referred to and transfer should take place when the patient's condition has been stabilized.

Conclusion

In conclusion, A&E nurses need to be fully aware of the knowledge that underpins the practice of nursing patients with neurological conditions if favourable patient outcomes are to be achieved. Subsequent life-threatening injuries need to be identified and treated as a priority. Management is aimed at early recognition of neurological dysfunction with timely medical/nursing interventions employed to reduce the high incidence of morbidity and mortality associated with such groups of patients.

Recommended Further Reading

American College of Surgeons (1997) Advanced Trauma Life Support for Doctors (ATLS): A Student Course Manual, 6th edn. Chicargo, Ill: American College of Surgeons.
Guberman A (1994) An Introduction to Clinical Neurology. Boston: Little Brown.
Hickey JV (1992) The Clinical Practice of Neurological & Neurosurgical Nursing, 3rd edn. Philadelphia: JB Lippincott.

References

Advanced Life Support Groups (1997) Advanced Paediatric Life Support (UK): Student Manual. London: BMJ Publications.
American College of Surgeons (1997) Advanced Trauma Life Support for Doctors (ATLS): A Student Course Manual, 6th edn. Chicargo, Ill: American College of Surgeons.

American Heart Association (1997) Paediatric Advanced Life Support 1997–99. USA: American Heart Association.

Cartwright K, Reilly S, White D, Stuart J (1992) Early treatment with parenteral penicillin in meningococcal disease. British Medical Journal 305: 143–7.

Department of Health (1993) The Health of the Nation: One Year On . . . A Report on the Progress of the Health of the Nation. London: Department of Health.

Guberman A (1994) An Introduction to Clinical Neurology. Boston: Little Brown.

Hickey JV (1992) The Clinical Practice of Neurological & Neurosurgical Nursing, 3rd edn. Philadelphia: JB Lippincott.

Hodgetts TJ, Brett A, Castle N (1998) Review: the early management of meningococcal disease. Journal of Accident and Emergency Medicine 15: 72–6.

Hopkins A (1993) Clinical Neurology: A Modern Approach. Oxford: Oxford University Press.

Illingworth R (1995) Subarachnoid Haemorrhage. London: Stroke Association.

Mcnamara M (1999) Shaping the role of the clinical placement coordinator. Emergency Nurse 7(1): 26–30.

National Meniningitis Trust: Fact Sheets 1–6. Stroud: NMT.

Petty R (1997) Review Article: Status epilepticus. Care of the Critically Ill 13(5): 189–92.

Robinson R, Stott R (1989) Medical Emergencies: Diagnosis and Medical Management, 5th edn. Oxford: Heinemann Medical.

Roper N, Logan W, Tierney J (1996) The Elements of Nursing. Edinburgh: Churchill Livingstone.

Royal Society for the Prevention of Accidents (RoSPA) (1997) Road Accidents Great Britain. London: RoSPA.

Russell A (1997) How nurses can support people with epilepsy. Nursing Times 93(27): 50–1.

Ryan J, Nash S, Lyndon J (1998) Epilepsy in the accident and emergency department: developing a code of safe practice for adult patients. Journal of A&E Medicine 15: 237–43.

Scholtes FB, Renier WO, Meinardi H (1994) Generalized convulsive status epilepticus: causes, therapy and outcome in 346 patients. Epilepsia 35: 1104–12.

Shorvon S (1994) Status Epilepticus. Cambridge: Cambridge University Press.

Stroke Association (1998) Caring for Today, Researching for Tomorrow. London: Stroke Association.

Treadwell L, Mendelow D (1994) Audit of head injury management in the Northern Region. British Journal of Nursing 3(3): 136–40.

Waldmann CS, Thyveetil D (1998) Review Article: Management of head injury in a district general hospital. Care of the Critically Ill 14(2): 65–70.

Warlow C (1996) Carotid Endarterectomy. London: Stroke Association.

Chapter 8
Psychological Aspects of Care

Jean Haire

Introduction

Those attending an A&E department with psychological problems are likely to do so out of desperation. They have reached a crisis in their lives that is affecting their whole physical and mental well-being. A crisis is an individual concept, therefore the meaning and cause is variable. Psychological responses are subjective phenomena and how one person copes with a personal tragedy or accumulative stress can be very different from another. Some individuals experience such depths of despair that they do not know where to turn next, they feel their lives are in turmoil and many contemplate or attempt suicide.

There are no boundaries for people attending A&E. The A&E department functions on a 24-hour open-house policy and therefore it is often the place where people find themselves at times of desperation and despair. How effectively, as A&E nurses, do we meet the needs of this client group and how skilled are we to assess, prioritize and plan onward care for patients who are experiencing such psychological pain?

This chapter discusses important issues that arise when assessing patients who present in A&E and are psychologically distressed. It also discusses how psychological trauma can cause disabling physiological changes that, in turn, can cause further suffering and anxiety. It does not examine mental illness or diagnostic mental disorders but refers to mental health in relation to psychological well-being.

It is the intention of this chapter to give an overall synopsis of crisis management of patients attending an A&E department suffering from a psychological illness. It is intended to offer guidelines and information on symptoms and treatments to A&E nurses, enabling an effective and prompt assessment of the needs of this group with onward referral to appropriate agencies. It also highlights some of the psychosociological factors that contribute to mental health and well-being.

Assessing the Patient in A&E with Psychological Problems

Triage

The purpose of triage is to assess the patients' clinical priority by identifying their immediate problems and to avoid any deterioration in their condition through delay in treatment. Patients presenting in A&E with psychological problems may not have a life- or limb-threatening illness, unless it is associated with a serious attempt at self-harm, but have a real need for a prompt assessment and prioritization. Delay in assessment can not only cause further mental suffering to individuals as they become more anxious or feel they are not worthy, but some patients could become restless and agitated causing disruption within the A&E department. When confronted by somebody who is evidently distressed it can sometimes be difficult to assess and prioritize his/her immediate needs. Further difficulties can be encountered as many triage areas lack privacy by being open to the main waiting area and patients who already find it difficult to talk of their problems may feel further impeded.

Patients may present as tearful, sobbing or simply numb of feelings and not able to say anything. Assessments can be very complex and emotive as patients talk of their personal distress that has brought them to A&E. A&E departments are noisy, busy places where many patients require urgent life-saving decisions and actions. It maybe difficult to listen or calm an anxious patient in such a hyperactive environment and the assessment process may be helped if it can take place in a quieter area of the department. Psychological distress and mental ill health can sometimes cause patients to behave in an unpredictable manner. There may be bouts of anger or aggression, and although a quieter area is recommended, it should not be an isolated area where the assessing nurse would be vulnerable or feel his or her safety could be at risk.

Many A&E departments use the Manchester Triage system, which has appropriate flow charts to ensure a safe and concise priority assessment. Departments not using the Manchester Triage system should have in place guidelines, possibly drawn up with the psychiatric services, that will help to elicit the essential information and prioritize the patient's needs during this initial phase of assessment and triage.

Assessment

The main purpose of the A&E nursing assessment is to elicit the essential information that has precipitated the psychological distress and to assess any presenting symptoms, both psychological and physiological. It is not an in-depth mental health or social assessment, as this will be completed by the specialist teams, but an understanding of the presenting factors and needs of the patient at this time. The A&E nurse should encourage the patients to talk about the problems that have brought them to A&E. However, whilst it is important that the patients feel unhurried and listened to and allowed to tell their stories, it is not necessary to hear their whole life histories. The A&E assessment should involve a brief summary of the essential facts that are relevant. The whole process of assessment is helped if the nurse can build a rapport with the patient from the beginning by being open and friendly while being sensitive to the person's distress. Introductions are important along with a non-patronizing and non-judgemental manner. In the case of some patients, essential information may be gained only from accompanying friends or relatives, while others may talk about their problems only if the friends or relatives are not present.

Situations will vary and consideration will need to be given to the individual circumstances at the time. It is also important for the assessing nurse to note the source of referral to A&E; e.g. whether the patient self-attended, was brought by friends or relatives, was sent by the GP or arrived with the police or by ambulance. This helps to complete the assessment picture as to whether the patient came voluntarily seeking help or was encouraged to do so by others.

Guidelines for Assessment in A&E

Medical History

A brief history of the relevant medical illness and current symptoms should be taken. This includes physical and mental ill health. It is important to establish whether today's problems are new (i.e. a reactive psychological state to a distressing event such as a recent bereavement/assault) or an accumulation of symptoms over a period of time that has led to a longer-term illness. The nurse should complete a set of baseline observations. Further investigations would be required if any abnormalities were found identifying an organic cause for the symptoms. All medications taken by the patient should also be listed.

General Appearance and Presentation

A person's general appearance can be indicative of how he/she is feeling. For example:

- Is the person well dressed or wearing stained and crumpled clothing?
- Are there obvious signs of self-neglect or poor hygiene?
- Are there suggestive signs of alcohol or drug abuse?
- Is the person overweight or anorexic?
- Does the person look depressed, anxious or nervous?
- How is the person sitting (head down, slumped shoulders)?

However, although it is important to make note of the person's general demeanour and presentation, it is also important not to jump to the wrong conclusions; i.e. the person who is distressed and smelling of alcohol does not necessarily have alcohol-related problems.

Behaviour

Patients who are distressed or have mental health problems can express a range of behaviours and emotions that can suddenly and unpredictably change; one minute they can be sobbing and the next angry or aggressive. It is important for the assessment nurse to remember that emotional outbursts that may be directed towards staff are not personal. Staff safety cannot be underestimated; however, this does not mean that every distressed patient is going to have an angry or violent outburst. What is important is that the nurse should not feel uneasy or at risk. The nurse must assess each situation on an individual basis and if such circumstances do arise then immediate assistance from colleagues should be sought.

The nurse should note if the person:

- is agitated;
- is crying or tearful;
- is behaving in a hostile or aggressive manner;
- is reluctant to talk, making little or no eye contact;
- is talking excessively or is incoherent;
- is displaying unusual body movements such as a tremor;
- appears nervous or irritable.

Physiological Symptoms or Changes

It is essential to rule out any organic cause and the A&E nurse should complete a set of baseline observations. Further interventions may be required as many physiological changes, which can be anxiety induced, need to be eliminated as not being caused by other pathology.
These may include:

- frequent headaches;
- palpitations;
- shortness of breath (hyperventilating);
- outbreak of sweats;
- generally run down, frequent colds/flu type symptoms;
- hair loss;
- panic and anxiety attacks;
- changes of sleep pattern, insomnia or constantly tired;
- lack of appetite or excessive eating.

The assessment nurse also needs to ensure that there is no evidence of self-harm, including self-mutilation or self-poisoning.

Lifestyle Changes

There are many associating factors that can lead people to feel depressed or believe that they are no longer able to cope. Major lifestyle changes can be the cause, or at least influential, in how individuals cope with the stress of day-to-day living. A personal crisis is a very individual phenomenon and people can react in various ways. Other contributing factors such as previous learnt experiences, coping mechanisms, support networks, cultural attitudes and family medical history are all relevant in formulating an individual's coping abilities and general well-being.

For example:

- change of employment status – loss of income, redundancy;
- housing status – loss of home; repossession, no fixed abode, hostel;
- financial difficulties – large debts;
- relationship changes and loss – divorce, bereavement;
- increased use of or dependency on alcohol or drugs.

These guidelines are by no means a checklist for a psychological assessment in A&E but offer key points within a broad framework to help the nurse complete the assessment. It should also be remembered that assessment may further be complicated by the use of alcohol or drugs. Many patients who present in a distressed state or have mental health problems may be intoxicated and this can affect their behaviour. This may result in them remaining in A&E for a considerable length of time until they become sober, ensuring a thorough and objective assessment.

Depression

A&E nurses are often confronted with patients who could be described as being in crisis or suicidal, and such individuals will often present in A&E in despair, feeling they cannot go on. Depression can range from a feeling of being low in mood to a severe clinical depression that can be life-threatening. Equally, as there are many degrees of depressive states, there are as many reasons and causes why some people become depressed. Reactive depression can be the body's physiological and psychological response to a personal crisis or traumatic event such as a bereavement or serious accident. The individual's equilibrium has been thrown into chaos and accumulative stress can lead to the person feeling overloaded with pressure or depressed in mood, which may result in a depressive illness. Time is needed to heal, grieve and find emotional and psychological support that will help in the restoration of physical and psychological home-ostasis. People may need medication for insomnia or anxiety and therapeutic support such as counselling. Some people may lapse into depression that can often be triggered by other life crises. People who suffer from a clinical depressive state, which is often more severe and long term, may have abnormal chemical or hormonal pathology. Suicidal despair along with a serious state of self-neglect is not uncommon. Individuals suffering from such severe depression are often brought into A&E following suicide attempts or having been found in a serious state of self-neglect. Many patients are found wandering the streets in a state of stupor or semi-stupor and will either arrive by ambulance or be brought by police. The latter may involve sectioning under the Mental Health Act.

Signs of depressive illness may include:

- low self-esteem, feelings of worthlessness and that all is hopeless;
- loss of interest in the outside world, relationships or previous interests;
- loss of interest in self, unkempt appearance and poor hygiene;
- constant tiredness or apathy – nothing is worth the effort;
- tearfulness or crying;
- uncommunicative or slurred speech, talking in monosyllables;
- physiological changes – loss of appetite, sleep disturbance;
- dependency on or addiction to alcohol or drugs;
- loss of or change in previous lifestyle, job, status, relationships;
- poor posture, little or no eye contact with others;
- thoughts of or attempts at self-harm.

Self-harm

Deliberate self-harm (DSH) can present in varying degrees of serious-ness. It is important to remember that the actual physical act of DSH does not always reflect the degree of psychological disturbance or the seriousness of the intent. For example many people, particularly the young, may be ignorant of the effect of drugs such as paracetamol because the drug is so easily available and accessible, and an impul-sive and emotional act can have fatal results. Conversely, what may appear to be a minor overdose or act of self-mutilation may be accompanied by serious suicidal intent. It is therefore essential that all patients who self-harm have a full medical and psychological assessment and it is always safer to assume that any degree of DSH is a serious attempt. Some patients may use more than one method; for example, the patient who has presented with a minor self-inflicted wrist laceration may also have taken a serious overdose. Consequently nurses need to be vigilant in their assessment but also sensitive and non-judgemental. It is relatively easy to recognize a bleeding wound or displaced fracture and associate it with the degree of pain that the patient must be experiencing. However, it is far more difficult to recognize and acknowledge pain when there are no physical changes and the pain is related to the individual's subjective feelings. Further complexity may follow if the patient is hostile or aggressive. He/she may be refusing any medical intervention or generally refusing to cooperate. He/she may be drowsy, confused, intoxicated or unconscious, with no evidence available as to what has been ingested. Relatives and friends may also feel angry, tearful or guilty and the nurse may have to deal with varying family dynamics or cultures when supporting the relatives of such patients.

Self-inflicted Injuries and Mutilation

All A&E departments will see patients who have fallen into the category of 'regular attenders' as certain patients will attend with repeated episodes of self-mutilation. Usually these involve the wrists and forearms, although other body parts may be used, to a varying degree from superficial to deep lacerations. Wounds are usually treated with steri-strips, glue or suturing. Occasionally there may be some tendon involvement that will require further investigations and treatment, but generally the self-damage does not require a surgical opinion. Other body parts may include the abdomen and legs. These are often lacerated or commonly burnt with cigarettes. More serious wounds may include self-inflicted stab wounds or the swallowing of objects such as razor blades or safety pins. Other self-inflicted injuries include gassing and carbon monoxide poisoning, overdoses of drugs and the ingestion of chemicals such as cleaning detergents or multiple injuries from jumping off high buildings or bridges. It is not uncommon for more than one method of DSH to be used and attempts are often associated with intoxication from drugs and/or alcohol.

Drugs Commonly Taken in Self-Poisoning

Asprin (Salicylic Acid)

Absorption of aspirin may be delayed, especially if enteric-coated tablets are taken, and blood levels taken in the first 6 hours could therefore be misleading. The main features are hyperventilating, tinnitus, deafness, dizziness, nausea and vomiting, confusion and gastric bleeding. In severe poisoning fits and coma may occur.

Treatment in A&E

Gastric emptying can achieve a worthwhile effect if performed within 2 hours of ingestion or even 4 hours if enteric-coated tablets have been taken. Repeated doses of activated charcoal will reduce absorption and enhance the elimination of the drug. Rehydration will help to enforce urinary salicylate excretion. Diazepam may be required if fitting occurs.

Paracetamol

Very commonly used in overdoses, as few as 20–30 tablets (10–15 g) can cause irreversible liver and kidney damage. Nausea and vomiting is the early feature but this usually settles within 24 hours. Should nausea and vomiting continue, associated with abdominal pain and discomfort, the development of hepatic necrosis must be suspected. Liver damage is maximal 3–4 days after ingestion.

Treatment in A&E

Gastric emptying can be carried out if performed within 2 hours of ingestion. Acetylcysteine (Parvolex) and methionine protect the liver if given within 12 hours of ingestion.

Benzodiazepines (Diazepam, Lorazepam, Temazepam)

Benzodiazepines depress the central nervous system and can cause drowsiness and respiratory depression.

Treatment in A&E

Supportive treatment should be undertaken as required, particularly for the airway. Flumazemil, a benzodiazepine antagonist, may be considered.

Analgesics (opiates)

Narcotic analgesics can cause varying degrees of coma and respiratory depression along with pinpoint pupils. Patients could die of acute cardiovascular collapse before reaching hospital (particularly if alcohol is taken).

Treatment in A&E

Supportive ventilation should be administered as required. Gastric emptying can be effective if performed within 2 hours of ingestion. Naloxone is given as the antidote although it has a short duration of action and close monitoring and repeated injections may be required.

Tricyclic Antidepressants

Overdose of the tricyclic and related antidepressants can cause cardiac arrhythmias, convulsions, ventilatory depression, hypotension, hypothermia and dry mouth. Dilated pupils and urinary retention can also occur.

Treatment in A&E

Symptomatic treatment and ventilatory support should be given as required along with cardiac monitoring. Gastric lavage can be effective if performed early but activated charcoal by mouth, given as soon as possible, will help to reduce some absorption. Diazepam can be used to control convulsions and arrhythmias respond best to the correction of hypoxia and acidosis.

Intervention

Gastric Lavage

Emptying the stomach by gastric lavage is now thought to be of little benefit unless it is attempted two hours following ingestion and even then there are varying medical opinions as to its effectiveness. In some cases, if the patient is showing marked signs of toxicity and has taken a potentially lethal amount of salicylates or tricyclics, gastric lavage may be attempted later than two hours following ingestion but this is usually in extreme circumstances. Gastric lavage is no longer used for mild to moderate poisoning because it carries a high risk of inhalation of stomach contents. Should the procedure be performed, the patient must have a cough or gag reflex confirmed and if there is a reduced level of consciousness the airway must be protected by a cuffed endotracheal tube.

Induced Emesis

Induced vomiting, as a means of emptying the stomach, again has doubtful value. There is no evidence to suggest that it prevents absorption even if performed within 2 hours of ingestion and it should never be considered if the substance taken is corrosive.

Activated Charcoal

Activated charcoal has been found to be very effective in reducing absorption in the stomach. It can be given by mouth or via a stomach tube and binds the poisons together, reducing their effect. The sooner charcoal is given following ingestion the more effective it is. It is relatively safe and particularly useful in the prevention of poisons that are toxic. Repeated doses can also enhance the elimination of some drugs after they have been absorbed.

Panic Attacks

Panic attacks are a real illness, with both a physical and a psychological component. Patients present in the A&E department experiencing very real physical symptoms that are associated with biological changes, which enhances their fears of a serious illness or even impending death. This makes panic attacks difficult to recognize in A&E because the patient tends to focus exclusively on their very real physical symptoms of chest pains or difficulty in breathing.

Panic attacks are very common and can cause severe suffering and disruption to the individual's life. However they are neither dangerous nor life-threatening. Some individuals can experience repeated attacks, and although stressful situations or events can bring on an attack many attacks can occur quite spontaneously and without apparent reason. Attacks can last anywhere between one minute and an hour, and can be very exhausting and frightening for the patient. Patients may self-attend A&E or be brought by ambulance experiencing a variety of physical and psychological symptoms.

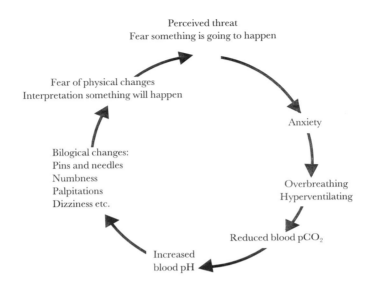

Figure 8.1 Cycle of anxiety and fear.

Symptoms may include:

- difficulty in breathing, dry mouth, hyperventilating (which disturbs the blood chemistry resulting in muscle spasms/tetany) and tingling or numbness;
- chest pain, palpitations, tachycardia (due to increased anxiety) and hyperventilation;
- dizziness, faintness, shaking, coldness, clammy skin, nausea, vasoconstriction in stomach and skin;
- feeling of dread, of dying, of going crazy or losing control.

Patients who present with real physical symptoms must be investigated for an organic cause before a diagnosis of panic attack can be made. However, nursing and medical interventions such as ECG recordings or blood samples may further exacerbate the feelings of something being seriously wrong. Although such tests are necessary, it is therefore essential that the nursing and medical staff constantly reassure the patient, explaining the results of the tests and why the patient is experiencing the physiological symptoms.

A treatment regime is set out in Table 8.1.

Table 8.1 Treatment of panic attacks in A&E

Category	Intervention	Rationale
Emotional support	Stay with the patient during the attack constantly reassuring him/her	Panic attacks are associated with fears of severe illness and dying. The presence of another person is comforting
	Move patient to a quieter area in A&E if possible	Reduce stress and anxiety
Slow patient's breathing	Use of a paper bag /demonstrate slow breathing exercises/breathe with the patient	Return body to normal homeostasis reducing tachycardia, cramps, palpitations etc.
Medication (severe attack or of long duration)	Emergency treatment for severe panic attack is diazepam (Valium) 5 to 10 mg orally	A benzodiazepine will usually stop or relieve symptoms. Acute use has little risk of dependency
Patient teaching	Patient needs reassurance regarding the physical symptoms and that the illness is treatable and controllable	Helps to reduce symptoms by understanding the body's reactions, sense of relief to know what the symptoms mean
Referral	Explain how a referral to the psychiatric staff who are experts in the field of panic attacks may help with symptom control and counselling	Patients will be more willing to accept expert help. Lose the stigma of a psychiatric referral

Post-traumatic Stress Disorder

Post-traumatic stress disorder (PTSD) is a severe psychological illness that can manifest itself as serious and disturbing physical symptoms, disabling the person from being able to carry on with daily living.

The number of people who suffer from PTSD at any one time is equal to about 1% of the general population. In 1987 researchers carried out a survey of psychological disorders exhibited by the population of St Louis, Missouri. A total of 2500 randomly selected residents were studied with 28 people diagnosed as suffering from PTSD (Kinchin,1998).

PTSD is associated with being involved in an event outside the range of usual experience and is likely to be extremely distressing. Healthcare workers and those working in the emergency services can be particularly vulnerable to PTSD simply because of the nature of their work. The 1980s became known as the 'decade of disasters' because of one tragedy after another. Disasters such as Piper Alpha, Hillsborough, Zeebrugge, Kings Cross and Clapham, to name but a few, remind us of the devastation and destruction to people's lives. More recently incidents such as Dunblane and the Soho bombing leave behind the most horrific memories. From each disaster and its aftermath there are lessons to be learnt for those involved in major incident and disaster planning. Included in this is the significant psychological effect that incidents and disasters can produce in some people, both those directly affected, the front line professionals and the emergency services subsequently involved. Sadly, however, personal disasters and traumatic incidents are not just seen on a large scale but may happen on a daily basis. People involved in a traumatic event or personal crisis will often find themselves in an A&E department. Individuals may develop the symptoms of PTSD following a personal tragedy that has affected or had a significant impact on their lives. Sufferers may include the victims or witnesses of an attack, rape, sexual or physical abuse, car crash victims, those witnessing the death of another or those who survive an accident when others die. The damaging effects of psychological trauma for the survivors, victims and helpers is now fully recognized and since 1980 the collective symptoms of PTSD have been diagnosed as a psychiatric disorder.

The criteria for a diagnosis of PTSD to be made are:

- The person must have experienced, witnessed or been confronted with an event or events that involve actual or threatened death or serious injury or threat to the physical integrity of him/herself or others.

- The person experiences recurrent and intrusive distressing recollections of the event such as dreams and nightmares or feelings that the event is reoccurring, including flashbacks, illusions or hallucinations.
- The person persistently avoids stimuli associated with the trauma.
- The person experiences symptoms of increased arousal such as irritability, outbursts of anger, hypervigilance or physiological reactions to any exposure that resembles the event, e.g. sweating, nausea.
- Symptoms last for more than one month.
- Symptoms cause severe disturbance and distress to the person's social, occupational and daily routine.

Patients may attend A&E having been immediately involved in a serious incident or may attend because of the symptoms they are experiencing which they may or may not associate with a previous traumatic incident. Those people who attend A&E following a serious incident should be told of the possible symptoms that they might experience prior to discharge. It is important for them to know that they may experience some of the symptoms of PTSD following any traumatic event and that this is a normal reaction. However, if the symptoms persist or affect day to day living their general practitioner should be contacted.

There are many health education leaflets and organizations that may be of help or support following a tragic event, e.g. the Samaritans, Victim Support and Cruse. It is therefore advisable for every A&E department to have access to local support agencies. In severe cases referral to the psychiatric or counselling services may be necessary as recovery from a traumatic event or PTSD can be a long and difficult process.

Alcohol and Drug Misuse and Abuse in A&E

Many patients attending A&E are intoxicated from alcohol and drugs. Patients may present in a collapsed state or have serious withdrawal problems. Patients who arrive in a collapsed state need to be kept safe, with regular observations and maintenance of their airway, until they are less intoxicated and a full assessment can be completed. However, it is essential to ensure that the primary cause of the collapse is alcohol or drug related and that the patient has not collapsed for another reason.

Other patients may attend as a result of alcohol-related incidents such as assaults, head injuries or accidents. Violence and disturbed behaviour is not uncommon as intoxication can change mood, cognition and perception and some patients may become aggressive or disruptive, particularly if they have to wait. Staff safety is paramount and it may be necessary to call hospital security or request the assistance of the police if the situation becomes high risk.

Alcohol and drug misuse can have serious physiological and psychological effects on an individual. Patients may present in A&E with physiological withdrawal from alcohol or drug dependency. They may self-present wanting relief from their physical symptoms or requesting help through a detoxification programme.

Alcohol Withdrawal

Alcohol produces an acute effect on the membranes of neurones causing a disorder that inhibits transmission of nerve impulses and so depresses the nervous system. Repeated exposure to alcohol counteracts the acute effect and more alcohol is therefore required to gain the desired effect. When alcohol is withdrawn or reduced in quantity, the central nervous system undergoes a phase of overactivity leading to medical emergencies such as alcohol-induced fits, severe dehydration and delirium tremens. Hallucinations, both auditory and visual, are not uncommon and patients are often confused, disorientated and agitated.

There are various degrees of alcohol withdrawal, from a mild hangover to a serious life-threatening condition. The condition of the patient determines the care required in the A&E department and a sensitive and understanding approach will help with the assessment and develop confidence for future management. Alcohol abuse may be secondary to other factors and a psychiatric assessment may be required.

Drugs

Patients may present with similar symptoms to those of alcohol withdrawal. Abdominal cramps, nausea and vomiting are common. Some individuals may also present inventing various medical symptoms in the hope of obtaining opiates and strong analgesics. Pethidine addicts have been known to present with the 'symptoms' of renal colic and if successful in obtaining the drug will leave the department shortly afterwards. Often addicts will use fictitious names and move from one A&E department to another with opiate-seeking behaviour.

Referral made from the A&E department to alcohol and drug teams is often the patient's access to resources that can help with dependency. Thus the A&E nurse is often the first person that the patient will make contact with in the hope to access some of these services. Nurses must not be judgemental regarding the person's condition or dependency. First impressions can be lasting and it may have taken a great deal of courage and determination for the patient to acknowledge his/her problem and seek help. Patients with dependency problems are not hopeless cases and can often do well given the support and education they need.

The Role of the Psychiatric Liaison Nurse in A&E

With greater emphasis being placed on care within the community for mental health patients it is highly likely that A&E departments will see an increase in the number of patients presenting with psychological and psychiatric problems. However, even with today's nurse training taking its roots from philosophy and advocating a far more integrated and holistic approach to nursing care, it is recommended that patients presenting in A&E departments with a serious psychological crisis or a psychiatric illness receive the expertise of a suitably trained person. The Psychiatric Liaison Nurse (PLN) forms part of the A&E team and works in conjunction with A&E staff to offer optimal treatment for the patient. Not every person who presents in A&E with mental health problems requires hospital admission or assessment by the duty psychiatrist yet a detailed mental health assessment, which includes risk assessment of self-harm, is essential in formulating a plan for the patient's specific needs and onward care. This assessment may be immediate in the department following referral from A&E staff, or delayed if the patient requires assessment and stabilization of any physiological conditions such as priority treatment for an overdose or self-mutilation.

The PLN also plays an integral part in sectioning patients under the Mental Health Act in A&E should this be considered necessary. The PLN will liaise with all the relevant people including the psychiatric services, social work teams, the patient's family or friends if applicable and possibly the police. If it is considered that a patient is at high risk of self-harm or absconding, he/she will need close and constant observation in A&E until all assessments for sectioning have been completed. The patient may require transfer out of the hospital to another specialist unit in which case the PLN may act as an escort, ensuring continuity of care until the patient has been admitted to the receiving hospital.

The PLN forms an integral part of the multi-disciplinary team and is the key link with other services such as psychiatric specialist teams, social work teams and community mental health teams. The PLN is also an excellent resource in A&E for teaching and staff education, not only on mental health issues but also in defusing violent or potentially volatile situations. Some PLNs also have training in counselling and debriefing. The role of the PLN in A&E, working alongside the A&E staff, therefore offers a collaborative approach to optimum care that aims to meet the patient's physical and mental health needs.

Sectioning Patients in the A&E department

Application and completion of mental health sections can often be a lengthy process. Ideally, A&E departments should have a psychiatric assessment room or a specific area where the patient can wait or be assessed away from the main area. A patient may experience an acute episode which can often be very distressing or behave in a manner that is socially unacceptable. Patients may also become violent and require restraining or sedation.

The Mental Health Act 1983

The Mental Health Act 1983 relates more to those working in the field of mental health. However, staff working in A&E do become directly involved with the management of psychiatric patients and, from time to time, patients will come into A&E having been placed on a mental health section or will be sectioned whilst in the A&E department. The Mental Health Act 1983 is divided into 10 parts and each part has several sections.

This chapter will only discuss those sections that are directly related to A&E and that are most commonly used.

Section 2. *Admission for Assessment*

This section authorizes the compulsory detention of a patient for up to 28 days. Two medical recommendations are required for this section: one is usually from a psychiatric consultant or senior registrar and the second from a doctor who may possibly know the patient (usually the patient's family doctor). In A&E this can be difficult and another senior psychiatric doctor may therefore become involved. A third person is required for the detention of a patient; this is often an approved social worker. Application can be made by the next of kin but this can sometimes lead to difficulties as relatives may find it distressing to be asked to sign forms for a compulsory detention order.

Criteria for section under this Act require that the person should be:

• detained in the interests of his or her own health or safety or with a view to the protection of others;
• suffering from mental illness which warrants the detention of the patient in hospital for assessment or requiring assessment following medical treatment.

Patients cannot be detained under the Act for drug or alcohol dependency alone.

Section 4. *Admission for Assessment in Cases of Emergency*

Section 4 is used in a genuine emergency and usually when there is insufficient time to get a second medical recommendation. One doctor, usually one who knows the patient, may make this medical recommendation. An emergency arises when those involved cannot cope with the mental state or behaviour of the patient or there may be significant risk of mental or physical harm to the patient, others or property, or physical restraint of the patient is required.

Application may be made by the next of kin but for reasons stated in Section 2 it is desirable for an approved social worker to be involved. The applicant must have seen the patient within the past 24 hours and the patient must be admitted to hospital within 24 hours of the medical examination or recommendation for detention.

Section 136. *Police Power to Remove to a Place of Safety*

The police have the authority to remove a person who appears to be suffering from a mental illness and is found in a public place. A place of safety is usually a matter for local agreement, but generally it is desirable for the police to take the person to a police station or an A&E department where immediate contact can be made with the local social services and an appropriate doctor. The patient maybe detained for up to 72 hours for the purpose of making arrangements for treatment and care. Once examination by an approved doctor and social worker has taken place, the provisions for section 136 no longer apply and if further detention is required an alternative section is invoked.

Conclusion

Not everybody will experience psychological ill health following a traumatic event or personal tragedy or will experience cumulative pressure resulting in a stress-related illness. Many people experience intense emotional and physical stress but have the inner ability to cope and continue living their lives as normally as possible. This is not to say that their lives may not be changed but that responses to psychological stress and illness are very individual. External circumstances such as sociological and economic factors, associated with learnt responses and behaviours, are all influential in how people perceive themselves in the world and how they may react physically and psychologically to stressful stimuli.

It is hoped that this chapter has highlighted some of the painful and powerful emotions, along with the physiological changes, that many people encounter when experiencing a psychological crisis or illness. Symptoms can escalate and may result in further mental and physical deterioration that may lead to compulsory hospital admissions and/or long term psychiatric treatment.

The A&E nurse is usually the first person the patient will see when arriving in A&E. It is also worth bearing in mind that people who present in A&E departments with a genuine psychological illness are likely to present in crisis. The first interaction and assessment by the nurse is the key to how the patient may respond and be receptive to all subsequent treatment or future presentations.

Suggested Further Reading

Bradley J (1992) The Psychiatric Emergency. London: Medical Protection Society.
Brown T, Scott A, Pullen I (1990) Emergency Psychiatry. Edinburgh: Churchill
    Livingstone.
Wright B (1986) Caring in Crisis, A Handbook of Intervention Skills. Edinburgh:
    Churchill Livingstone.

References

Department of Health (1990) Code of Practice Mental Health Act 1983. London:
    HMSO.
Kinchin D (1998) Post Traumatic Stress Disorder, The Invisible Injury. Oxfordshire:
    Success Unlimited.
Mackway-Jones K (1996) Emergency Triage, Manchester Triage Group. London: BMJ
    Publications.

Chapter 9
Nursing Care of Orthopaedic Conditions

Judith Welsh and Jeanette Smith

Introduction

This chapter will assist nurses to assess, plan and implement treatment of adult acute bony injuries presenting to accident and emergency (A&E) departments. The chapter will cover the healing bone; specific types of fractures and associated incidence; common causes; presenting signs and symptoms; nursing care (including pain assessment, pressure area care and 'fast tracking'); specific treatment aims (including immobilization, application of plaster of Paris [POP] and surgical intervention).

Underlying Theories

In understanding the nursing care of people who have sustained fractures it is important to outline the body's own healing defences. The human body is designed with very efficient self-repair mechanisms, namely the inflammatory process and bone healing. The role of healthcare staff is to subsequently enable the body to do its work unhindered and provide the individual patient (and his/her relatives) with information and support about how these natural processes can be optimized.

The aims of treatment are:

- to restore alignment;
- to restore function;
- to preserve vascular and neurological function;
- to avoid further soft tissue damage;
- to prevent infection;
- to prevent complications of treatment.

Therefore, using the example of a fracture dislocation of the ankle, the first priority is to reduce the dislocation. This takes precedence over everything else provided the patient is otherwise stable. Strong analgesia is required to achieve this and it is not generally advised that such patients be sedated for reduction. Once the reduction has been effected then X-ray is needed to confirm the extent of damage and which treatment is most likely to maximize function. Meanwhile application of a plaster backslab will hold the leg in position and so prevent further soft tissue damage. Pedal pulses and sensation will need to be monitored for signs of vascular or neurological damage. Any wounds should be covered with iodine swabs to reduce the risk of infection. Prophylactic IV antibiotics and tetanus are also essential if any wounds are present. High-flow oxygen may be considered to reduce the incidence of fat embolism in major leg fractures.

Specific complications of fractures fall into early, delayed and late stages. In A&E the important complications are the immediate category. However, the immediate care given has an impact on some of the later complications. From the list in Table 9.1 it can be seen that most complications can be anticipated and hence prevented by good initial nursing care, although current surgical techniques allow much earlier mobilization than in former years, which reduces the incidence of many problems.

Table 9.1 Complications of fractures

Immediate	Delayed	Late
Vascular injury	Infection	Avascular necrosis
Inadequate blood supply	Stiff joints	Shortening of limb
Nerve injury	Mal-union	Growth-plate damage
Damage to joints	Delayed union	Osteoarthrosis
Fat embolism		Residual deformity
Gas gangrene		
DVT		
PE		
Tetany		

Inflammatory Process and Bone Healing

This is crucial to the initial stages of bone healing (Figure 9.1) and for this reason non-steroidal anti-inflammatory drugs (NSAIDS) are not recommended as the analgesia of choice for new fractures as they may interfere with normal in-built healing mechanisms.

Any physiology textbook will explain this process in greater detail than is possible here. Briefly, however, the substances released by the injured tissues result in the area being invaded by large quantities of red and white blood cells and platelets. The usual clotting mechanisms act to halt the bleeding and the capillary walls become more

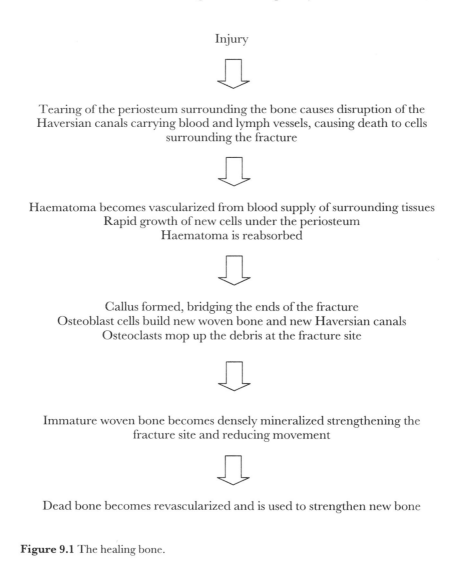

Injury

Tearing of the periosteum surrounding the bone causes disruption of the Haversian canals carrying blood and lymph vessels, causing death to cells surrounding the fracture

Haematoma becomes vascularized from blood supply of surrounding tissues
Rapid growth of new cells under the periosteum
Haematoma is reabsorbed

Callus formed, bridging the ends of the fracture
Osteoblast cells build new woven bone and new Haversian canals
Osteoclasts mop up the debris at the fracture site

Immature woven bone becomes densely mineralized strengthening the fracture site and reducing movement

Dead bone becomes revascularized and is used to strengthen new bone

Figure 9.1 The healing bone.

'leaky' to allow white blood cells into the tissues to phagocytose dead cells and debris. This results in haematoma formation.

Within the haematoma small blood vessels and fibroblastic cells proliferate, forming a soft tissue callus around the fracture site. As this matures the cells become osteoblasts, transforming the tissue into woven bone. This callus can be seen on X-ray. As the osteoblasts work away the woven bone becomes consolidated into lamellar bone and calcium salts are laid down. After this the site 'remodels' and the bulging bony area reduces until it looks much as it did prior to fracture. This final process can take up to two years.

What is the relevance of this to the A&E nurse? First, this highlights the need to get the fracture well aligned before the ends of the bone become sticky and healing in the wrong position starts, as a poor position will lead to poor function. Second, this process shows the rationale for keeping patients in plaster until the callus has sufficient strength to carry its normal load.

Osteoporosis

This is a common bone-thinning condition predominantly affecting post-menopausal women, although men and younger women can also be affected. The balance of removal and replacement of bone that occurs in healthy bone becomes imbalanced and the bone loss outweighs replacement. This results in a thin and weakened bone matrix that is susceptible to fracture, often from minimal trauma.

The main causes of osteoporosis include:

- lack of oestrogen: oestrogen protects bones by maintaining calcium levels and so when oestrogen production stops at menopause, hysterectomy or oophorectomy this protection is lost and bone thinning starts;
- lack of calcium: bone strength and skeletal maintenance are dependent on calcium;
- medication: certain drugs such as oral corticosteroids can increase the risk of osteoporosis.

Nurses have an important role in patient education to prevent or minimize osteoporosis, and although prevention should start as early as possible in life it should also be encouraged in the elderly to prevent further deterioration. Health education should address:

- diet: high calcium intake, vitamin D to aid calcium absorption and reduced sodium intake (because high sodium intake causes increased loss of calcium in urine);
- exercise: improved physical fitness and weight-bearing exercises help maintain bone mass;
- smoking and high alcohol intake increase osteoporosis in both sexes;
- hormone replacement therapy (HRT) can be prescribed to replace oestrogen lost by the menopause;
- prevention of falls: fractures increase with osteoporosis, so minimizing falls will assist in fracture prevention. Patients and relatives should be aware of safety in the home and regular hearing and vision tests should be encouraged.

Immobilization

The aims of limb immobilization are:

- to restore alignment, preserve nerve and blood supply and avoid further soft tissue injury. It is intended to prevent angulation and displacement of fragments and prevent movement that may disrupt bone healing;
- to relieve the pain associated with fractures. It is not unusual to find that a patient with a fractured wrist that has been reduced and put in a well-fitting plaster will not require any more than paracetamol for pain relief after the first day;
- to limit gravitational swelling, by elevation;
- to limit swelling and haematoma formation, by using compression bandaging.

There are several methods of immobilization:

- elastic or compression bandaging;
- limb supports, e.g. futura splints;
- slings: broad arm, high arm, collar and cuff;

- plaster: initially plaster of Paris then lightweight synthetic casts, cast bracing and orthoplast splints further into the healing process;
- continuous traction;
- skin traction effected by applying a U-shaped piece of cushioned, non-slip fabric held in place with bandages and a maximum of 5 lb traction weight applied;
- skeletal traction effected by surgeons inserting a pin through a bone. A greater weight can be applied using this method.
- operative procedure: internal fixation and external fixation.

The method chosen depends on the site and type of fracture, the patient's lifestyle and the individual preferences of the orthopaedic surgeon.

Traction is now used less frequently owing to the complications resulting from bed rest and the long period of hospitalization that can be required to allow full natural healing to occur. However, it remains useful where fractures are unstable and unsuitable for plastering prior to operative treatment, e.g. fractured shaft of femur. Application of traction, like plastering, requires nursing expertise and skill as mal-union can result if it is applied incorrectly.

If a fracture is stable (i.e. there is no displacement of the bone ends) then the treatment will be conservative, with the patient remaining in plaster until the fracture is healed. Ultimately some form of cast bracing may also be used. For unstable fractures plaster provides a method of holding alignment and providing pain relief and comfort until surgery can be performed. Plaster slabs are always used for this task as they can be applied with minimal movement of the limb and ensure that associated swelling does not affect the blood supply to the limb whilst still allowing X-ray investigation to confirm position. Different departments have their own preferences but backslabs, gutterslabs and volar slabs are all satisfactory options.

Fixation is a surgical intervention and the choice of fixation is the choice of the operating surgeon. Internal fixation is used when high-quality reduction and fixation is required, e.g. in the elderly, the multiply injured patient and patients with pathological fractures. Early mobilization is possible but the infection risk is higher. External fixation holds the fracture more firmly than other immobilization methods and is particularly useful in compound fractures where skin damage makes use of internal fixation undesirable. However, it carries a risk of non-union.

Plastering

Application of plaster is a skill and should be performed only by nursing staff who are competent. Many orthopaedic textbooks describe the process and the types of plaster that should be used for a specific injury. However, there is no substitute for demonstration and practice.

Initial plasters are always incomplete (either plaster 'slabs' or full 'split' casts) to allow for initial swelling of the injured part. This prevents problems with circulation and nerve damage, both of which are a significant problem following plaster application. For this reason plasters should be checked within 48 hours and early fracture clinic follow-up arranged. The importance of elevation of the limb, to minimize swelling, and the signs of neurovascular problems associated with a tight plaster must be explained. Patients should be given written plaster instructions in addition to verbal explanations and advised to return to A&E for nurse review if there are any problems with the plaster.

As bone healing commences and swelling reduces it is possible to either 'complete' the plaster cast or replace it with a synthetic cast. The choice will depend on how stable the fracture is. Plaster of Paris has the advantages of being cheap, flexible and easy for most staff to use but it is heavy for patients. Synthetic materials are lightweight and very firm, but are more expensive and difficult to apply and therefore are usually only applied by trained plaster technicians following fracture clinic review. Plasters have great potential for causing problems, due to either poor application of the cast or non-compliance with instructions by the patient. The desire to be clean sometimes gets the better of the instruction not to get the plaster wet and the impulse to walk or put a foot to the ground when on crutches leads to cracked casts.

Walking Aids

Patients with lower limb fractures will require a walking aid to assist mobilization. This usually takes the form of crutches or a walking frame. A walking stick can be used if partial or full weight bearing is possible. Initially, non-weight bearing is usual to allow the healing process to begin at the fracture site and permit the plaster to dry.

Later in the healing process a walking plaster may be applied allowing partial or full weight bearing of the affected limb.

It is essential that any walking aids are measured correctly and nursing staff should therefore be competent to do so. If necessary a physiotherapist can be involved. Clear verbal and written instructions in the correct usage of walking aids is essential and the nurse's job is not complete until he/she is satisfied that the patient will be safe following discharge from A&E.

Assessment of Limb Injuries in A&E

Nurse triage of patients on arrival allows for a quick assessment to determine the path that the patient will follow through A&E. The Manchester Triage Group's 'Emergency Triage' (1997) is a concise flowchart system with simple questions to ascertain the triage category (Figure 9.2).

Pain is a major contributing factor to a patient's presentation and a difficult factor to quantify as it presents in many different ways in

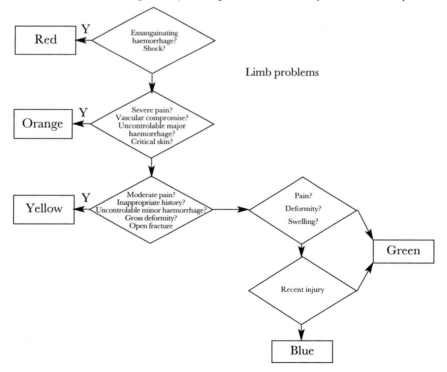

Figure 9.2 Emergency triage for limb problems. Source: Reprinted from: Emergency Triage, Manchester Triage Group (1997). ©BMJ Publishing Group.

an individual. Pain assessment tools attempt to measure pain and enable evaluation of pain-relief measures. The Manchester Triage 'pain ruler' (Figure 9.3) is a recognized and easily used tool, combining verbal descriptions, visual analogue and behaviour tools. It is consequently suitable for all ages and cultures.

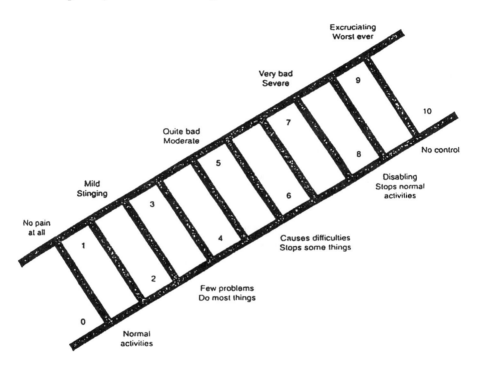

Figure 9.3 The pain ruler. Source: Reprinted from: Emergency Triage, Manchester Triage Group (1997). ©BMJ Publishing Group.

Fractures and Dislocations

The different types of fracture are:

(1) simple/closed – skin intact;
(2) compound/open – skin pierced;
(3) complicated – involving other vital structures;
(4) comminuted – bone splintered into several pieces;
(5) greenstick – found in children only. The bone bends and cracks but does not break in two;

(6) pathological – resulting from underlying disease (often metasta-
    tic cancer);
(7) transverse – fracture runs at right angles to bone;
(8) oblique – fracture line runs at less than 90° to the long axis;
(9) spiral – fracture line runs in a spiral fashion;
(10) impacted – one fragment driven into another;
(11) depressed – a segment of cortical bone pushed below the level of
    surrounding bone;
(12) crush – occurs in cancellous bone;
(13) stress – found in bones subjected to persistent stress;
(14) fracture dislocation – the fracture is associated with a dislocated
    joint or the fracture leaves the joint unstable.

Dislocations

These are defined as the two joint surfaces being so far displaced that
there is no apposition between them and may involve serious ligamentous and joint capsule damage. The most common dislocations are of
the shoulder and fingers, less commonly of the hip. Patients should never
be sent home with a joint dislocated. Fracture dislocations are more difficult to manage and the most common of these is a fracture dislocation of
the ankle. Distal pulses and circulation must be monitored and if
compromised reduction of the dislocation must be undertaken immediately. These are emergencies and treatment for these patients is a priority over all other patients except those triaged as immediate.

Fractures of the Arm

General Principles

Most fractures of the arm result from a fall onto the affected arm or
direct violence. The part that breaks is either that of greatest weakness or that part which comes into contact with the direct violence.

Treatment depends on degree of displacement as this is the factor
that makes complications more likely. Minimal displacement is
defined as < 1 cm and minimal angulation is defined as < 45°.

Patients tend to present supporting the injured arm with the other
hand. If the fracture is severely displaced or angled there will be obvious deformity and increasingly severe bruising. Any mobility at the
fracture site will give an indication of the exact position of the fracture.

Confirmation of the injury is by X-ray, which rarely poses an inter-pretation difficulty. Adequate X-rays are those that show the full length of the bones in question and their proximal and distal joints.

Humeral Fractures

Fractures of the proximal humerus can involve the anatomical neck of humerus, surgical neck, greater tuberosity or lesser tuberosity. Combinations of these are common. If no displacement is present then treatment is collar and cuff application until pain has settled (approximately 1–3 weeks), when mobilization should be commenced. With minimal displacement a broad arm sling is applied when disimpaction is not required or collar and cuff where disimpaction is needed. Some surgeons may also request a body bandage for added limb immobilization. When the bone ends are displaced and if closed reduction fails to restore alignment then internal fixation or shoulder replacement (if avascular necrosis occurs) will be necessary. These patients will need admission.

Fractures of the humeral shaft tend to displace due to pulling of the deltoid muscle. These require closed reduction and application of a plaster U-slab to hold the position with a broad arm sling worn under the clothes to support this. Mid-shaft fractures often develop non-union problems and therefore are considered for early internal fixation. Other considerations for operative treatment include immo-bile patients, patients who have sustained bilateral or multiple frac-tures or those with radial nerve palsy after limb manipulation.

Elbow Fractures

Supracondylar fractures of the humerus occur in the distal third of the humerus. The olecranon and medial and lateral epicondyles preserve their normal equilateral triangular relationship but the patient will be tender over the distal humerus. X-rays will be difficult to interpret.

As nerves and vasculature run close to the joint these are the structures most likely to be damaged if there is any bony displace-ment and this is the main indication for manipulation. Distal circula-tion and sensation must be assessed on a regular basis. Once reduced, an above-elbow plaster of Paris is required and a check X-ray performed. If reduction fails then skin traction is indicated with possible internal fixation.

Humeral condyle and olecranon fractures occur when the elbow is forcibly pulled or sustains a direct blow. Again nerve and vascular damage are the main concerns. If the fracture is undisplaced a padded sling and follow up are the appropriate treatment. If there is any displacement this needs reduction and, as a last resort, internal fixation.

All elbow fractures require regular assessment of distal pulses and sensation and subsequent follow up will need to include weekly X-rays to ensure there has been no slippage of the fracture.

Forearm Fractures

The radius and ulna are held together by the annular ligament, an intraosseus membrane, radio-ulnar ligaments and the triangular fibro-cartilage which provides extra stability. Fractures are caused by a fall onto an outstretched hand or direct violence. The anatomical design means that fracture of a single bone may result in some axial rotation, which will also need correction.

Fracture dislocations can occur when one bone breaks and angulates and the second inevitably dislocates at the elbow or wrist. When the radius breaks it may angulate but can also rotate relative to the ulna. This is caused by the muscles, which allow pronation and supination. Open reduction and internal fixation is usually required as a priority. Where both forearm bones break, mid-shaft reduction is more difficult.

Treatment/Nursing Intervention

- Comfort comes first – supporting the arm with pillows or folded blankets with administration of appropriate analgesia.
- X-ray to confirm diagnosis.
- Check colour, sensation, movement and warmth.
- If treated conservatively, plasters need to be full and checked regularly by X-ray for slippage. A broad arm sling will also be necessary.
- Patients scheduled for open reduction should be put in a plaster backslab for comfort until surgical intervention.

Specific Complications

- Slippage of the fracture may occur when treated conservatively.

Wrist Fractures

These are the most common fractures of the arm, usually caused by falls, and are more common in the winter from slips on ice. Classically the patient presents with a tight, swollen wrist. The most common fracture is a Colles' fracture which gives the wrist the classic 'dinner fork' deformity.

Treatment/Nursing Intervention

- Safety first – remove all rings and bracelets. Check the radial pulse. Check colour, sensation, movement and warmth.
- Then comfort – support the affected arm with pillows or blankets followed by appropriate analgesia.
- X-ray will confirm the type of fracture.
- Where there is no displacement of the fractured bone ends a below-elbow plaster and a broad arm sling are required with fracture clinic follow up.
- Displaced fractures require reduction. The urgency of this depends on whether adequate circulation is reaching the fingers. Reduction may be done under haematoma block (local anaesthetic injected into fracture site), Bier's block (local anaesthesia of the affected arm), IV sedation or general anaesthetic. The arm must then be held in its reduced position whilst a plaster cast is applied.

Specific Complications

All of the following may occur:

- slippage of reduced fractures – this is not unusual;
- persistent deformity or mal-union;
- delayed rupture of extensor pollicis longus due to attrition of the tendon by roughness at the fracture site;
- Sudeck's atrophy – usually noticed when a patient comes out of plaster and has swollen fingers with reduced flexion. This requires intensive and prolonged physiotherapy;
- carpal tunnel syndrome – caused by compression of the median nerve.

Hand Fractures

The scaphoid bone is the most common carpal bone to fracture. Clinically this is detected by tenderness in the anatomical snuffbox and may not show on initial X-ray. Therefore treatment is limb support (with either a plaster of Paris cast or support bandage) and further X-ray after 10 days to confirm/exclude diagnosis.

Specific Complications

These are:

- avascular necrosis;
- Sudeck's atrophy;
- non-union.

Fractures of other carpal bones are rare and will also require treatment with plaster of Paris. Metacarpal fractures are more common, with 5th metacarpal fractures most prevalent. Such a fracture is often referred to as the 'punch fracture' as this is one of the main causes. Treatment of all metacarpal fractures is similar and depends upon the degree of angulation.

If angulation is minimal, support is provided using a plaster of Paris volar slab, or wool and crepe bandage with a high arm sling to minimize swelling, and fracture clinic follow up. Direct pressure to the fracture site can reduce moderate angulation prior to plaster application. If severe angulation cannot be reduced the patient may need admission for internal fixation.

Phalangeal fractures are the result of direct trauma to the finger. 'Neighbour' or 'buddy' strapping is sufficient to support simple fractures. This is achieved by strapping the injured finger to the neighbouring finger with non-elastic strapping. Gauze is put between the fingers to protect the skin. A high arm sling should be worn and gentle mobilization of the fingers commenced as pain allows. Patients should be shown how to reapply strapping, as it needs to remain in place for 2 weeks. After this time normal use should be encouraged.

Dislocations should be reduced by direct manual traction using a local anaesthetic ring block to minimize pain. Once the correct position has been restored neighbour strapping and a high arm sling will be sufficient. Patients wearing slings must be advised to remove the sling regularly and exercise the shoulder and elbow joints to prevent stiffening.

Thumb Fractures

The most common injury to the thumb is a Bennett's fracture, caused by longitudinal force to the thumb (e.g. by boxing) or hyper-abduction (e.g. by a skiing fall). The main feature is the joint involvement. The thumb fractures and subluxes but involvement with the trapezium bone is maintained.

Expert reduction and repositioning is essential to prevent joint osteoarthritis. Reduction under general anaesthetic by manual traction followed by plaster of Paris application should be attempted, but if a perfect position is not achieved then internal fixation using screws or wiring must be considered. If the manual reduction and POP is successful, close follow up is required to check that the fracture has not slipped or that the cast has not loosened. If the base of the thumb metacarpal has fractured but with no subluxation or joint involvement then treatment with POP (Bennett's cast) will be sufficient.

Dislocation of the metacarpo-phalangeal joint (MPJ) requires manual traction to relocate and either a POP (Bennett's cast) or thumb spica should be applied to secure.

Rupture of the ulnar collateral ligament causes subluxation of the MPJ. The rupture occurs after forced abduction of the thumb (previously known as gamekeeper's thumb because one mechanism of injury was the twisting of animals' necks!); again manual reduction is required to regain position and a scaphoid POP should be applied to maintain the position.

Pelvic Injuries

The pelvis is a remarkably stable structure composed of two innominate bones (fused ilium, ischium and pubis) and the sacrum. The stability is due to a continuous osseo-ligamentous ring and the strength of the ligaments, particularly the posterior ligaments. Consequently enormous force is required to disrupt this structure which protects several viscera, major blood vessels and the lumbar-sacral plexus. This degree of force constitutes major trauma.

Apart from pathological fractures, indirect trauma cannot cause isolated disruption at one site so a second area of damage should always be looked for. Any X-ray will underestimate the degree of bony displacement and internal structure damage owing to the elastic recoil of the ligaments. Internal structures may have been impaled by bone ends/shards or been severely crushed. There are three mechanisms of injury:

- external rotation – caused by a severe blow to the posterior aspect of the pelvis, an anteriorly directed compression force or indirect force caused by torsion of the femur. This mechanism of injury causes the pelvis to open like a book. This is colloquially known as a 'sprung pelvis';
- lateral compression – caused by forces applied from behind and in front of the iliac wing or a blow to the greater trochanter. This produces anterior and posterior damage on the same or opposite sides. The anterior damage will be disruption of the symphysis pubis, fractures of both pubic rami on one side or fracture of all four pubic rami ('saddle' fracture). The posterior damage will be an impacted fracture of the sacral body, a posterior fracture of the ilium or a posterior sacral ligament rupture. The presence of a posterior compression fracture suggests that the hemipelvis has hinged on the ligaments and so the ring is reasonably stable;
- vertical shear (Malgaigne) – when shearing forces are applied obliquely across the pelvis bony failure does not occur in compression and ligamentous support is less able to resist disruption. When the force is applied antero-posteriorly the potential for instability in the lateral and vertical planes is increased. This can be unilateral or bilateral. This is a very unstable pelvis.

Clearly the history of such patients suggests a mechanism involving great force, which may include a fall from a great height, RTAs with high impact speeds, and building site and other industrial accidents. Isolated pelvic fractures are rare, except in the elderly after falls where one pubic ramus may be fractured. It is therefore imperative to observe for other injuries.

Treatment/Nursing Intervention:

- Treat isolated fractures of the pubic rami (both unilateral and bilateral) with bed rest and analgesia followed by gentle physiotherapy.
- Follow Advanced Trauma Life Support (ATLS) guidelines for dealing with multiple injuries.
- Identify the early complications:
  - haemorrhage and shock;
  - damage to the urinary tract;
  - damage to other internal structures;
  - damage to the hip joint.
- Identify stability of the pelvis.
- Consider timing of definitive treatment, which will depend on associated injuries. A stable pelvis may be needed to facilitate reconstructive surgery of vasculature or urethra. Ideally the pelvic injury should be managed conservatively and any necessary surgery performed by an orthopaedic surgeon experienced in pelvic injuries.
- The choice of pelvic fixation is pelvic slings and traction or external 'pelvic' fixators placed anteriorly. In using these in the resuscitation room,the senior doctor's familiarity with the equipment is more important than any other consideration. The final option is internal fixation.
- Expect these patients to be admitted to intensive care units or transferred to a specialist hospital after their general condition has been stabilized.

Associated Injuries

McLaren (1990) lists the percentages below:

- musculoskeletal: 89%;
- chest: 60%;
- neurological: 40%;
- gastrointestinal: 30%;
- urogenital: 12%;
- cardiovascular: 6%.

Special Considerations

- 20% of all cases of blunt multiple trauma will have pelvic fractures.
- Blood loss can range from 0.5 to 5 litres. Haemorrhage is from veins around the sacro-iliac joints torn by disruption of these joints. Surgical exploration of any associated retroperitoneal haematoma will release the tamponade effect and result in catastrophic haemorrhage.
- 12% of pelvic injuries have urogenital trauma. Early catheterization should be attempted and concern should arise when the catheter cannot be inserted, and when catheterization produces only blood or nothing at all.
- Compound pelvic fractures, associated major vessel injury or associated major head injury have a mortality rate of 50%. (Combined data from McLaren, 1990; Paton, 1992; Dandy, 1993; Robertson and Redmond, 1994.)

Lower Limb Fractures

Legs are bigger than arms and each has to be able to carry the weight of the whole body. Consequently patients with leg fractures are much more likely to be admitted than patients with arm fractures. The size of the bones and their strength means that considerable force is required to cause a fracture, with all the attendant soft tissue trauma that this implies. Generally falls and trauma cause leg fractures but as the mechanism of injury is so diverse this has been noted with each fracture type.

Because the bones are so vascular, blood loss is a significant risk and therefore all patients will require baseline recording of vital signs. Those whose condition is unstable should have regular nursing observations, the frequency of which should be based on the stability of their overall condition and associated interventions.

Intravenous access is required for fluid and analgesia administration with nurse evaluation of intervention effectiveness. Fat embolism is a significant risk in young adults with long bone fractures and is caused by the release of fat particles from the bone marrow at the fracture site. Signs include shortness of breath, confusion, mild pyrexia, tachycardia, decreased urine output and petechiae. Regular nursing observations are therefore needed with blood gas monitoring as required. The best prevention has been found to be high-flow oxygen for the first 24 hours, starting in the ambulance and continuing within the A&E setting (Emergency Nurses Association, 1995).

Fractured Neck of Femur

The main causative factor for this injury is osteoporosis. Patients are usually elderly and have fallen with some rotational force at the hip joint. Patients are also usually female, first because women suffer more from osteoporosis and secondly because women tend to live longer than men.

The Department of Health audit and statistics for England 1995-96 recorded an incidence of 65,937 fractured necks of femur. This figure illustrates the proportion of the public affected and the financial implications for the NHS. Indeed, for many of these patients this injury will be the first indication that they are no longer able to cope alone at home. It is highly likely that such patients will need a detailed discharge package and the sooner this is started the better. This will involve the A&E nurse assessing the patient's current social circumstances upon arrival.

Patients present with pain and bony tenderness over the affected hip and some shortening and external rotation of the affected leg due to the degree of fracture displacement. Gentle internal rotation of the leg will cause pain in the groin and is a way of confirming the diagnosis prior to X-ray.

The majority of patients require surgery to allow early mobilization, which aims to reduce the complications of bed rest. The type of fixation chosen depends on the level of the fracture, the degree of displacement and the risk of avascular necrosis. These are described using Garden's classification:

Type 1 – incomplete fracture;
Type 2 – complete fracture with no displacement;
Type 3 – complete fracture with partial displacement;
Type 4 – complete fracture, fully displaced (Garden, 1961).

Nursing care in A&E should involve all the standard pre-operative procedures, including:

- baseline neurological observations;
- assessment of the neurovascular status of the limb, i.e. checking colour, warmth, sensation and movement of all parts of the limb distal to the injury and confirming and marking the position of the pedal pulse;
- analgesia – preferably an IV opiate titrated until pain controlled, with anti-emetic cover;
- clear and concise explanations of all procedures planned, as sudden and unexpected injury can cause great pain and distress, especially to the elderly who are easily disoriented and worry about being a burden and becoming dependent on others;
- assessment for signs of other injury caused by the fall and an attempt to identify reasons for any collapsing episode, e.g. low blood pressure, cardiac arrhythmia. An ECG is mandatory pre-operatively but if theatre is not scheduled within 24 hours and if there is no history of collapse, this can wait until ward admission
- X-rays – radiographers will often perform a routine pre-operative chest film if a fracture of the neck of femur is identified;
- admission – this tends to be fast tracked by the A&E nurse and integrated care plans are instituted (see Figure 9.4). Such a nursing initiative aims to reduce the amount of time that an elderly person spends on an A&E trolley and so reduces the risk of pressure sore development.

Because of the age group that this injury affects all patients are at high risk of developing pressure sores and poor nutritional status. These risks need to be assessed using an appropriate nursing tool (e.g. the Waterlow Score – Figure 9.5 p. 250) where subsequent nursing interventions are based on risk calculation.

Specific Complications

There are specific complications for this client group and injury type:

- Consider the patient's general condition and the disruption to his/her daily routine. Be aware of confusion, loss of independence, urinary incontinence, urinary infections, chest infections, deep vein thrombosis and pressure sores.

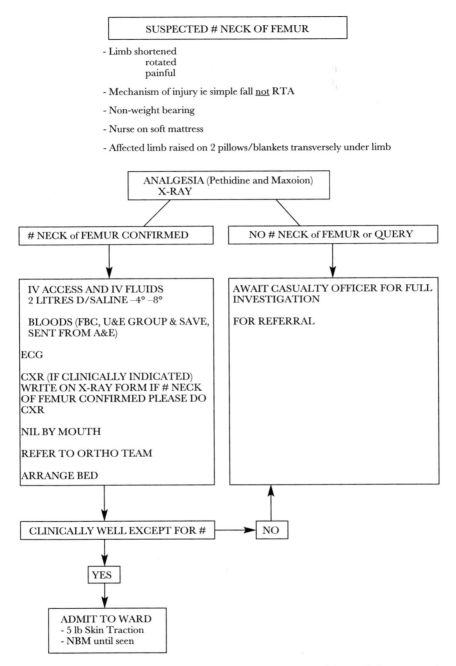

Figure 9.4 Example of fast track proforma for fractured neck of femur (S. Leverett and J Smith, University College Hospital, London July 1996). # = Fracture.

WATERLOW PRESSURE SORE PREVENTION/TREATMENT POLICY

RING SCORES IN TABLE, ADD TOTAL. SEVERAL SCORES PER CATEGORY CAN BE USED

BUILD/WEIGHT FOR HEIGHT	★	SKIN TYPE VISUAL RISK AREAS	★	SEX AGE	★	SPECIAL RISKS	★
AVERAGE	0	HEALTHY	0	MALE	1	TISSUE MALNUTRITION	★
ABOVE AVERAGE	1	TISSUE PAPER	1	FEMALE	2		
OBESE	2	DRY	1	14–49	1	e.g.: TERMINAL CACHEXIA	8
BELOW AVERAGE	3	OEDEMATOUS	1	50–64	2	CARDIAC FAILURE	5
		CLAMMY (TEMP↑)	1	65–74	3	PERIPHERAL VASCULAR DISEASE	5
		DISCOLOURED	2	75–80	4	ANAEMIA	2
		BROKEN/SPOT	3	81+	5	SMOKING	1
CONTINENCE	★	MOBILITY	★	APPETITE	★	NEUROLOGICAL DEFICIT	★
COMPLETE/ CATHETERISED	0	FULLY	0	AVERAGE	0	e.g.: DIABETES, M.S, CVA,	4–6
OCCASION INCONT	1	RESTLESS/FIDGETY	1	POOR	1	MOTOR/SENSORY	
CATH/INCONTINENT OF FAECES	2	APATHETIC	2	N.G. TUBE/ FLUIDS ONLY	2	PARAPLEGIA	
DOUBLY INCONT	3	RESTRICTED	3	NBM/ANOREXIC	3		
		INERT/TRACTION	4			MAJOR SURGERY/TRAUMA	★
		CHAIRBOUND	5			ORTHOPAEDIC - BELOW WAIST, SPINAL	5
						ON TABLE > 2 HOURS	5
						MEDICATION	★
						CYTOTOXICS, HIGH DOSE STEROIDS ANTI-INFLAMMATORY	4

SCORE	10+ AT RISK	15+ HIGH RISK	20+ VERY HIGH RISK

Figure 9.5 The Waterlow risk assessment scoring system. Reproduced by kind permission of Judy Waterlow SRN, RCNT. www.judywaterlow.fsnet.co.uk

- Avascular necrosis is a risk when the blood and nutritional supply to the femoral head is disrupted due to the fracture. This can lead to ischaemia and damage to the femoral head and hip joint. A total joint replacement or hemiarthroplasty will be used rather than a pin and plate if this is a real risk.
- Non-union may occur if a fracture site fails to unite after surgery. Hence a patient may re-present to A&E some time later with complaints of pain, immobility and shortening. Further surgery may be required. This will take the form of new internal fixation or bone grafting of the fracture site.

Fractured Shaft of Femur

This is a major injury caused by major trauma, especially following road traffic accidents. Consequently patients tend to be young and Department of Health statistics for England for 1995–96 indicated that 4700 injuries of this type occur per annum. A complicated recovery will lead to these younger patients not being able to return to their former income-generation roles with resultant financial and psychological problems for the patient. It is therefore important that A&E treatment does nothing to contribute to complications in recovery.

Patients may present in severe pain, pale and short of breath due to blood loss, with a swollen thigh and some external rotation and shortening of the affected limb. It is highly likely that there will be other related injuries owing to the mechanism of major trauma.

Treatment/Nursing Intervention

- All major trauma should be assessed using standard ATLS protocols.
- Baseline nursing observations are needed and pulse, blood pressure, respiration rate and oxygen saturation should be measured and recorded quarter-hourly to monitor the degree of shock and response to associated fluid replacement. As a result of this injury, in excess of a litre of blood may leave the circulation and move into the injured tissues.

- Blood tests taken must include cross-matching at least four units of blood in addition to baseline full blood count and blood biochemistry.
- IV access is essential for fluid replacement and analgesia (opiates with an anti-emetic).
- Fluid replacement should ideally be colloid, followed by cross-matched blood. Fluid balance must be monitored and insertion of a urinary catheter is needed for accurate measurement of fluid output.
- X-rays are required and are likely to include major trauma films of the cervical spine, chest and pelvis.
- Traction will be necessary to provide counter-traction against the strong pull of the large thigh muscle groups, reducing shortening and displacement. This is usually skin traction and via either a Thomas or a Donway splint, depending on local preference.
- The orthopaedic team should make a decision for further treatment. This may involve skeletal traction or intramedullary nailing.

Specific Complications

The following complications may be seen:

- haemorrhage;
- fat embolism;
- infection – if the fracture is compound this is a high risk. Thorough cleaning of wounds and prophylactic IV antibiotics are needed;
- delayed union, mal-union and non-union are all long-term risks. If patients have to re-present then bone grafting or a change of fixation will be needed;
- limb shortening may occur, which can be corrected by shoe raises. Extensive physiotherapy will be needed to ease muscle wasting and knee stiffness.

Supra-condylar Fractures of Femur

These occur in elderly osteoporotic patients after a fall and in any age group as a result of high-speed RTAs. The latter case is associated with posterior dislocation of the hip and acetabulum fractures. Direct force needs to be applied to the knee to cause this type of fracture. Department of Health figures for 1995–96 suggested that there are 2000 such fractures sustained annually within England.

Patients will present with severe pain and a swollen, deformed knee.

Treatment/Nursing Intervention

In addition to the general principles of leg fractures:

- If this is a major trauma injury take into account all the points noted earlier in relation to a fractured shaft of femur.
- Analgesia and positioning of the leg for comfort is important until a treatment regime is decided.
- For an elderly patient take into account all the care points noted earlier for patients with a fractured neck of femur.
- The treatment choice depends on the degree of displacement: six weeks of skeletal traction for minor displacement, followed by cast bracing; internal fixation for fractures that do not respond to closed reduction or are badly displaced.

Specific Complications

- The pull of the gastrocnemius muscle can pull fragments of the fracture backwards, putting the popliteal artery at risk of damage. Remember to assess tibial pulses and perform circulation checks of the lower leg and foot.
- Knee stiffness will occur as a result of immobilizing the joint and will require intensive physiotherapy, although full movement may never return.
- Non-union is a later stage problem due to a variety of causes including excessive traction or muscular pull holding the fractured ends apart.

The femoral condyles can be fractured separately and may cause a swollen knee due to associated blood vessel damage. This must be aspirated prior to following the above treatment regime. Complications are similar.

Fractured Patella

Direct trauma, falls and muscular contraction cause this type of fracture.

Patients will present with a swollen, tender knee which is difficult to extend. There may be a palpable gap in the patella, a deformed appearance and blood in the joint (haemarthrosis).

Treatment/Nursing Intervention

- Comfort comes first – analgesia should be given and support provided in a comfortable position with pillows or blankets.
- X-ray should include the femur and hip joint as injuries to these are associated with a fractured patella.
- Haemarthrosis needs to be aspirated by medical staff using an aseptic technique.
- Undisplaced fractures can be put into a cylinder plaster for six weeks, instructing the patient to keep the leg elevated and to use crutches for mobilization. Patients also need to be instructed to perform colour, sensation, movement and warmth checks of the foot and skin checks of the malleoli between fracture clinic appointments.
- Displaced fractures require internal fixation with wires to hold the fragments together. If it is not possible to achieve joint alignment because of the number of fragments, a partial or full patellectomy will be performed and damage to the quadriceps repaired. After this the treatment regime for undisplaced fractures can be used.

Specific Complications

- Muscle weakness of the leg may occur – exercises and physiotherapy are required.

Lower Leg Fractures

Fractures to the tibia and fibula mostly occur in young people as a result of sporting injuries, falls, RTAs and direct trauma. Patients may present in pain and unable to weight bear with some swelling over the fracture site. Displaced fractures tend to be very mobile over the affected area.

Treatment/Nursing Intervention

- Comfort comes first – analgesia should be given, and pillows or blankets used to support the leg in a comfortable position. Entonox may be needed as extra pain relief.
- Assess circulation and mark pedal pulse.
- Badly displaced fractures must be reduced in A&E prior to plaster application and X-ray assessment.
- X-ray confirms diagnosis.
- If the fracture is undisplaced a long-leg plaster of Paris backslab is applied and the patient admitted for elevation and ongoing assessment. In the absence of complications, the plaster may be changed and the patient sent home partially weight bearing on crutches to be followed up in the fracture clinic.
- Displaced but stable fractures will also require a long-leg plaster of Paris backslab and admission. However, this injury will require manipulation under anaesthetic to correct the displacement. Post-operatively the patient may be discharged non-weight bearing on crutches and followed up in the fracture clinic.
- Displaced unstable fractures need fixation – either internal or external.

Specific Complications

These are:

- infection – many tibial fractures are compound. Prevention of infection by debridement of the wound and prophylactic IV antibiotics are essential before wound closure. Post-operatively patients are taught to observe for signs of infection and to return for reassessment if any problems present. In this instance a window may need to be cut in the plaster to allow for wound assessment;
- Volkmann's ischaemia – there is an increased risk of this in proximal tibial fractures. Swelling occurs around the fracture site, which reduces the blood supply to surrounding muscles causing ischaemia and necrosis of nerves and muscles. Signs include pain, paraesthesia, limb pallor, paralysis and absence of pulse. This requires an emergency fasciotomy to relieve the problem. This is a major reason for ensuring that colour/sensation/movement/warmth checks are maintained;

- damage to the popliteal artery owing to the fracture – this is high-lighted following circulation checks which will show limb pallor, numbness, coldness and a weak pulse. In this instance the plaster or other splinting should be removed and any displacement reduced. If there is no improvement, surgery will be needed to fix the fracture and repair the damaged artery. Patients can arrive in A&E with this complication before any treatment has been started.

Fibula Fractures

These can occur in isolation from tibial fractures as a result of direct force being applied. Patients will find it painful to fully weight bear and there will be slight swelling over the fracture site.

Provided there is no tibial involvement identified on X-ray, treatment is conservative. It involves application of a below-knee plaster cast and the patient is sent home non-weight bearing with crutches, prior to fracture clinic follow up.

Ankle Fractures

These are more common in younger people and are caused by rotation of the ankle, inversion and eversion injuries from sports, compression injuries from falls and sudden braking in road traffic accidents. Patients may present with deformed, bruised, swollen and tender ankles and are non-weight bearing owing to pain.

Treatment/Nursing Intervention

- Comfort comes first – analgesia should be given and the patient's leg supported/elevated in a comfortable position with pillows/blankets. Entonox may also be required.
- Check colour, sensation, movement and warmth and mark pedal pulse.
- Assess the skin over the malleoli as this can become ischaemic due to pressure of bone ends on the skin.
- X-ray will confirm diagnosis.
- A single, stable malleolar fracture can be conservatively treated in a below-knee plaster and the patient sent home non-weight bearing on crutches with instructions to keep the leg elevated until fracture clinic follow up.

- Displaced and unstable malleolar fractures require admission for internal fixation with screws.
- Fracture dislocation of the ankle is an emergency and requires immediate treatment.

Specific Complications

These are:

- joint stiffness due to immobilization – this requires physiotherapy;
- swelling – this is common even months post-treatment and is often a prime concern for patients;
- instability – this may occur as a result of ligament weakness. Wearing ankle supports or strapping may help.

Calcaneum Fractures

These fractures often occur in situations involving scaffolding and ladders and are caused by a fall or jump from a height and landing on the heel or heels. Patients may present with heels that are tender to the touch and may be bruised, widened, flattened and shortened. More often they will complain of pain on weight bearing. Mechanism of injury and thorough nursing assessment usually suggest the diagnosis.

Treatment/Nursing Intervention

- Comfort comes first – elevation of the legs with heels off the trolley or pillows (rather than supported) and adequate analgesia.
- X-ray to confirm diagnosis.
- There is some debate about further treatment but expect admission for bed rest and strict elevation and no plaster until the swelling has reduced.
- A walking plaster and crutches will be provided for discharge and fracture clinic follow up arranged.
- Some consultants prefer not to admit such patients and will discharge them with double tubigrip support and crutches for rest and elevation at home. A plaster will be applied later at the fracture clinic.

- If the fracture is displaced or involves the tarsal joint, further treatment will be needed and the patient should be admitted until this decision has been made.

Specific Complications

These are:

- joint stiffness – especially if there is joint involvement, when intensive physiotherapy will be required;
- osteoarthritis – talocalcaneum joint may be affected. Physiotherapy is essential but surgery may become necessary;
- look for associated injuries – check both knees and the lumbar region of the spine. Fractures in these areas are commonly associated with this mechanism of injury.

Foot Fractures

There are many similarities between the anatomy of the hand and the foot and treatment for some fractures is similar.

Metatarsal fractures are often caused by a heavy weight dropping onto the foot. Soft tissue damage often occurs and this requires thorough cleaning and assessment in its own right.

Undisplaced metatarsal fractures can be treated with a supportive bandage, e.g. double tubigrip or crepe bandage toe to knee, and the patient should be non-weight bearing on crutches. Rest and elevation must be emphasized to the patient to minimize gravitational swelling and fracture clinic follow up is necessary.

Multiple displaced metatarsal fractures require admission for internal fixation. High elevation and strict bed rest are essential to minimize swelling prior to surgery.

'Stubbing' injuries commonly cause fractures and dislocations of the toes. If dislocation is confirmed a local anaesthetic ring block is required before applying direct traction to relocate the joint. Neighbour strapping is necessary to support the injured toe. The patient can be partially weight bearing and crutches are not necessary.

Conclusion

This chapter has covered the assessment, planning and implementation of care for adult patients with bony injuries in the first few hours after injury. The aims of treatment are simple and easy to remember, but each injury is unique to the person who has been injured and it is this that makes caring for patients with bony injuries such a challenge. To achieve the aims of care within the comprehension and lifestyle constraints of each individual is not a simple task. When family and friends of the patient are added to the equation, it can be even more challenging and rewarding to care for such patients. It is hoped that this chapter has provided the tools for a high standard of nursing care to adults with bony injuries.

Suggested Further Reading

Paton DF (1992) Fractures and Orthopaedics, 2nd edn. Edinburgh: Churchill Livingstone.
Royal College of Nursing/Society of Orthopaedic Nursing (1991) A Practical Guide to Casting. Hull: Smith & Nephew.
Robertson C, Redmond AD (1994). The Management of Major Trauma, 2nd edn. Oxford: Oxford University Press.

References

Dandy DJ (1993) Injuries to the trunk. In Essential Orthopaedics and Trauma, 2nd edn. Edinburgh: Churchill Livingstone.
Department of Health (1999) Hospital Episode Statistics: Ordinary Admissions and Day Cases Combined: Completed Episodes by Primary Diagnosis, NHS Hospitals, England, 1995-96. London: DOH.
Emergency Nurses Association (1995) Musculoskeletal trauma. In Trauma Nursing Core Course, Provider Manual, 4th edn. Illinois: Emergency Nurses Association.
Garden RS (1961) Low angle fixation in fractures of the femoral neck. Journal of Bone Joint Surgery 43B: 647.
McLaren MI (1990) Pelvic fractures. In Orthopaedic Surgery. The Medicine Group (UK): 1816–22.
McRae R (1997) Practical Fracture Treatment, 3rd edn. Edinburgh: Churchill Livingstone.
Manchester Triage Group (1997) Emergency Triage. London: BMJ Publishing Group.
Paton DF (1992) Fractures of the pelvis. In Fractures and Orthopaedics, 2nd edn. Edinburgh: Churchill Livingstone.
Robertson C, Redmond AD (1994) Spinal and skeletal injury. In The Management of Major Trauma, 2nd edn, Handbooks in Emergency Medicine. Oxford: Oxford University Press.
Waterlow J (1985) A risk assessment card. Nursing Times 81(48): 49–55.

Chapter 10
Burns and Scalds

Liana Wakeford

Introduction

The management and care of an individual following burn trauma has changed dramatically over the last 20 years, leading to decreased morbidity and improved survival, function and cosmetic results in the long term (Marvin, 1991). In severe incidents, burn injuries can present complex problems, often requiring specialist intervention. Minor burns, however, are seen every day in accident and emergency (A&E) departments. This chapter will ensure that the A&E nurse has a good basic knowledge of the mechanism of a burn injury, how burns are classified and the assessment and nursing care of the burn-injured patient, from the time the patient arrives in the department to the time he/she leaves. The nurse will also gain insight into the medical care of the burn-injured patient and when it is appropriate to refer to a specialist burns unit.

Epidemiology

A common estimate of the annual incidence of burns worldwide is 4.7 per 1000 population. Many burns and scalds are serious enough to need outpatient treatment and about one in 12 needs hospitalization (Lawrence, 1996). At least 600 deaths related to burns are recorded annually (Arturson, 1993).

International statistics show that the number of productive years lost from burns is greater than that from cancer or heart disease because of the young age of victims (Arturson, 1993). The workplace is responsible for about 12% of burns; the remainder result from mishaps at school, assaults, self-inflicted injuries and road traffic accidents (Lawrence, 1996).

About 80% of burns occur in the home and the most common cause of burn injury is scalding with water (Orr and Hain, 1994). Before starting school, one child in 130 is likely to have been admitted to hospital as a consequence of sustaining a burn or scald (Arturson, 1993). There are many studies into children and thermal injuries as it is a common reason for paediatric attendances in A&E, with approximately 50% of paediatric burns occurring within the kitchen (Orr and Hain, 1994).

The incidence and severity of flame burns from domestic fires has decreased in England and Wales since the 1940s because of the reduction in 'clothes alight' burns through effective legislation, an increase in central heating as opposed to open fires and safer clothing fashions (Wood et al., 1986). Infection is a major cause of morbidity and mortality in severely burned patients, causing 50–70% of all fatalities in those patients who survived the first 48 hours (Manson, 1994).

Common Causes of Burns/Scalds

Burns and scalds are relatively common injuries seen in the A&E department and there are several types and causes of these injuries, the severity of the injury depending upon the thickness of the burn.

Thermal

Thermal burns are caused by dry heat such as flames from house fires or hot surfaces such as irons and ovens. Burns caused by fire can be very severe, sometimes leading to death, and they can also be complicated by inhalation burns. Scalds are caused by moist heat such as hot fluid or steam and are also classed as thermal burns. Although most scalds will result in superficial skin loss, boiling water will cause full-thickness burns in seconds (Wardrope and Smith, 1992). Incidentally, injuries caused by molten substances such as fat from chip pans, tar or bitumen are classed as burns, not scalds (Lawrence, 1996). A rare, but nevertheless potentially limb-threatening thermal injury is frostbite.

Radiation

Sunburn, unfortunately also a predominant cause of skin cancers, is caused by radiation. Such burns are always superficial but very painful. Radiotherapy treatment and exposure to radioactive substances can also cause burns but these patients are rarely seen in an A&E department. 'Welder's flash' is a radiation burn of the eye where the intense light radiation from the welding arc causes small burns of the corneal epithelium (Wardrope and Smith, 1992).

Friction

Friction generates heat and can induce superficial burns, for example carpet burns or burns caused by contact with a moving part of machinery. Motorcyclists wearing leather garments can often find that they have friction burns following an accident that has involved them being dragged across the ground.

Electrical

Electrical currents pass along planes and structures of least resistance such as veins, arteries and muscle tissue causing thrombosis and deep tissue necrosis (Edwards, 1996). Electrical burns can therefore be complex and are further subdivided into:

- flash burns caused by electrical arcing – this may also ignite clothing;
- electrothermal and low-voltage burns commonly caused by domestic electrical equipment which is either faulty or has been used carelessly. The charge causes an entry wound that is generally full thickness, with underlying tissue damage and a similar exit wound where the charge has been earthed. If the charge has crossed the heart or the brain, unconsciousness and cardiac arrhythmias including ventricular fibrillation can occur.
- high-voltage burns caused by electric shocks from a live railway line, pylons or lightning are very dangerous injuries and often fatal.

Chemical

Chemical burns occur mostly in the workplace (Edwards, 1996), schools, science laboratories, or at home (Brown, 1992). Such burns are usually caused by strong acids or alkalis and occasionally phosphorus and phenol. These injuries can be complicated by systemic absorption leading to toxic effects, possibly causing the wound to deepen progressively (Gower and Lawrence, 1995) and specialist treatment is often needed. Chemical burns can be caused by skin contact, inhalation, ingestion or injection of the chemical agent. The chemical nature of the substance is generally the cause of the burn rather than heat production. Cement is responsible for most deep chemical burns as cement is alkaline in nature.

Inhalation

Tissues of the respiratory tract are damaged by smoke, heat and noxious chemical inhalation. Inhalation injuries can be further divided into carbon monoxide poisoning, inhalation injury above the epiglottis and inhalation injury below the epiglottis. These are all serious problems and will be described in more detail later in the chapter.

The Structure of Skin

The skin is the body's first-line protective barrier against infection and trauma and is the largest organ of the body. It possesses an array of sensory receptors and is self-repairing. Skin plays an essential role in temperature regulation. Damage to skin affects its owner in many ways, both physiologically (affecting the sensation of touch and temperature regulation) and emotionally by altering the person's body image.

Structure

There are two principal layers to skin. The exterior layer known as the epidermis is stratified squamous epithelial tissue, consisting of sheets of cells that become flatter and scalier near the surface. Beneath the epidermis is the dermis, which comprises fibrous and elastic tissue tunnelled by blood vessels, nerve fibres, hair follicles, lymph vessels, sebaceous glands and sweat glands. Under the skin is a layer of fat covering muscle, which overlies bone.

Function

The main function of skin is to protect the body from injury and infection. The sebaceous glands discharge sebum into the hair follicles and onto the skin. Sebum produces some waterproofing, lubricates the skin, keeps it pliable and prevents cracks and fissures. Sebum also acts as a bactericidal agent, protecting the body from invasion of micro-organisms.

Skin also has other important functions. It retains fluid to prevent dehydration and assists with fluid balance maintenance. The skin regulates body temperature by controlling the evaporation of water from sweat glands and vasodilatation and constriction of the capillaries.

Cholesterol compounds in the skin react with sunlight to produce vitamin D. The human body can react to its environment and respond to danger because skin senses pressure, pain, touch and temperature. When skin is damaged, however the individual becomes a target for infection and disease.

Classification of Burns

The depth of a burn is determined by the agent causing the burn, the temperature of that agent, the duration of exposure to the agent, the conductivity of the tissue and the thickness of the tissue involved (Trofino, 1991). If the heat absorption by tissue is greater than the heat dissipation, cellular temperature rises higher than is conducive to cell survival. At between 44° and 51°C the rate of cellular destruction doubles with each degree rise in temperature. Above 51°C rapid tissue destruction occurs with only a brief exposure. At 70°C, one second of exposure produces a full-thickness burn injury (Bayley, 1990).

There are four clinical classifications of depth of burns:

- *Superficial*: These involve only the epidermis. The skin continues to function relatively normally. There will be erythema (bright pink/red appearance) of the burned area and possibly blistering as fluid leaks from dilated dermal capillaries, followed by peeling as in sunburn. As the nerve endings in the upper reaches of the dermis remain intact, superficial burns are very painful. If pressure is applied to the affected areas, they blanch and quickly refill after release. Complete and rapid healing usually occurs within three to seven days. Scarring does not occur as epidermis regenerates normally.
- *Partial thickness*: Both the epidermis and dermis are involved in a partial thickness burn, leaving less cutaneous tissue although the

epidermal cells lining the hair follicles and sweat glands are preserved. The area is pink/red or white and often mottled, feels thickened, does blanch when pressure is applied but is slow to refill. There are usually large, thick-walled blisters which often increase in size. The burn has increased sensitivity to pain and temperature as nerve endings are exposed. The wounds are wet and weeping with heavy exudate. Healing can take up to three weeks although some partial thickness burns may need skin grafting to avoid leaving a scar (Brown, 1992), especially if function is impaired or contractures start to develop from the scar tissue (Edwards, 1996).

- *Deep dermal*: Deep dermal burns extend to subcutaneous tissue. The thermal and fluid-balancing properties are impaired or destroyed and the barrier to infection is removed. They are characteristically white and mottled with a moist blistered texture. Capillary refill does not occur and the area can become oedematous. Pain is not felt as the nerve endings are destroyed. Skin grafting is necessary to maintain the function of the affected area.
- *Full thickness:* These burns involve destruction of the epidermis and dermis, and may extend to underlying subcutaneous fat, muscle and bone. The depth is characterized by a dry leathery appearance and may be cherry-red, brown, black, tan, dark brown or pearly white (Edwards, 1996). There is no capillary refill and complete loss of sensation occurs due to the neurovascular destruction. These wounds are very vulnerable to infection (Bruce, 1989) and will not heal spontaneously; surgical intervention such as skin grafting or skin flaps is required. Skin grafts will leave scars and possibly contracture problems (Harulow, 1995).

Presenting Signs and Symptoms/Complications

The main problems in the early phase of treatment are respiratory complications and burn shock (Arturson, 1993).

Respiratory Complications

If the patient has received facial burns, it must be assumed that an inhalation injury has occurred. Other signs of inhalation injury are soot in the nostrils and singed nasal hair. Exploration of the mouth will often reveal thermal damage, with inflammation of the oral and pharangeal mucosa. Inhalation of hot gases can produce burns as far down as the terminal bronchi. Steam is capable of carrying sufficient heat into the lungs to produce thermal damage to the alveoli which, although rare, carries a very poor prognosis (Wood et al., 1986).

Carbon Monoxide Poisoning and Smoke Inhalation

In house fires the burning of many everyday materials such as plastic and gloss paint give off noxious fumes such as carbon monoxide. Carbon monoxide has no taste or smell and is produced by incomplete combustion of carbon. Most people who die in a fire will have been overcome by carbon monoxide before they sustain their burn injury. This is especially common in fires within confined spaces. Carbon monoxide has 200 times more affinity for haemoglobin than oxygen, causing inadequate oxygen perfusion. Carbon monoxide also combines with myoglobin in the muscles resulting in muscle weakness. These two factors in combination are the major cause of fatalities during a fire (Budassi Sheehy et al., 1989).

The clinical signs of a patient with carbon monoxide poisoning will vary depending on the length of exposure. Mild exposure can present in a range of symptoms from no abnormal symptoms to alterations in consciousness level. Classically patients with carbon monoxide poisoning are cherry-pink in colour. Severe carbon monoxide poisoning will present in the form of an unconscious patient with a bounding pulse. Carbon monoxide levels of 5% are commonly found on admission in burned patients, with unconsciousness developing at 30% (Harvey Kemble and Lamb, 1987). The mere presence of smoke also causes hypoxia, cerebral oedema, confusion, coma and collapse. Hypoxia may occur as a result of the depletion of available oxygen in the environment when combustion occurs in a confined area. When smoke or chemical irritants are inhaled severe pulmonary oedema and bronchospasm can be produced. Until recent legislation, polyurethane foam was widely used as a filler in furniture and caused cyanide poisoning when burnt.

Burns of the Upper Respiratory Tract

Thermal injury to the upper airway is usually associated with facial burns. Whenever there are facial burns or scalds, the need for airway support must always be actively considered as oedema can progress rapidly and can totally occlude the airway in minutes. Hoarseness or changes in the character of the voice and particularly the onset of respiratory stridor are warning signs of an impending obstruction and the need for urgent medical/nursing intervention.

Burns of the Lower Respiratory Tract

Incidences involving steam or explosions involving hot or toxic gas can, although rarely, result in lower respiratory tract injury. An explosion in a confined space may cause pressure effects to the lung tissue such as pneumothorax, pulmonary oedema from alveolar damage and surgical emphysema of the mediastinum. Inhalation injury of the alveoli is generally smoke damage due to the toxic and corrosive nature of the chemicals involved. Overall, the presence of a severe inhalation injury increases the patient's mortality probability by about 30% (Mathur, 1986). At a later stage, corrosive damage to the alveoli due to smoke inhalation may cause a decrease in lung compliance and impairment of gas diffusion (Settle, 1997).

Burn Shock

Within minutes of a burn occurring, oedema begins to develop beneath the damaged areas. The amount of oedema that occurs depends partly on the circumstances (i.e. temperature and the time of exposure) and partly on the elasticity and tissue tension of the area affected. The composition of the oedema is essentially plasma but with less protein than usual. The rate of fluid lost is at its highest in the first 8–12 hours in a burn-injured patient. This gradually decreases and eventually ceases at around 36–48 hours post-injury (Wood et al., 1986). The timing varies depending on age, though is quicker to settle in younger patients, and the process is slower in deeper/larger burns. In burns of up to 30% of the body surface area the leakage is from around the injured area, but when it is over 30% the leakage becomes generalized. Following a major burn injury, cardiac output falls within half an hour to one-third of normal despite attempts at fluid replacement. However, replacement of circulating fluid volume by transfusion can reduce a later fall in cardiac output 6–8 hours after the injury. With fluid replacement therapy, cardiac output returns to normal by 24–36 hours.

The clinical signs of severe burn shock include an ashen pallor, cold and clammy skin with collapsed veins, little evidence of capillary filling and a rapid pulse. As the shock progresses the pulse becomes weak and thready. Hypotension is a late sign. Respirations are initially rapid and shallow, becoming gasping and 'air hungry'. Urine flow is inadequate for effective renal function. Initially the patient may be alert and anxious, but as shock progresses he/she becomes restless and disoriented. He/she may complain of feeling cold, extremely thirsty and needing more air. Loss of consciousness is often a pre-terminal event (Settle, 1997).

Renal Function

Renal function is impaired to some extent in most patients who sustain thermal injuries of 10% of the body area or more (Barrett, 1986). Due to the action of angiotensin, catecholamines and antidiuretic hormones, renal blood flow and urine output diminish after a severe burn. If fluid replacement has been inadequate, acute tubular necrosis may occur. In deep burns affecting muscle or bone such as high-voltage electrical burns, myoglobinuria or haemoglobinuria may ensue which, if left untreated, can lead to rapid renal failure. It is therefore important to correct hypovolaemia quickly and efficiently to prevent unnecessary renal impairment. If the urine becomes dark in colour, myoglobins and haemoglobins are present within the circulation indicating deterioration in renal function (Bird, 1999).

Wounds

As opposed to other types of wounds, burns are more complex. Considerable loss of area and mass can occur without being immediately apparent, misrepresenting the fact that there has been profound disruption in the functional capacity of the skin. Damage caused to blood vessels affects not only the circulation to the injured area but also that of areas distal to the site (for example, a full thickness burn to an upper limb will impede the blood supply to the peripheral part of that limb: 'compartment syndrome'). This can later result in ischaemia and aggravation of problems (Harulow, 1995). The loss of plasma from the capillaries leads to an increase in the ratio of red blood cells to plasma in the blood. The blood becomes more viscous and the circulation in the capillaries may slow down or stop. Poor tissue perfusion leads to an increase in the burn depth as a result of reduced oxygen supply to the tissues.

Burn wounds are notoriously difficult to assess accurately and are often best dealt with by a regional burns unit that has the expertise and experience to assess correctly. On arrival in the A&E department, simple erythema can easily be mistaken for burn area and included in the final calculation of the percentage of the body surface area burned. However, it later becomes more obvious what is and what is not burned. Similarly, areas of partial thickness burns can have patches which are full thickness but difficult to see with the inexperienced eye.

Electrical Burns

Electrical burns always appear less severe than they actually are if they are viewed purely on their local pathology. The electrical current enters the body at its point of contact, then travels along the planes of least resistance and exits at the earth contact. The entry and exit sites are the only visible signs of injury but the amount of actual injury is indicated by several factors:

- the voltage (voltages as low as 45 volts have been known to be fatal);
- the amperage (the current determines the amount of heat generated). Ventricular fibrillation has been induced on the heart by 100 amps;
- the resistance (blood vessels provide the least amount of resistance to the current followed by nerves, muscle and skin. Tendons, fat and bone provide the greatest resistance but all provide a pathway for the current);
- the duration of exposure (for example, a current of 100 mA for 3 seconds is equivalent to 900 mA for 0.3 seconds). Therefore, exposure to low voltage can cause considerable tissue damage and possibly ventricular fibrillation (Bird, 1999).

Thrombosis of blood vessels can result in ischaemia of the tissue supplied by that vessel, although it may be some distance from the site of injury (Bosworth, 1997). The current is most concentrated at the point of entry, with the skin offering the least resistance to flow.

The result is that the entry wound is often a full thickness burn. As the current passes through the casualty there will be an exit wound, which is also usually full thickness. Currents can leave and re-enter the body several times, causing multiple entry and exit wounds. Current passing through the thorax can cause cardiac arrythmias by affecting the electrical pathways in the heart. If it passes through the head and affects the respiratory medullary centre, respiratory arrest may occur.

Electrical burns are most easily recognized by the presentation of the tissue trauma. These injuries can range from two small wounds to, in extreme cases, loss of limbs. There are three categories of skin loss due to electrical current:

- exit and entry wounds;
- thermal burns caused by combustion of clothing;
- multiple entry and exit wounds.

Exposure to lower voltages will cause local full thickness wounds but rarely deeper tissue damage. However, the duration of exposure is of great significance. If the current was AC the victim may have been unable to release the source of the current owing to tetany, resulting in more extensive tissue damage.

If a person is struck down by lightning it is often fatal, although this is extremely rare. More commonly a nearby object such as a tree is struck with most of the energy dissipated through the tree before the energy reaches the individual. The electricity then usually passes over the surface of the individual, rarely through him/her. The resulting injuries can be superficial injuries to the skin, often with bizarre distribution and possibly ruptured tympanic membranes and damaged corneas (Bird, 1999).

Compartment Syndrome

When burns are full thickness and cover the circumference of a limb, or if a proximal part of a limb is oedematous with absent or decreased distal pulses, compartment syndrome may develop. Compartment syndrome is caused by insufficient circulation to the peripheral part of the limb resulting in ischaemia and possible amputation. An escharotomy to such circumferential burns can help to prevent compartment syndrome if the circulation has been compromised.

Ocular Burns

The most common causes for burns to the eye and/or surrounding area are chemicals, radiation or thermal injury. As with most burns, the severity of the injury depends on the causative agent and the length of exposure.

The most damaging agents to the eye are chemicals, particularly those that are alkaline in nature. The corneal tissue is easily penetrated by alkaline substances, which amalgamate with cell membrane lipids and result in cell disruption and tissue softening. Ultimately a rapid rise in pH can cause damage severe enough to lead to ischaemia. Acids are less penetrating, precipitating tissue proteins which then form a barrier to deeper penetration thereby localizing the damage to the point of contact. Minor chemical burns to the eye are likely to heal quickly with minimal scarring.

Thermal burns to the eye usually involve damage to the lids and other surrounding structures. Minor burns such as those caused by ash result in superficial damage and can be treated as corneal abrasions. However, severe burns such as those caused by molten metal or glass may require reconstructive surgery.

Ultraviolet light causes radiation burns to the eye as the light is absorbed by the cornea resulting in local cell death. Eventually the damaged epithelial cells slough off, exposing the nerve fibres underneath the epithelium. Symptoms often begin 6–8 hours after the initial exposure and patients will often arrive in A&E in the early hours of the morning. The condition resolves spontaneously after 24–36 hours post-injury.

Toxic Shock Syndrome

Toxic shock syndrome (TSS) may complicate burns and scalds in young children and is a clinically diagnosed disease of children and young adults. Children are particularly susceptible to TSS because they have limited prior exposure to toxin-producing strains of staphylococci. TSS can occur in children with either superficial or deep burns and the symptoms include pyrexia, diarrhoea, vomiting, tachycardia, tachypnoea and irritability within 1–5 days after the injury. Within 12–48 hours they develop further central nervous system involvement, hypotension and multisystem failure. Prompt recognition is essential. Children with TSS often present at district general hospitals as this complication can occur in clean small burns (Davies and Griffin, 1996).

Nursing Assessment/Initial Management of a Burn-injured Patient

Along with physically assessing a burn injured patient, the following must be established:

- history and mechanism of the injury;
- time of occurrence;
- any first aid measures already started and their effectiveness;
- any relevant medical history.

History and Mechanism of the Injury

The nature of the incident must be ascertained. How was it started? Was there an explosion? Was the patient in an enclosed space? Were smoke or fumes present? Was there fire or did he/she fall into a hot bath? Were any chemicals involved? If so, what chemicals were they? Are the burns electrical burns? If so, was it AC or DC and what was the voltage of the current? How has the patient been since the incident? Have there been any episodes of unconsciousness? Have there been any breathing complications? Has the patient needed cardiopulmonary resuscitation?

Time of Occurrence

How much time has passed since occurrence? This will indicate whether or not the burns will still be burning. If the incident has occurred within minutes of attendance, more complications may develop that are not initially evident. How long was the patient exposed to the burning agent?

First Aid Measures

Has anyone tried to cool the burns or are they still hot? Are there any amateur dressings stuck to any burns? Has the ambulance crew intubated a patient whose airway is compromised? Has the patient received any oxygen or intravenous fluid from the ambulance crew? Have the parents of a child cooled their child to a state of hypothermia? Has the patient already received analgesia? Has the chemical causing the burn been washed off?

Relevant Past Medical History

Has the patient had a history of respiratory problems such as asthma, cystic fibrosis or airways disease? Does he/she have any cardiac, renal or endocrine impairment? Does he/she take any medication regularly? Does he/she have any allergies? When did he/she last have a tetanus booster?

As with all assessments of patients within the A&E setting, the first consideration must always be A, B, C and D:

* A – *A*irway with cervical spine support;
* B – *B*reathing;
* C – *C*irculation;
* D – *D*isability.

This initial stage of assessment usually occurs very rapidly, especially if the patient self-presents to the triage desk, as he/she obviously does not have his/her A, B or C compromised. However, as a thermally injured patient can present with any state from a 'walking wounded' minor injury to a very severe and life-threatening injury, it is appropriate to cover all aspects of assessment.

Airway (with cervical spine support)

Fires kill more people by asphyxia than by burns (Wood et al., 1986). Initially the assessment must focus on establishing and maintaining the patient's airway (Arturson, 1993). This is particularly significant if an inhalation injury is suspected. If it is clinically obvious that airway obstruction is likely, immediate endotracheal intubation should be performed. The nurse should check the patient's nostrils and mouth for any signs of burning such as singeing of nasal hair, soot in the nose or mouth and erythema or blistering of the mouth or nose. The patient should be assessed for signs of hoarseness, changes in voice and inspiratory stridor, which could indicate an impending obstruction. If there is a delay in recognizing that an airway is compromised complete obstruction can occur due to rapid swelling of the airway, which would make intubation very difficult to achieve. Therefore early recognition of upper airway obstruction is life saving.

Breathing

During the assessment the nurse must be alerted to any history of inhalation of noxious fumes, hot gases or steam. As the assessor moves into the breathing phase, the patient must be observed for signs of rapid, laboured breathing associated with bronchospasm, expiratory wheeze and/or a 'brassy' sounding cough. Depending on the delay in attendance, pulmonary oedema may be present, which is characterized by bloodstained, watery secretions when coughing. The nurse should note the depth, rate and ease of respiration. Are there deep burns that are restricting the mechanism of breathing? Carbon monoxide and cyanide poisoning should always be suspected in severely burned patients. If a high voltage has passed through the patient's thorax, does he/she have a pneumothorax or any other lung trauma which may affect gaseous exchange?

Circulation

Here the nurse must assess for symptoms of hypovolaemic shock: pallor, clammy skin, restlessness. Regular blood pressure, pulse, respiratory rate and Glasgow Coma Score should be recorded. If the patient has sustained an electrical injury, a twelve-lead ECG and continuous cardiac monitoring is required. If the patient is an adult with 15% or more burn surface area, or a child with 10%, fluid resuscitation is required. Urine output must be measured in the severely burned patient, a urinary catheter must be passed and the colour and volume of the urine recorded hourly. If the urine becomes discoloured, fluid administration should increase to maintain a urine output of between 75 and 100 ml/hr.

Disability

Having established that the patient is stable, although this could change at any moment depending on the severity of the patient's injury, the burn injuries themselves are assessed. By now the nurse should have categorized the patient as a major injured person or a minor injured person. A patient with major burns is one who fits into any of the following criteria:

- There are burns involving more than 15% of the body area in an adult, 10% in a child.
- There are full thickness burns of more than 5% of body area.
- There are burns involving the airway.
- There are deep burns in particularly vulnerable areas (eyes, hands, genitalia).

A head-to-toe survey can now be carried out and it is essential to remember that a log roll is needed to examine the back and spine in the severely burned patient, according to the mechanism of injury.

In order to assess and treat thermal injuries effectively, the A&E nurse needs to have a sound knowledge of skin structure and the implications of injury (Harulow, 1995). A combination of factors needs to be considered when assessing the severity of a thermally injured person:

- extent and depth of the burn;
- the body part concerned;
- the causative agent;
- the risk factors involved including age and medical history;
- other injuries incurred.

Difficulties are often encountered when estimating the severity of an injury because of two factors: burn depth and burn surface area. Harulow (1995) reported examples of gross underestimation of burn area and mismanagement of full thickness injuries because of both this problem and generally inexperienced staff.

Extent and Depth of Burn

Burn Depth

Sound knowledge of the function of skin and its structures is needed to assess accurately the extent of damage caused by a burn wound. The depth of a burn is estimated using the descriptions given earlier. Estimating burn depth therefore relies on the clinical appearance of the wound, sensitivity to pain and capillary refill. This method replaces the previously used first-, second- and third-degree burn classification, which was a less specific method and often led to confusion.

Burn Surface Area

The expanse of the burn surface area has significant implications for the functional capability of skin. Vast quantities of fluid can be lost when the network of capillaries in the dermis is destroyed, through wound secretion and evaporated loss, localized oedema and in more extreme cases generalized oedema in surrounding uninvolved areas. The larger the surface burned, the more fluid is lost and the risk of hypovolaemic shock becomes greater. A patient with major burns will develop severe hypovolaemia within three to four hours. Essentially, the percentage of burn area must be established when assessing a burn-injured patient as this directly reflects the amount of fluid resuscitation needed.

Various tools have been created in an attempt to standardize the assessment of the burn surface area:

(1) *Rule of nines/fives* The rule of nines or fives is used as a convenient and rapid initial assessment to determine the severity of the burn and whether it should be classed as a major or minor injury. The rule of nines applies to adults, the rule of fives applies to children. Each part is given a percentage of body area (as a rough guide only) and the burns can be plotted on a body map and a percentage estimated.

- **Rule of 9s (adults)**
  - 9% head;
  - 9% each upper limb;
  - 18% front trunk;
  - 18% back trunk;
  - 18% each lower limb;
  - 1% perineum.

- **Rule of 5s (children)**
  - 20% head;
  - 10% each upper limb;
  - 20% front trunk;
  - 20% back trunk;
  - 10% each lower limb (Wardrope and Smith, 1992).

For areas of the body which have small areas of burn-injured tissue, it is useful to remember that the palmar surface of the patient's hand is approximately 1% of the body surface area.

(2) *Lund and Browder Chart*: The Lund and Browder chart provides a more detailed assessment tool to establish burn surface area. The percentage can be adjusted according to age, which gives a more accurate estimation. These charts are now printed and widely available and both nursing and medical staff should be encouraged to use them to avoid inaccuracies in these first important stages of treatment.

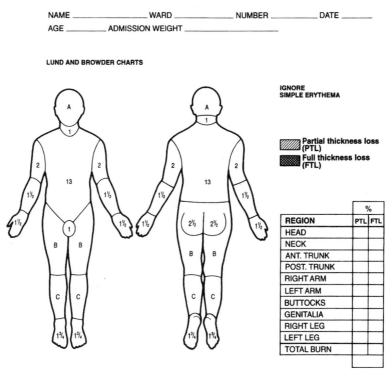

NAME _____ WARD _____ NUMBER _____ DATE _____
AGE _____ ADMISSION WEIGHT _____

LUND AND BROWDER CHARTS

IGNORE
SIMPLE ERYTHEMA

Partial thickness loss (PTL)
Full thickness loss (FTL)

	%	
REGION	**PTL**	**FTL**
HEAD		
NECK		
ANT. TRUNK		
POST. TRUNK		
RIGHT ARM		
LEFT ARM		
BUTTOCKS		
GENITALIA		
RIGHT LEG		
LEFT LEG		
TOTAL BURN		

RELATIVE PERCENTAGE OF BODY SURFACE AREA
AFFECTED BY GROWTH

AREA	AGE 0	1	5	10	15	ADULT
A = ½ OF HEAD	9½	8½	6½	5½	4½	3½
B = ½ OF ONE THIGH	2¾	3¼	4	4½	4½	4¾
C = ½ OF ONE LEG	2½	2½	2¾	3	3¼	3½

Figure 10.1 Lund and Browder chart.

Major burns indicate the need for intravenous fluid replacement and preparation should be made to refer the patient to a specialist burns unit. Burns over 30% need immediate attention. A very crude estimate of the probability of death is the percentage of the surface area burnt plus the age of the patient: if 100 is reached the prognosis is poor.

It is difficult in the initial stages of assessment to distinguish between a superficial burn and simple erythema and even the use of ice packs can cause erythema of areas that have not been injured. Including erythema in an estimation of burn surface area could therefore be seen as inaccurate as most erythema disappears within 24 hours. However, given the difficulty in differentiation it is probably better to overestimate than disregard an area that may in fact be injured.

Body Part Concerned

In determining the severity of a burn the location on the body needs to be taken into consideration. For example, burns of the eyes, face, feet, hands and perineum are rarely considered to be minor burns (Trofino, 1991).

Causative Agent

As stated earlier, in thermal burns the higher the heat and the longer the exposure the deeper the wound will be. In electrical burns the greater the current, the longer the exposure and the extent of local tissue resistance the more internal damage there will be.

Age and Medical History

Age is always a major factor in determining the severity of a burn. Patients under the age of 2 and over the age of 60 have a higher mortality than other age groups with a similar-sized injury (Trofino, 1991). Factors such as poor mobility due to other medical conditions will indicate that exposure time may have been greater. Some serious burns can be as a direct consequence of another illness such as a collapse in a hot bath and in emergency situations the trauma of the injury could exacerbate any pre-existing conditions. As with all wounds the tetanus status of the patient must be established and any allergy and regular medication must be noted.

Other Injuries Incurred

The circumstances of the burns may suggest whether there are any other injuries. People involved in house fires often jump out of windows, with consequent fractures and other trauma. People who have electrical burns can sustain fractures owing to the tetanic contraction of muscle groups and can also sustain other injuries from being thrown in a jolt. Burns sustained during a road traffic accident may have multiple associated injuries which may take precedence in the treatment plan.

It is unfortunately necessary to remember that one of the presentations of non-accidental injury is burns, so careful documentation of mechanism of injury is important.

Nursing/Medical Interventions in A&E

Ideally the management of a burn should start at the scene of the incident and during transportation to hospital. This is obviously not always possible unless an ambulance has been called or the people involved have adequate and up-to-date first aid knowledge.

Care of a Patient with Major Burns

All traces of the burning agent must be removed; this is especially important with chemical burns. The removal of corrosive chemicals from the skin is just as urgent as extinguishing the flames of blazing clothes. If the accident and emergency department is suitably equipped, chemicals/toxic substances should always be washed off in a decontamination facility. If this is not available there will usually be policies to follow, which all staff should be familiar with. Often the Fire Brigade has such facilities and will use them at the site of the incident. Chemicals/toxic substances must never be washed off in the department other than in a decontamination room because of the risk of harm to staff and other members involved within the vicinity of the treatment area. Wearing gloves when caring for such a patient if he/she has not been decontaminated is not adequate protection as the gloves may perish. There is also a risk of inhalation of the noxious substance.

All the patient's clothing should be removed.

Resuscitation

Airway: with Cervical Spine Support

The airway must be secured as early as possible in a patient with major burns. Local oedema can progress very rapidly to obstruct the airway completely. Stridor is a late sign, therefore do not wait for a stridor to appear before requesting consideration of endotracheal intubation. If the airway appears to be safe then humidified high-flow oxygen should be administered. When the need for intubation has been established, it should be performed by the most experienced anaesthetist available as mucosal oedema may cause gross distortion of the pharynx and larynx and often it is impossible to visualize the vocal chords, rendering the intubation difficult and hazardous.

Breathing

If full thickness burns on the chest are restricting breathing, an urgent escharotomy is needed. The cutaneous nerves of such burns have been destroyed so an escharotomy is a pain-free procedure performed by splitting the full thickness area with a scalpel.

Circulation

The nurse should secure or assist with obtaining immediate venous access. The usual sites of cannulation may be affected by burns and hypovolaemia, resulting in peripheral vasoconstriction which may also add to difficulty in cannulation. In these circumstances a large-bore cannula (at least 16-gauge) must be inserted into any available vein. The following list may be useful as it begins with the safest first:

- Use a large arm vein, such as the antecubital fossa, or the cephalic vein at the wrist in areas that are not burned – bear in mind that if the vein is situated distally to a burned area then the circulation may be very poor.
- Use the external jugular vein in an area that is not burned.
- Use either of the above if there are only superficial burns in that area.
- Get senior help.
- Cut down on the arm veins (Wardrope and Smith, 1992).

If there has been no success with the above, then the following may be used (note that these should be used only if there is no alternative and they must also be used only in the initial resuscitation):

- the femoral vein (to achieve an adequate flow rate a large-bore cannula will be needed);
- the internal jugular/subclavian veins with Seldinger technique;
- the long saphenous vein cut down in the upper thigh.

In the case of children a senior A&E doctor will need to be present and/or an experienced paediatrician or anaesthetist, and an intra-osseous needle is likely to be needed.

Fluid Replacement

Initial fluid replacement is usually in the form of a colloid and/or an electrolyte solution, depending on the preference of the department concerned. However, the type of fluid, as long as it contains 130–150 mmol Na/l, is less important than the need to commence an infusion (Wood el al., 1986). Usually there will be guidelines from a specialized burns unit. Plasma is the best fluid replacement as it is the closest to the fluid that has been lost and should be used as soon as available. The expected plasma requirement for the period of up to four hours post-burn is between 0.5 and 0.65 ml x kg body weight x percentage of burn (Settle, 1997).

The most common formula used to calculate the amount of fluid needed in a burns patient is the following:

(Total percentage of burn x weight in kg) ÷ 2

The calculation dictates the amount of fluid replacement required within the first four hours of burning. For example:

A patient who has a burn surface area of 25% and weighs 75 kg will need 937.5 ml of fluid over 4 hours (25 x 75 = 1875 ÷ 2 = 937.5).

This total is a guide only and can be adjusted according to hourly urine output, the general condition of the patient and subsequent blood results.

Investigations

An electrocardiograph should be performed in all severely burned patients to check for arrhythmia or ischaemic changes.

During the resuscitation phase blood samples must be taken for:

- urgent cross-match;
- haematology – haemoglobin concentration, haematocrit (this is an important indicator of fluid replacement required), white cell count and platelet count;

- biochemistry – urea, creatinine, electrolyte concentrations and plasma osmolarity (to give a baseline to monitor for renal failure);
- urine should be tested for blood as an indicator of damage and osmolarity as an indicator of hydration status.

The treatment of the burns themselves at this stage has been to remove all clothing and ensure the burning agent has been completely removed. Urgent escharotomy may be needed for burns constricting breathing and circumferential full thickness burns on the limbs.

Drugs

Analgesia

Once the initial resuscitation and assessment have been completed, analgesia must be given. As described earlier, full thickness burns are completely pain free whilst partial and superficial burns are extremely painful. A patient with full thickness burns is likely to have partial and superficial burns around the circumference of the burn as well as elsewhere on the body. The best form of analgesia is small intravenous boluses of an opiate as the response to analgesia can be measured and respiratory depression can be avoided. Opiates will also help to alleviate some of the fear felt by the patient.

Tetanus toxoid

This should be given if the patient is unlikely to have had a booster in the last 10 years. If he/she has never had a course of tetanus toxoid, the immunoglobulin will need to be given.

Carbon Monoxide Poisoning

Carbon monoxide poisoning is treated by either a tight-fitting face mask or endotracheal intubation and ventilation with 100% oxygen. The patient may need hyperbaric oxygen until the carboxyhaemo-globin saturation levels are less than 5% and the neurological symptoms have improved as much as possible.

Pulse oximetry is used widely in most emergency situations. A study by Vegfors and Lennmarken (1991) compared measurements obtained with a pulse oximeter against measurements from a carbon monoxide monitor in a patient with carbon monoxide poisoning. Their study confirmed that pulse oximetry may be misleading during carbon monoxide poisoning as the pulse oximeter does not differentiate between oxyhaemoglobin and carboxyhaemoglobin. Oxygen competes with carbon monoxide for the same site on the haemoglobin molecule. Carboxyhaemoglobin can absorb as much light as oxyhaemoglobin and can therefore register on a pulse oximeter as oxyhaemoglobin. Diagnosis of carbon monoxide poisoning therefore relies on clinical evidence and should be confirmed by measuring the carboxyhaemoglobin concentration on a multiple band CO-oximeter.

Hyperbaric oxygen therapy should be considered in the following circumstances:

- The patient is or has been unconscious.
- The patient has neurological symptoms.
- The patient has at any stage had a carboxyhaemoglobin saturation level greater than 30%.
- The patient has ischaemic electrocardiographic changes.
- The patient has metabolic acidosis.
- The patient is pregnant.
- Children (whose injuries should be taken very seriously).

Carboxyhaemoglobin dissociates with a half-life of 19 minutes if the patient is breathing 100% oxygen. This should be considered before a patient is transferred to a hyperbaric centre.

Summary

To summarize the priorities when a severely burned patient arrives in A&E:

- Check airway and breathing.
- Assess severity of the burn injury (surface area).
- Start an intravenous fluid regimen.
- Provide analgesia.
- Catheterize the bladder.
- Reassess the burn wound and the patient's general condition.

Once the initial resuscitation phase is over and if a method such as the 'rule of nines' was used to estimate the burn injury surface area, now is the time to use a more accurate method such as the Lund and Browder chart.

Care of the Major Wound

If the patient will be transferred to a burns unit, the wound should be covered with clear plastic food wrapping, taking care not to restrict areas such as the chest or limbs by not applying the plastic food wrapping too tightly. This serves to reduce pain levels by removing the airflow, protects the wound from colonization *en route* to the unit and is unlikely to stick to the wounds. The burns unit will then be able to make its own assessment of the wound easily. Do not apply dressing agents such as 1% silver sulphadiazine cream to any burns that require assessment by a burns unit as the burns specialists will not be able to assess accurately the underlying wounds.

Care of a Patient with Minor Burns

Dressings

The purpose of a burn dressing is to absorb exudate from the wound and, as far as possible, to prevent colonization of the wound by pathogenic bacteria (Settle, 1997). To fulfil these purposes dressings should be absorbent and act as a barrier to external contaminants.

Hand Dressings (Bags)

Hands which have partial thickness burns can be placed in a polythene bag containing an appropriate anti-bacterial cream such as silver sulphadiazine (Flamazine). The bag can be secured to the patient by bandaging it to the patient's wrist. The patient should be encouraged to elevate the hand(s) to prevent excessive swelling. Although these bags are unpleasant to look at, the wounds are kept in an ideal moist environment, there are no dressings to stick to the wounds and a certain amount of dexterity can be maintained, hence reducing the amount of restriction in activities of daily living. The bags encourage the patient to use the hand, which acts as a form of physiotherapy and helps to prevent tight scarring.

1% Silver Sulphadiazine

As infection can be a major problem for burn-injured patients, 1% silver sulphadiazine is often used for burn dressings to prevent gram-negative sepsis (Settle, 1997). Many A&E departments use 1% silver sulphadiazine as a generalized treatment for most burns. However, its use is controversial and many burns units rarely use it. First-line treatment may alternatively involve paraffin jelly-impregnated tulle as wounds are difficult to reassess at future wound re-dressings because 1% silver sulphadiazine discolours the skin and prolonged use has been known to cause over-granulation. Referral to the local regional burns unit for their preference in choice of dressing is therefore advocated. There have also been previous concerns that 1% silver sulphadiazine can have a cytotoxic effect on leukocytes and may contribute to local immune dysfunction, with adverse effects on wound healing (Zapat-Sirvent and Hansbrough, 1993).

Other Dressings

Hydrocolloid and transparent film dressings have been shown to be useful on minor burns (Wright et al., 1993; Thomas et al., 1995) although these can leak if there is excessive exudate, further increasing the risk of infection. Petroleum jelly-impregnated tulle such as 'Jelonet' or 'Unitulle' applied liberally to the burn wound to reduce adherence to the wound, and covered with gauze, is another popular alternative.

Rationale for Referral to a Specialist Burns Unit

Transferring a critically ill patient a long distance should be attempted only when the patient has been resuscitated and can be considered stable.

In the United Kingdom, patients with more than 85% surface area burnt have a very poor prognosis, thus careful consideration should be made as to the ethical implications of transferring such patients. Factors such as the unnecessary discomfort of a hospital-to-hospital transfer, whether or not the patient will survive the journey, and the distance relatives will need to travel to get to the burns unit when they will already be very distressed should all be nursing considerations.

Only a rough guide can be given as to the rationale for transfer to a specialist burns unit as these differ from unit to unit. Factors such as age, other injuries or complications should also be taken into consideration when the decision to transfer is made. Burn surface areas of 15% or more in adults and 10% in children are considered major burns and require admission. Deep burns of more than 5% of the body area and deep burns involving the hands or face will also need the services of a burns unit at some stage, but not necessarily immediately (Wardrope and Smith, 1992). Policies vary in each regional burns unit, but written guidelines regarding the admission and care of a patient with burns should be available. The regional burns unit is always available should advice be needed.

Conclusion

It is clear from this chapter that a thorough understanding of burns and their effect on a patient is vital in order to care effectively for a burn-injured patient. Having read this chapter, the A&E nurse should be able to assess and plan the nursing care of the burn-injured patient. A skill particular to the A&E nurse is to be able to predict future events in order to anticipate what the patient will need. This chapter has aimed to provide the A&E nurse with the necessary information to be able to make such predictions and prioritize their patient's care accordingly.

Suggested Further Reading

Bird D (1999) Electrical injuries. Emergency Nurse 7(2): 27–31.
Bosworth C (1997) Burns Trauma Management and Nursing Care. London: Baillière Tindall.
Edwards K (1996) Burns. Emergency Nurse 4(3): 9–13.
Settle JAD (1997) Burns: The First Five Days. Hull: Smith & Nephew in partnership with the Royal College of Nursing.

References

Arturson G (1993) Management of Burns. Journal of Wound Care 2(2): 107–112.
Barrett M (1986) Renal function following thermal injury. Care of the Critically Ill 2(5): 197–201.
Bayley EW (1990) Wound healing in the patient with burns. Nursing Clinics of North America 25(1): 205–222.
Bird D (1999) Electrical injuries. Emergency Nurse 7(2): 27–31.
Bosworth C (1997) Burns Trauma Management and Nursing Care. London: Baillière Tindall.
Brown AFT (1992) Accident and Emergency Diagnosis and Management. Oxford: Butterworth Heinemann.
Bruce E (1989) Thermal injuries in paediatrics. Paediatric Nursing December: 8–9.
Budassi Sheehy S, Marvin JA, LeDuc Jimmerson C (1989) Manual of Clinical Trauma Care – The First Hour. St Louis, MO: Mosby.

Davies T, Griffin N (1996) The consequence of toxic shock syndrome in an 18-month old boy with 20% scalds. Journal of the Royal Society of Medicine 89 (February): 115–116.

Edwards K (1996) Burns. Emergency Nurse 4(3): 9–13.

Gower JP, Lawrence JC (1995) The incidence, causes and treatment of minor burns. Journal of Wound Care 4(2): 71–74.

Hall M (1997) Minor burns and hand burns: comparing treatment methods. Professional Nurse 12(7): 489–491.

Harulow S (1995) Assessment of burn injuries. Emergency Nurse 2(4): 19–22.

Harvey Kemble JV, Lamb BE (1987) Practical Burns Management. London: Hodder & Stoughton.

Lawrence JC (1996) First-aid measures for the treatment of burns and scalds. Journal of Wound Care 5(7): 319–322.

Manson WL (1994) Systemic sepsis in burns. Care of the Critically Ill 10(2): 63–65.

Marvin J (1991) Cited in: Bosworth C (1997) Burns Trauma Management and Nursing Care. London: Baillière Tindall.

Mathur N (1986) Inhalation injury in major burns. Care of the Critically Ill 2(5): 195–196.

Orr J, Hain T (1994) Burn wound management: an overview. Professional Nurse December: 153–156.

Settle JAD (1997) Burns: The First Five Days. Hull: Smith & Nephew in partnership with the Royal College of Nursing.

Thomas S, Lawrence J, Thomas A (1995) Evaluation of hydrocolloids and topical medication in minor burns. Journal of Wound Care 4(5): 218–220.

Trofino RB (1991) Nursing Care of the Burn Injured Patient. Philadelphia: FA Davis.

Vegfors M, Lennmarken C (1991) Carboxyhaemoglobinaemia and pulse oximetry. British Journal of Anaesthesia 66: 625–626.

Wardrope J, Smith JAR (1992) The Management of Wounds and Burns. New York: Oxford University Press.

Wood C et al. (1986) Accident and Emergency Burns: Lessons from the Bradford Disaster. Oxford: Royal Society of Medicine Services.

Wright A, MacKechnie D, Paskins J (1993) Management of partial thickness burns with Granuflex 'E' dressings. Burns 19(2): 128–130.

Zapat-Sirvent R, Hansbrough J (1993) Cytotoxicity to human leukocytes by topical antimicrobial agents used for burns. Journal of Burn Care and Rehabilitation 14:2(1): 132–140.

Chapter 11
Paediatric Care

JULIE DIGHT

Introduction

In 1991 The Department of Health (DoH, 1991a) recognized that approximately one-third of all patients attending A&E departments in the UK are under 16 years of age. This equates to about 3 million children.

Despite the DoH (1991b) guidelines that all A&E departments should provide an RSCN or equivalent on every shift, and separate paediatric waiting and treatment areas, there is little evidence that this is the case. In 1992, Shelley discovered that of 189 hospitals with large A&E departments, three-quarters of them had no separate waiting room and only 15% had a qualified paediatric nurse on the staff. The Audit Commission (1996) found that none of the A&E departments that they studied met the standard of having a paediatric nurse available 24 hours a day. It is therefore likely that every A&E nurse will come into contact with children on every shift at work and encounter the unique problems that they and their parents bring, despite having little or no formal training in paediatric issues.

This chapter aims to give an overview of the more common ailments and injuries that children present with within the A&E setting, but is by no means a comprehensive guide to every possible paediatric complaint that may be encountered. It will begin by covering paediatric trauma and paediatric resuscitation. The text will explore pain control and fluid regimes as they relate to children, which are frequently not adequately addressed in the A&E department. Legislation affecting paediatric nursing in A&E will also be addressed. A basic knowledge of normal growth and development is assumed throughout.

288

Cardiac and Respiratory Arrest

For the pulseless, apnoeic child rushed to A&E following an out-of-hospital arrest, the prognosis is poor. Powers (1994) recognized that mortality rates exceed 90% with the majority of the survivors suffering some degree of neurological deficit as a result of prolonged hypoxia. However, the survival rates in children experiencing only a respiratory arrest are between 40% and 50% with the long term prognosis being much better.

Children and infants rarely experience cardiac arrest as a result of cardiac disease and most cardiac arrests are secondary to a hypoxic event (Campbell and Glasper, 1995). It is therefore important that A&E nurses are able to recognize potentially life-threatening conditions in order to initiate appropriate treatment.

The predisposing factors of cardiac arrest are respiratory failure and cardiac failure. Central nervous system (CNS) failure will, also, eventually lead to cardiac arrest. However, the CNS should never be assessed until the primary survey (Airway, Breathing, Circulation [ABC]) has been completed. There are no neurological conditions that take priority over ABC.

There are many anatomical and physiological features that predispose children to respiratory and cardiac failure:

- Infants have narrow nasal passages that can easily become obstructed by mucus, foreign bodies and oedema and therefore are at risk of respiratory failure as they are nose breathers.
- A child's airway is narrow and short so a minimal amount of oedema or mucus can dramatically reduce the diameter of the airway and cause increased airway resistance.
- The epiglottis is large and can easily cause obstruction with minimal oedema (e.g. in epiglottitis).
- The glottic opening is high in relation to the oesophagus so the risk of aspiration is higher.
- Children have large tongues that can cause airway obstruction if the head is poorly positioned.
- The cricoid cartilage is the narrowest part of the airway until middle childhood so any foreign bodies can be aspirated quite deeply and are therefore harder to remove.
- A shorter airway means pathogens have a shorter distance to travel before they reach the terminal airways, thus increasing the

likelihood of pulmonary or systemic infection. An immature
immune system also makes children more susceptible to infection.
- The cartilage supporting the airway is poorly developed in children so hyperextension or flexion can easily obstruct the airway.
  Infants are particularly susceptible to hyperextension or flexion
  during the first few months of life as they have poor control of
  their heads.
- The chest wall and sternum have a greater proportion of cartilage to
  hard bone so the chest wall can collapse inwards when airway resistance and work of breathing increase. This will decrease the child's
  tidal volume, thus further compromising effective ventilation.
- Intercostal and accessory muscles are poorly developed in infancy
  and cannot help the child to breathe more effectively when respiratory distress develops.
- Infants are therefore dependent on diaphragmatic function to
  maintain adequate ventilation and factors such as abdominal
  distension that impede this functioning can lead to respiratory
  distress.
- A child's higher metabolic rate means that his/her oxygen
  demand and consumption are increased and so cardiopulmonary
  disorder quickly leads to hypoxia and acidosis.
- A child's stroke volume is small and fixed so that cardiac output is
  dependent on heart rate. Bradycardia is poorly tolerated.
- In a child's autonomic nervous system, parasympathetic activity is
  dominant so his/her response to stress can result in a bradycardia.
- Seizures, raised intercranial pressure, metabolic disturbance and
  narcotic administration are also more likely to lead to cardiopulmonary arrest in paediatrics than in adults.

Chameides, 1988; Powers, 1994; Glasgow and Graham, 1997

To recognize potential respiratory failure the nurse needs to look at
the work of breathing, effectiveness of breathing and the effects of
respiratory inadequacy on other organs.

Work of Breathing

Tachypnoea at rest, intercostal or sternal recession, inspiratory or
expiratory noise, grunting, accessory muscle use and nasal flaring
indicate an increase in work of breathing. These signs will be absent

in a child who has had respiratory distress for some time as he/she becomes fatigued. Children who have reduced respiratory drive from poisoning or raised intercranial pressure will not present with increased work of breathing so respiratory failure is assessed and identified using the following two points.

Effectiveness of Breathing

Listening to a child's chest for air entry and observing the degree of chest expansion can help establish effectiveness of breathing. Pulse oximetry can be used to measure the arterial oxygen saturation but the equipment becomes less effective when the child is saturating at less than 70%, when the child is shocked and when the child has been exposed to carbon monoxide.

Effects of Respiratory Inadequacy on Other Organs

Hypoxic children are drowsy or agitated and initially become tachycardic. If the hypoxia is prolonged, vasoconstriction occurs and the child will become cyanosed. The severely hypoxic child will eventually be bradycardic. Both cyanosis and bradycardia are preterminal signs and respiratory arrest is imminent.

In recognizing potential circulatory failure (shock) in a child it is important to assess cardiovascular status and effects of circulatory inadequacy on other organs.

Cardiovascular Status

The shocked child will initially be tachycardic as the heart tries to compensate for the decreased stroke volume. However, the shocked child will maintain his/her blood pressure and hypotension is a late and preterminal sign. Absent peripheral pulses, poor capillary refill and weak central pulses are earlier signs of shock.

Effects of Circulatory Inadequacy on Other Organs

Circulatory failure will result in acidosis, causing an increased respiration rate without intercostal recession. The child's skin will appear mottled, pale and cool. Agitation followed by drowsiness is caused by poor cerebral perfusion and urinary output will fall to less than 1 ml/kg/hour in children and less than 2 ml/kg/hour in infants as a result of inadequate renal perfusion. Table 11.1 outlines systemic responses to blood loss in a paediatric patient.

Table 11.1 Systemic responses to blood loss in the paediatric patient

	<25% blood volume loss	25–45% blood volume loss	>45% blood volume loss
Cardiac	Weak thready pulse: increased heart rate	Increased heart rate	Hypotension, Tachycardia to Bradycardia
CNS	Lethargic, irritable confused	Reduced level of consciousness, dulled response to pain	Comatose
Skin	Cool, clammy	Cyanotic, decreased capillary refill, cold extremities	Pale, cold
Kidneys	Decreased urine output	Minimal urine output	No urinary output

Source: Alexander and Proctor (1993).

Both respiratory and circulatory failure will affect the function of the CNS owing to poor perfusion. However, it should be remembered that conditions with direct neurological effects such as meningitis and raised intercranial pressure from trauma may themselves cause respiratory and circulatory failure. For example, abnormal breathing patterns such as Cheyne-Stokes or apnoea accompanied by coma is an indication that the child is unresponsive primarily because of brain dysfunction rather than CNS failure due to respiratory or circulatory inadequacy. Similarly, hypertension with bradycardia is due to brain dysfunction as the brain is herniating through the foramen magnum or 'coning'. A final example of the differences exhibited in direct CNS failure is that the child will have stiff posturing rather than the floppy limbs that a child with respiratory or circulatory failure would display.

Knowledge of normal vital signs in children and infants is also important as they differ dramatically from those of adults. Table 11.2 outlines normal ranges for vital signs in paediatric patients.

Table 11.2 Normal ranges for vital signs in paediatric patients

Age	Respirations/min	Heart rate/min	Systolic blood pressure (mm Hg)
<1 yr	30–40	110–160	70–90
2–5	25–30	95–140	80–100
5–12	20–25	80–120	90–110
>12	15–20	60–100	100–120

Source: Glasgow and Graham (1997).

For the child that does experience a respiratory or cardiac arrest, The Resuscitation Council UK (1997) has provided clear guidelines on the procedure that should be followed. The Council defined that an infant is a child under the age of 1 year and a child is aged between 1 and 8 years. Unless specified the following guidelines apply to both an infant and a child.

The algorithm for paediatric basic life support is shown in Figure 11.1 and for paediatric advanced life support in Figure 11.2.

The following information is given to support the algorithms:

- When checking responsiveness, gently stimulate the child and speak to him/her loudly. Infants and children with suspected neck injuries should never be shaken.
- To open a child's airway use the head-tilt chin-lift method to place the child's head in the sniffing position unless a cervical spine injury is suspected, when the jaw thrust method should be employed.
- Attempt only to remove obvious airway obstructions. Blindly sweeping around the child's mouth may damage the soft palate or push a foreign body further into the airway.
- To check for a pulse in a child, feel for the carotid pulse in the neck. For an infant, feel for the brachial pulse on the inner aspect of the upper arm.

Paediatric Basic Life Support

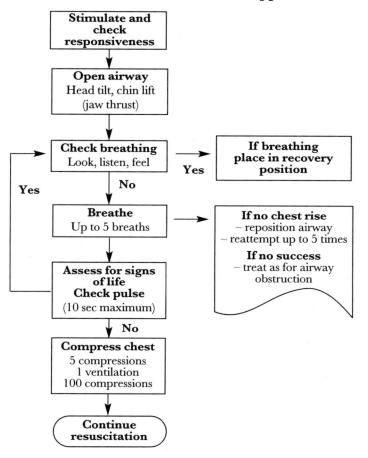

Figure 11.1 *Source:* Resuscitation Council UK (1997).

Chest compressions for a child:

(1) Locate and place the heel of one hand over the lower half of the sternum ensuring that you do not compress on or below the xiphisternum.
(2) Lift the fingers to ensure that pressure is not applied over the ribs.
(3) Position yourself vertically above the child's chest and with your arm straight, press down on the sternum to depress it approximately one-third of the depth of the child's chest.
(4) Release the pressure, then repeat at a rate of about 100 times a minute (a little less than 2 compressions per second).

Paediatric Advanced Life Support

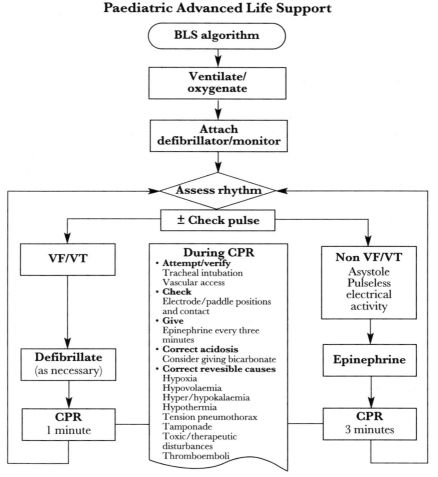

Figure 11.2 *Source:* Resuscitation Council UK (1997).

(5) In children over the age of approximately 8 years it may be necessary to use the 'adult' two-handed method of chest compression to achieve an adequate depth of compression.

Chest compressions for an infant:

(1) Locate the sternum and place the tips of two fingers, one finger breadth below an imaginary line joining the infant's nipples.
(2) With the tips of two fingers, press down on the sternum to depress it approximately one-third of the depth of the infant's chest.
(3) Release the pressure, then repeat at a rate of about 100 times a minute.

- When oxygenating a child provide positive pressure ventilation with a high inspired oxygen concentration, ensuring that the mask is a correct fit, covering both the mouth and nose but not the eyes.
- When attaching the child to a cardiac monitor, place the electrodes in the conventional position. When defibrillating a child place the paddles on the chest wall, one below the right clavicle and the other at the left anterior axillary line. For an infant it may be more appropriate to apply the paddles to the front and back of the infant's chest.
- In asystole or pulseless electrical activity, which are more common in children, epinephrine should be administered. The first dose should be 10 µg/kg (0.1 ml/kg of 1:10,000 solution) if direct venous or intraosseous access has been establish or 100 µg/kg (1ml/kg of 1:10,000 or 0.1 ml/kg of 1:1000 solution) via the endotracheal tube if venous access has not yet been established. A child's weight can be estimated by using the formula 2 x (age in years + 4) = weight in kg.
- The repeat dose of epinephrine should be 100 µg/kg intravenously.
- In the rare case of defibrillation being necessary, defibrillate the heart with up to three shocks: 2 J/kg to a maximum of 200 J, 2 J/kg again, then 4 J/kg to a maximum of 360 J. If VF or VT persists and further shocks are needed, continue at 4 J/kg.

The Paediatric Trauma Patient

The multiply injured child brought to A&E must be rapidly assessed using the structured approach of the Advanced Paediatric Life Support programme (APLS). When the patient first arrives the aim is to carry out a primary survey and resuscitation followed by a secondary survey. As previously mentioned, Airway/Breathing/Circulation must be assessed first followed by Disability and Exposure. In a trauma situation airway management must include cervical spine control. Whilst undertaking an assessment of ABCDE and initiating resuscitation it may be necessary to correct some of the damage that has occurred such as a tension pneumothorax or obvious haemorrhage in order to achieve successful resuscitation.

Alexander and Proctor (1993) believed that multisystem injury in a child is the rule rather than the exception and so all systems should be assumed to be injured until proved otherwise. There are also unique anatomical features in the paediatric patients that must be considered when assessing them in trauma situations:

- Children have a smaller body mass so linear forces from car bumpers and falls mean that a greater force is applied per unit of body area. Their bodies also have less fat, less elastic connective tissue and close proximity of multiple organs, which result in a higher frequency of multisystem injury.
- A child's pliable skeletal system means that internal organs can suffer significant damage without bony injury being present. For example, pulmonary contusions are common, rib fractures are not. A paediatric patient who has sustained rib fractures suggests a high-speed impact trauma and serious multiple organ damage is likely.
- A child's body surface area to body volume ratio is highest at birth and gradually decreases as the patient matures. As a result hypothermia will develop quickly and as thermal energy loss is a significant stress factor in a child it should be prevented as far as possible to reduce the likelihood of further complications (e.g. bradycardia).
- Young children tend to be emotionally unstable and this can lead to regressive behaviour in a painful, stressful or threatening situation. They also have a limited ability to interact with unfamiliar individuals in such situations and therefore their cooperation is not guaranteed. Establishing a good rapport and being supportive and understanding towards the child is very important to aid examination and history taking.

Assessment of Airway, Breathing and Circulation has already been discussed earlier in this chapter. Glasgow and Graham (1997) described management of the paediatric cervical spine as being similar to that of an adult patient in that a hard collar of the correct size, sandbags and tape must be used to totally immobilize the cervical spine. However, in a distressed and combative child a collar only need be applied. Infants need to have sandbags placed on either side of the head, which are secured with tape across the forehead and attached to the trolley to limit movement. Spinal cord injury should be assumed until proved otherwise. However, this is rare with only 5% of all spinal injuries occurring in the paediatric age group (Alexander and Proctor, 1993).

Assessment of Disability is covered later in the chapter in the section on head injuries. Exposure of the child is then carried out, taking care not to let the child become too cold whilst this is occurring. The child's temperature should be recorded and continually monitored throughout. The use of mercury and glass thermometers to measure an oral or rectal temperature is no longer recommended. Other means of recording temperatures such as tympanic membrane sensors, digital thermometers and disposable paper thermometers are more widely used through axillary and tympanic routes.

For the shocked child fluid resuscitation is vital. All trauma patients should have high flow oxygen administered through a reservoir mask. Once intravenous access has been established a fluid bolus of 20 ml/kg of warmed fluid can be administered. If the child does not respond to the bolus it can be repeated; 40 ml/kg is half the estimated vascular volume in a child and a child who has failed to respond to two initial boluses is continuing to bleed. Blood transfusion of 20 ml/kg must then be commenced. A common error in a paediatric trauma situation is a failure to replace enough of the volume deficit. It is relatively unimportant whether a crystalloid or a colloid is used so long as the fluid replacement is of an adequate volume (French, 1995; Glasgow and Graham, 1997). Table 11.3 shows the Paediatric Trauma Score (PTS), which should be used to determine the severity of the child's condition.

Table 11.3 Paediatric trauma score (PTS)

Component	Severity point +2	Severity point +1	Severity point −1
Size	>20 kg	10–20 kg	<10 kg
Airway	Normal	Maintainable	Unmaintainable
CNS	Normal	Obtunded	Comatose
Systolic BP	>90 mm Hg	90–50 mm Hg	<50 mm Hg
Open wounds	None	Minor	Major or penetrating
Skeletal	None	Closed fractures	Open or multiple fractures

Source: Tepas et al. (1987).

Analgesia should also be administered early on during a trauma resuscitation. Children experience acute pain from the injuries that they will have received as result of their accident, despite the myth that are unable to perceive pain. This misconception has led in the past to pain control in children being seriously mismanaged (Carter, 1994). Ideally, the nurse should question the child about his/her pain in order to establish its severity. The use of a pain assessment tool has proved to be useful in assessing paediatric pain and the most widely recognized is the Wong and Baker Faces Rating Scale (1988) which depicted simple faces showing various happy and sad expressions to represent the increase in severity of pain. Alder (1990) found this to be the most preferred assessment tool in the 3–18 years age group in comparison with other available tools. Several similar tools have also been developed incorporating more detail but there is little evidence that they are any more reliable then the Wong and Baker Scale.

Analgesics should be administered in relation to the amount of pain that the child is experiencing. A simple analgesic ladder such as the one shown below devised by Alder (1990) is helpful as it groups drugs of similar potency together. Milder analgesics can be introduced at first if appropriate before moving up the ladder to stronger analgesics. The ladder helps prevent drugs of similar potency being administered if one drug in the group is proving to be ineffective in managing pain. However, it should be remembered that drugs of similar potency that work in a different way may be effective and should not be ruled out before progressing up the ladder.

Non-opioids	Weak opioids	Strong opioids
NSAIDs	–	–
+/– adjuvants	+/– adjuvants	+/– adjuvants

Simple measures such as immobilizing broken limbs will also help considerably and should not be overlooked. Glasgow and Graham (1997) suggested the following pharmacological interventions:

- Morphine should be administered intravenously to children in severe pain after a trauma situation at a dose of 0.1 mg/kg, or 0.05 mg/kg in infants. Pethidine is of no greater value than morphine. Careful monitoring of vital signs is essential and naloxone can be administered to reverse the narcosis if necessary. Morphine is contraindicated in children with head injuries.
- Codeine 0.5–1.0 mg/kg is very effective in conjunction with paracetamol 15 mg/kg and can be used in children with head

injuries. Both can be given 4–6 hourly, with paracetamol being given alone for less severe pain.

- Non-steroidal anti-inflammatory drugs such as ibuprofen 5 mg/kg per dose and diclofenac 1 mg/kg per dose are extremely useful for musculoskeletal pain. They are, however, contraindicated in shocked or hypovolaemic patients as they may impair their platelet function and cause further bleeding.

Unfortunately, and as previously identified, resuscitation attempts are often unsuccessful. When a child dies suddenly and unexpectedly in the A&E department following either a cot death or a trauma, the focus of care shifts to the parents. Although the issue of relatives witnessing resuscitation situations remains controversial, Mitchell and Lynch (1997) believed that parents have more right than the medical staff to be present at an attempted resuscitation involving their child. They also recommended that staff should be trained to manage distressed relatives in the resuscitation room as part of ALS/PALS courses.

Whether the parents are present at the time of their child's death or not, the grieving process should begin in the resuscitation room when they are encouraged to hold their child. The nursing staff should arrange support for the family by contacting friends and other relations if they so wish. The health visitor, GP and coroner's office must be contacted. There are numerous support groups, some of whose addresses are listed at the end of the chapter, available to offer support to the child's family over the forthcoming months. Support for staff is also important. Grief following the death of a child is only to be expected and parents should be given the opportunity to talk through any emotions and feelings that they may have (Walsh, 1996).

The following sections will examine some common ailments that children present with. It is assumed that the child's airway, breathing and circulation have already been assessed and are not giving cause for concern at the time of arrival in the department. Fluid regimes and pain control previously discussed can be instigated where necessary.

The Febrile Child

Children become pyrexial for a variety of reasons, the most common being infection, inflammatory disease and dehydration. Other causes are identified as tumours, disruption of the temperature-regulating mechanism and toxins (Brunner and Suddarth, 1991). When a child's temperature rises very quickly convulsions may occur. Although febrile convulsions are usually very brief the episode can be extremely frightening for parents, who may believe that their child is dying.

A febrile convulsion is usually associated with viral illnesses such as tonsillitis, pharyngitis or otitis. They affect around 3% of children and are the most common paediatric neurological disorder. Generally, a first febrile convulsion will occur between the ages of 6 months and 3 years. The frequency of the episodes is likely to increase before the age of 18 months and they rarely occur once the child is over 5 years. Studies show that febrile convulsions occur when the child's temperature is rising rapidly rather than after a prolonged period of pyrexia. The child's temperature has usually reached at least 38.8°C when the convulsion occurs (Campbell and Glasper, 1995). The seizures tend to be brief, lasting less than 15 minutes, and generalized in nature. Occasionally the seizures are more complex, lasting longer and with focal features. This usually indicates an underlying neurological disorder that has been exacerbated by the pyrexia so a full history and thorough examination are vital.

If the child is still convulsing on arrival at the A&E department or if he/she begins to fit whilst in the department, airway management is paramount. Oxygen and suction must be to hand. The child should not be restrained but have his/her environment made safe so that no self-harm occurs during the convulsion. It is also important to reassure and support the child's parents. The child that continues to fit can be given an appropriate dose of rectal diazepam to control the seizure (Fawcett, 1998).

In the majority of cases the febrile convulsion occurs out of hospital and has ceased by the time the child presents in A&E. The child may well be in a post-ictal state but this will resolve. All children who have experienced a convulsion must have their temperature recorded. They will need close observation and control of the temperature with an antipyretic drug such as ibuprofen or paracetamol. Exposing the child's skin to air by removing some of his/her clothing and any blankets is beneficial, as is placing a fan in the cubicle with the child, ensuring that it is not pointing straight at him/her. It is inadvisable to sponge the child with cool water as this causes vasoconstriction and shivering, thus raising the body's core temperature.

Kelley (1994) reported that 30% of children who experience a febrile convulsion will experience further convulsions and the majority of these children will have a second episode within 12 months of the first event. This information needs to be explained to parents of children experiencing a febrile convulsion. They should also be reassured that febrile convulsions are unlikely to cause neurological deficits or physical problems in the long term. Some children do go on to develop epilepsy but they tend to be children with a family history of epilepsy or those who have experienced several prolonged seizures.

Parents need to be educated to control their child's pyrexia. It should be stressed that is impossible to prevent a child having a high temperature but that he/she can usually be controlled at home using the methods outlined earlier in this section.

The Poisoned Child

Bates et al. (1997a) concluded that in 1992, 52,000 under-16s attended A&E departments with a poisoning incident. Of those, 45,000 were under 5 years of age. Most needed little or no treatment. Only one-third of children attending with a suspected poisoning incident needed hospital admission. Twenty-two children died. Over 75% of poisoning incidents occur in a domestic environment, either at home or at a friend's/relative's home.

The 'high risk' age for poisoning incidents is in children between 12 and 36 months. Children are becoming independently mobile at this age and are eager to explore their environment. In doing so they naturally put things in their mouths. Children remain at risk until they reach 5 or 6 years of age. Until this time they have little concept of danger. They are still very curious about their surroundings and are unable to read well enough to understand labels on household products. After this age the incidence of poisonings lowers until the teenage years when poisonings are more likely to be deliberate than accidental (Bates et al., 1997a).

Although poisoning incidents are not normally severe, parents may find themselves waiting in the A&E department for several hours while their child is observed before being discharged home without any further treatment. This occurs because it is so difficult to get an accurate history from a child. Generally, the incident is not witnessed and the child is found with an empty bottle or with evidence of ingestion around the mouth. The amount ingested in a poisoning incident is most often overestimated. Treatment and investigations are based on the largest amount of a substance that could possibly have been ingested, even though the child has probably only taken one tablet or one mouthful.

It is important to gain as much information as possible pertaining to the incident from the child's parents including what was taken, how much, when and whether the child has vomited since ingestion. As with any other patient all regular medication and medical problems should be identified. The accurate weight of the child is extremely useful in establishing whether or not the maximum amount of the substance ingested will be toxic to that child. The A&E staff should be aware at all times that the child's parents may be very distressed and feel guilty about what has happened. They should be treated with tact and sensitivity, whilst treatment is carefully explained.

Most household products are of low toxicity but carry a risk of pulmonary aspiration if the child vomits, as the vomitus may be foamy. With this in mind Bates et al. (1997b) recommended that a child should not be made to vomit in the event of a poisoning incident. Most treatment consists of observation and, if indicated, administration of activated charcoal in order to prevent further absorption of the ingested substance.

It is impossible to list treatment for every substance that a child may accidentally ingest. Every department has access to the National Poisons Information Service, which can provide information on treatments and effects of substances. They can also provide posters for the department. The A&E attendance could subsequently be used as a health education opportunity to highlight ways to avoid further poisoning accidents.

The Burnt Child

Glasgow and Graham (1997) reported that around 50,000 children attend A&E annually with burns or scalds. Between 5000 and 6000 require admission. These figures have remained constant over the past decade. Of the 100 children who die every year as a result of their injury, the majority have suffered smoke inhalation. Deaths resulting from a scalding are rare. They also recognized that 10–15% of burns are non-accidental, making up 10% of physically abused children. Burns are most common in pre-school children, accounting for approximately 70% of paediatric burn victims. Peak incidence is in the second year of life. The authors also found that there was evidence suggesting that social deprivation and family stress were associated with burns in children.

Most burns are thermal in origin. Walsh (1996) concluded that over 50% of paediatric burns were caused by hot liquid, with the next most common causes being flames, irons and radiators.

Burns in children are often inappropriately managed. Irwin et al. (1993) reported that assessment and treatment protocols for burns in A&E were frequently not followed. Estimates of burn area and depth that determine the severity of a burn were either not done or were wrong.

The burn area is a calculation of the percentage of body surface area that has been burnt. It is widely acknowledged that the 'rule of nines' used for adults is inaccurate for children under 14 years as proportionally they have larger heads and smaller legs. Therefore, a Lund and Browder chart, which divides the body into sections giving each section a percentage of the total body surface area and also taking into account the proportional changes during growth, should be used.

Fowler (1998) recommended that two qualified staff estimate the extent and depth of paediatric burns as accurate estimation is essential. Table 11.4 shows how burn depth can be assessed.

Dimick and Rue (1988) recognized that the management of patients with minor burns is frequently a nursing responsibility. It entails more than simply applying a dressing. It involves making an accurate assessment of the child and his/her burn.

For the child who is being discharged home with subsequent follow-up, parents should be advised that the child needs to maintain a good fluid and calorie intake following even a minor burn to ensure that his/her protein and haemoglobin remain at an adequate enough level for wound healing to occur (Norman, 1997).

Diarrhoea and Vomiting

Children frequently experience episodes of diarrhoea or vomiting for which viral aetiology is most common. However, Lanros and Barber (1997) reminded nurses that diarrhoea or vomiting may be

Table 11.4 Assessing burn depth

Surface appearance	Superficial Partial thickness	Deep partial thickness	Full thickness
Colour	Pink/red	Mottled, red or mixed pink/white	White or sclerosed with blackened areas
Capillary	Excellent	Adequate but uneven	None
Condition	Dry no blisters	Moist, intact or broken blisters	Dry, leathery or waxy
Oedema	Minimal/none	Surface	Underlying tissues

Source: Daly and Meunier-Sham (1994).

an indication of more serious non contagious conditions such as pyloric stenosis, milk allergies, appendicitis, volvulus, brain tumour, toxic ingestions or intussusception. Worried parents may bring their child to A&E for assessment and advice.

Mild to moderate diarrhoea rarely requires hospitalization. If the child does not respond to simple treatments or the diarrhoea is severe, admission is necessary. However, children respond rapidly to fluid rehydration. In the case of mild diarrhoea, parents should be advised to encourage lactose free oral rehydration. Hygiene is paramount in preventing the spread of symptoms.

If the diarrhoea is caused by micro-organisms then the child is said to be suffering from gastroenteritis, which is a major paediatric problem accounting for numerous hospital admissions. The primary concern with infective diarrhoea is dehydration. Children are admitted for fluid rehydration and to ensure that electrolyte balance is maintained. If the organism causing the diarrhoea can be identified, appropriate antibiotics can be commenced (Campbell and Glasper, 1995). Vomiting can also occur with infective diarrhoea but is rarely of major concern. Vomiting alone is a very common symptom in children. It can simply be caused by overfeeding in infants.

When assessing a potentially dehydrated child, the nurse should try and establish fluid input and output totals for that day. The parents should be questioned on the frequency, timing and appearance of the vomit as this may aid diagnosis. The child's level of consciousness and general appearance should be noted and his/her vital signs recorded. Dehydrated children become pale and their skin dry and less elastic. Their eyes also become sunken, and in a young child whose fontanelle has not yet closed a depressed area may be evident. The nurse should also be aware of sweet breath that may indicate the presence of ketones and therefore the breakdown of fatty tissue (Spehac and Benson, 1994). As with diarrhoea, fluid replacement is necessary and an oral glucose-electrolyte solution given to an alert child is very effective. Prevention of aspiration is vital and the parents may need to be reminded to position an infant appropriately in order to minimize this risk.

Fractures

Lanros and Barber (1997) reported that two thirds of significant childhood injuries involve the musculoskeletal system. Children's bones are different from those of adults for two reasons. First, they have a higher proportion of collagen fibres to protein salts making them less rigid and therefore causing the greenstick fracture that is unique to children. Second, they have an epiphyseal plate or growth cartilage at the end of their long bones (Phelan, 1994). Any disruption or transection of this plate can lead to limb lengths being different as the fracture can interfere with the growth of the bone. The epiphysis is more prone to fracture than the long bones and does not fuse completely until after the age of 16. However, children are able to produce more periosteal recalcification following a fracture as they have a thicker periosteal covering. This enables them to smooth and remodel their bones.

The epiphyseal plate is located at the articulating end of a long bone between the metaphysis and the epiphysis. It is more vulnerable to injury as it has partial ligamentous attachments that can cause disruption to the plate from avulsion, shearing or compression forces. Careful assessment and management of epiphyseal plate fractures are essential because of the potential for long-term problems.

Mayeda (1990) reported that epiphyseal fractures are classified by Salter and Harris into five categories, from Type I to Type V. Potential for alteration in growth increases, the higher the grade of fracture.

Type I   Caused by shearing or avulsion forces.
           Results in separation of epiphysis from metaphysis without
           displacing the plate.
           May not be evident on initial X-ray.
           Characterized by pain, tenderness, and soft tissue swelling
           over the plate.
           Periosteal calcification evident 7 days post-injury.

Type II   Most common epiphyseal fracture.
           Epiphyseal plate slips with a fracture through the metaphysis.
           Visible on X-ray as a triangular metaphyseal fragment.

Type III   An intra-articular fracture of the epiphysis with slippage of
           the growth plate.
           Most commonly seen at the distal tibeal epiphysis and the
           lateral condyle of the distal humerus.

Type IV   An intra-articular fracture extending through the epiphysis,
           epiphyseal plate and metaphysis.

Type V   Rare.
           Compression causes a crush injury to the epiphyseal plate.
           Growth arrest is common.
           Difficult to see on initial X-ray.

Initial nursing assessment of a fracture to determine severity should
include the five Ps:

• pain and point of tenderness;
• pulse distal to the fracture site;
• pallor;
• parasthesia – sensation distal to the fracture site;
• paralysis – movement distal to the fracture site.

The mechanism of injury should also be established whilst immobilization of the affected limb, analgesia and reassurance are
provided.

Head Injury

Accidental head injuries occur frequently in children and play a large part in childhood morbidity and mortality. In a study in Scotland conducted over 10 years, over 20,000 children attended A&E following a head injury. Of those, one in 200 was admitted to hospital, one in 2100 developed intercranial bleeding and one in 19,000 died (Teasdale et al., 1990). Glasgow and Graham (1997) stated that head injuries occur more commonly in boys, 80% of head injuries are minor and most likely to be caused by a fall, 15% are classified as moderate to severe and the remaining 5% result in the death of the child.

It should be stressed to all nursing staff caring for a child with a head injury in an A&E department that examination and monitoring are more important than radiographic evidence. Nursing observations should include monitoring not only of the child's vital signs but of his/her general appearance; for example, is the child playing and interacting, is he/she coordinated and in a young child is the fontanelle bulging? To establish the level of consciousness, the Glasgow Coma Scale (GCS) should be used.

A child over 5 years of age can be assessed using a GCS assessment tool that would also be appropriate to use on an adult. For younger children, the coma scale is adapted to make allowances for their immature verbal response. Table 11.5 shows a GCS assessment tool for children.

A child's pupillary response must also be assessed for size, shape, reaction and equality. In a young child this may prove to be difficult. Wagner (1992) suggested that using a brightly coloured object to attract the child's attention aids evaluation of his/her pupils as he/she will look towards you. Getting an infant to suckle may also be helpful as they usually suck with their eyes open.

Another rapid way of establishing a child's level of consciousness is to use the AVPU method:

A = *a*lert;
V = responds to *v*oice;
P = responds to *p*ain;
U = *u*nresponsive.

Semarin-Holleran, 1994

Patients who are discharged home following a minor head injury should be given written instructions to back up what they have been

Table 11.5 Glasgow Coma Scale assessment tool for paediatric patients

Eye opening	>1 year	<1 year
Score = 4	Spontaneously	Spontaneously
3	To verbal command	To shout
2	To pain	To pain
1	No response	No response
Best motor response	>1 year	<1 year
Score = 6	Obeys	Spontaneous movement
5	Localizes to pain	Localizes to pain
4	Flexion withdrawal	Flexion withdrawal
3	Abnormal flexion (decorticate rigidity)	Abnormal flexion (decorticate rigidity)
2	Extension (decerebrate rigidity)	Extension (decerebrate rigidity)
1	No response	No response
Best verbal response	2–5 years	0–24 months
5	Appropriate words and phrases	Smiles, coos appropriately
4	Inappropriate words	Cries, but consolable
3	Persistent cries or screams	Persistent inappropriate crying or screaming
2	Grunts	Grunts, agitated, restless
1	No response	No response

told in the A&E department. Parents should be advised that children may experience unpleasant symptoms such as vomiting, headaches and dizziness. Less common symptoms are deafness and generalized seizures. It should also be stressed that the child with any of these symptoms must return for urgent medical reassessment.

Non-accidental Injury

Wynne (1992) recognized that the staff in the A&E department play a key role in identifying abused children and in initiating protective action. About 6000 children every year suffer some type of abuse. Walsh (1996) listed the following warning signs of child abuse:

- a delay in seeking treatment;
- inadequate explanation of the injury;

- the explanation is inappropriate for the extent or type of injury;
- signs of previous injury, such as fading bruises;
- defensiveness and hostility, or alternatively apathy and disinterest towards the child by the parent;
- silence and withdrawal on the part of the child;
- evidence of failure to thrive; if the child has not reached appropriate milestones for both physical or mental development;
- frequent parental attendances at A&E (often for non-specific reasons) with the child;
- signs of physical neglect.

Other 'red flags' were identified by Wynne (1992) as multiple fractures, fractured ribs, skull fractures, fractures in children under the age of two, any bruising in infancy, bruises to ears, cheeks, lower jaw, neck, chest and back, scalds in glove or stocking distribution indicating forced immersion, straight-edged burns and a torn frenulum.

The Children Act 1989 directly influences the management of child abuse. It encourages a partnership with families throughout child protection issues. It emphasizes that child protection policies are universal, including children's homes, foster homes and boarding schools. It stresses that action taken regarding child abuse should be decisive rather than precipitative to protect children from abuse or neglect, as there is potential for long-term damage to the child by taking precipitative action. These guidelines are set out in the *Working Together* document that leads to inter-agency management of child protection (Department of Health, 1991b).

Dimond (1993) recognized sections of the Children Act 1989 as being relevant to child protection issues. They were:

- Section 43: Child Assessment Order which gives legal authority for a detailed assessment to be carried out;

- Section 44: Emergency Protection Order which allows a local authority to take a child into care for protection;

- Section 46: Police powers which permit a constable to remove a child to a place of safety or prevent anyone else removing a child from a hospital or other accommodation.

A nurse who suspects that a child in his/her care has been abused would usually need to involve the social services. Departments should have clearly laid down procedures and close links with health visitors are essential.

The A&E nurse is only the initial link in protecting a child who has been abused. It is a stressful and highly emotive scenario and the sight of an abused child may leave the nurse feeling angry. However, displaying this anger will not help the child, who is him/herself already a victim of anger. Nivan (1992) advised that although stereotypes should not be made there is substantial evidence to link abuse to sociodemographic factors such as financial deprivation and until this issue is addressed the nurse can do little more than act for the child and try to prevent further harm being done.

Informed Consent

> Informed consent is a fundamental right of an individual, irrespective of age.
> (Royal College of Nursing, 1990, p. 33)

This is an important consideration in the A&E department for a nurse who must act as a child's advocate, ensuring that he/she fully understands the treatment that he/she is receiving. The Family Reform Act 1969 allows a person over the age of 16 years to consent to treatment. For a person younger than this the Act is less precise and consent depends upon the person's maturity.

The Royal College of Nursing (1990) stated that there are two legal principles involved when dealing with paediatric consent:

1) Consent can only be gained from a child who understands the nature, purpose and hazards of treatment. The ability to give consent is based on the age and cognitive development of the child, along with the nature of the treatment.
2) Parents have rights over their children. These rights range from the right to control their child to the right to advise their teenager.

An unaccompanied child should be questioned as to why there is no one accompanying him/her and it should be decided whether or not parental consent is required. However, the nurse needs the consent of the child to contact his/her parents and any objections need to be taken up with the doctor in charge of the child's care. Verbal consent from the child's parent over the telephone must be documented clearly. The child must be discharged home with written instructions so that his/her parents are aware of what treatment has been given and what follow-up is required.

Remember: Essential treatment must never be delayed, even if suitable consent cannot be gained.

Conclusion

This chapter concludes with a reminder that children are not little adults and should not be treated as such. They are unique beings with a wealth of anatomical and physiological differences that makes their care different to that of adults. This chapter has recognized that the majority of A&E departments have serious shortcomings in dealing with children. Smith (1998) concluded that there is an increase in the number of departments employing paediatric nurses but that long-term strategies need to be developed to ensure that staff dealing with children are adequately trained.

Other areas needing attention are play facilities and clinical areas designed for children. As the 21st century arrives, A&E departments need to be providing a facility that cares for the child and his/her family as a whole. Until the number of staff employed in A&E departments who are adequately trained to provide acute emergency care for children is proportional to the number of children attending the departments each year, this cannot be achieved.

Suggested Further Reading

Many of the texts in the reference list provide more in-depth coverage of the subjects addressed in this chapter.

References

Alder S (1990) Taking children at their word: pain control in paediatrics. Professional Nurse May: 398–402.
Alexander RH, Proctor HJ (1993) ATLS Course for Physicians Handbook. Chicago: American College of Surgeons.
Audit Commission (1996) By Accident or Design: Improving Accident and Emergency Services in England and Wales. London: HMSO.
Bates N, Edwards N, Roper J, Volans GN (Eds) (1997a) Paediatric Toxicology: Handbook of Poisoning in Children. London: Macmillan.
Bates N, Dines A, Volans G (1997b) Acute poisoning: initial management and sources of information. Emergency Nurse 5(3): 20–4.

Brunner LS, Suddarth DS (1991) The Lippincot Manual of Paediatric Nursing, 3rd edn. London: HarperCollins.

Campbell S, Glasper EA (1995) Whaley & Wong's Childrens Nursing. St Louis: Mosby.

Carter B (1994) Child and Infant Pain. Principles of Nursing Care and Management. London: Chapman & Hall.

Chameides L (Ed) (1988) Textbook of Advanced Paediatric Life Support. Dallas: American Heart Association.

Daly WL, Meunier-Sham J (1994) Burns. In Kelley SJ (Ed) Pediatric Emergency Nursing. 2nd edn. Connecticut: Appleton Lange, pp 351–64.

Department of Health (1991a) Welfare of Children and Young People in Hospital. London: HMSO.

Department of Health (1991b) Working Together under The Children Act 1989. London: HMSO.

Dimick A, Rue LW (1988) Outpatient treatment of burns. Alabama Journal of Medical Sciences. 25(2): 183–186. [Cited by Fowler A (1998) Nursing management of minor burn injuries. Emergency Nurse 6 (6): 31–7.]

Dimond B (1993) Non-accidental injury and the A&E nurse. Accident and Emergency Nursing 1: 225–28.

Fawcett J (1998) Auditing the treatment of childhood convulsions in A&E. Emergency Nurse 5(9): 29–32.

Fowler A (1998) Nursing management of minor burn injuries. Emergency Nurse 6(6): 31–7.

French JP (1995) Pediatric Emergency Skills. St Louis: Mosby.

Glasgow JFT, Graham, HK (1997) Management of Injuries in Children. London: BMJ.

HMSO (1989) The Children Act 1989. London: HMSO.

HMSO (1969) Family Reform Act 1969. London: HMSO. [Cited by The Royal College of Nursing (1990) Nursing Children in the Accident and Emergency Department. London: RCN.]

Irwin I, Reid C, McLean M (1993) Burns in children: do casualty officers get it right? Injury 24: 187–8.

Kelley SJ (Ed) (1994) Pediatric Emergency Nursing, 2nd edn. Connecticut: Appleton Lange.

Lanros NE, Barber JM (1997) Emergency Nursing, 4th edn. Connecticut: Appleton Lange.

Mayeda DV (1990) Orthopaedic injuries. In Barkin RM, Rosen P (Eds) Emergency Pediatrics: A Guide to Ambulatory Care. St Louis: Mosby, pp 418–49.

Mitchell MH, Lynch MB (1997) Should relatives be allowed in the resuscitation room? Journal of Accident and Emergency Medicine 14: 366–9.

Nivan C (1992) Psychological Care for Families. Oxford: Butterworth Heinemann.

Norman L (1997) Nutritional care in burns patients. In Bosworth C (Ed) Burns Trauma Management and Nursing Care. London: Baillière Tindall.

Phelan A (1994) Musculoskeletal trauma. In Kelley SJ (Ed) Pediatric Emergency Nursing, 2nd edn. Connecticut: Appleton Lange, pp 323–34.

Powers A (1994) Resuscitation of infants, children and adolescents. In Kelley SJ (Ed) Pediatric Emergency Nursing, 2nd edn. Connecticut: Appleton Lange pp 175–97.

Resuscitation Council UK (1997) The 1997 Resuscitation Guidelines for Use in the United Kingdom. London: Resuscitation Council (UK).

Royal College of Nursing (1990) Nursing Children in the Accident and Emergency Department. London: RCN.

Semarin-Holleran R (1994) Head, neck and spinal cord trauma. In Kelley SJ (Ed) Pediatric Emergency Nursing, 2nd edn. Connecticut: Appleton Lange, pp. 307–32.

Shelley P (1992) Children in Accident and Emergency. London: Action for Sick Children.

Smith F (1998) Caring for children. Emergency Nurse 6(6): 20–4.

Spehac AM, Benson CR (1994) Gastrointestinal emergencies. In Kelley SJ (Ed) Pediatric Emergency Nursing, 2nd edn. Connecticut: Appleton Lange, pp 453–90.

Teasdale GM, Murray G, Anderson E (1990) Risks of traumatic intercranial haematoma in children and adults: Implications for managing head injuries. British Medical Journal 300: 363–7.

Tepas JJ, Molitt DL, Talbert JL, Bryany M (1987) The paediatric trauma score as a predictor of injury severity in the injured child. Journal of Paediatric Surgery 22: 24–8.

Wagner M (1992) Neurologic emergencies in the young: evaluation and stabilisation. Emergency Medicine 6: 204–13.

Walsh M (1996) Accident and Emergency Nursing, a New Approach, 3rd edn. Oxford: Butterworth Heinemann.

Wong DL, Baker CM (1988) Pain in children: a comparison of assessment scales. Paediatric Nursing 14: 9–17.

Wynne J (1992) The construction of child abuse in the A&E department. In Cloke C, Naish J (Eds) Key Issues in Child Protection. Harlow: Longman.

Useful Addresses

Foundation for the Study of Sudden Infant Death,
35 Belgrave Square,
London SW1X 8QB.

National Association for the Welfare of Children in Hospital (NAWCH),
Argyle House,
29–31 Euston Road,
London NW1 2SD.

Stillbirth and Neonatal Death Association,
Argyle House,
29–31 Euston Road,
London NW1 2SD.

Compassionate Friends,
6 Denmark Street,
Bristol BS1 5DQ.

Chapter 12
Soft Tissue Injuries

Tina Marie Stokoe

Introduction

Lacerations in a busy accident and emergency (A&E) department may be classified as a minor injury. However, this may not be the case as each wound varies in its presentation. For example, the injury may be close to or involve some inner structures underlying the skin that would classify the wound as requiring urgent attention. It is therefore important for the A&E nurse to understand the anatomical and physiological principles of wound healing to ensure that a thorough assessment of the wound can be performed, determining the best type of wound closure method to be used. Thorough nursing assessment and wound management will subsequently enable the patient to be directly involved in his/her care and this will lead to optimal wound healing on discharge.

The first section of this chapter aims to give the reader an understanding of the principles of wound healing, the role of the A&E nurse in the assessment of wounds and the procedure for performing each type of wound closure. The second part of the chapter will discuss soft tissue injuries to the upper and lower limbs, including the different techniques of treatment and strapping for such injuries.

Wounds and Wound Closure

A laceration is a wound that penetrates the skin and has a torn and jagged edge. The best way to manage these wounds is to bring the wound edges together to heal by first (primary) intention. This may be achieved by the use of sutures, staples, glue or adhesive strips.

When a patient arrives in the A&E department it is important that a full assessment and evaluation of the patient's wound is performed because the combination of wound characteristics, anatomical site and any other factors surrounding the injury will affect the overall management of the wound.

The next step is to consider whether the wound requires any immediate first aid treatment; wound bleeding may be stopped by simple pressure using compression bandages and if the wound is situated on a limb elevation should be initiated. All nursing intervention should be fully explained to the patient and the plan and treatment of his/her care discussed to gain his/her cooperation and understanding of all pending treatment.

Assessment and History

A thorough nursing history and assessment of the wound is necessary to gain a full understanding of the extent of the injury so that a plan of care can be formulated. This will also help the nurse to adopt a holistic approach to caring for the patient and his/her injury, including the promotion of health and accident prevention.

The history and assessment should find out the following:

- how the wound developed;
- what object was involved in the injury (e.g. if this was glass it will need to be documented as wounds will require an X-ray prior to wound closure);
- whether the object was at high speed when the injury occurred;
- the time elapsed since the injury;
- mechanism of the injury;
- what type of first aid was carried out;
- the depth and haemostasis of the wound;
- the patient's tetanus status to determine whether the patient will require passive or active immunization.

An examination of the wound should then follow to eliminate any underlying complications and damage to other anatomical structures.

Examination

Undertake Clinical Observation of the Wound

This is necessary to assess the wound for bleeding, any evidence of foreign bodies and to determine whether any important structures are involved.

Perform a Neurovascular Assessment

This is to determine:

- *circulation*: the area surrounding the wound should be assessed for colour, noting any pallor or blanching, warmth and neuro-sensation. A further assessment of circulation may be carried out by identifying a palpable pulse and capillary refill through finger pressure (pressure should be maintained for 5 seconds and capillary refill should occur within 2 seconds);
- *movement*: this should be performed distal to the injury and any weakness or decrease in the range of movements over joints should be noted. This procedure will test the motor and tendon functions of the limb following injury.

By performing such an examination it can be determined whether any additional medical interventions are required (for example the repair of nerves, tendons or large vessels).

This process of assessment, history taking and examination will allow each laceration to be assessed individually and prioritized accordingly using a standard triage system. Once all the findings have been identified they must be documented in the nursing notes because an initial and immediate assessment provides a good baseline for subsequent review. If the A&E department is busy and there is likely to be a delay, wounds may require reassessment. Trott (1991) advocated that if there is an extended delay from the time of injury to the wound becoming repaired (over 3 hours) then a sterile saline moistened dressing should be applied to prevent drying of the wound (hence maintaining it as a primary wound). The optimum time for wound healing will be discussed later in the chapter.

Pain Assessment

The next stage of assessment is to determine the degree of associated pain. This can be achieved by undertaking a pain assessment using a recognized pain-scoring tool. This not only evaluates the patient's sensation but also identifies whether any analgesia is required.

Prior to discussing the various forms of wound repair and wound closure the natural process of wound healing will be discussed. This is because not all wounds will require repair and closure, particularly if they are uncomplicated and superficial and may therefore be left to heal without intervention.

Wound Healing

Wound healing can be described as having anything from four to six phases in its process.

Four stages of wound healing will be discussed here:

- *Inflammatory phase*: This involves haemostasis as it is the phase of wound healing where a blood clot forms in the wound that begins the process of apposing the wound edges. An anti-bacterial process also occurs here. At this phase a migration of white cells and neutrophils is released to the damaged site. Granulocytes, which are also responsible for controlling bacteria, are prevalent at this stage. These peak between 12 and 24 hours.
- *Migratory/destructive phase*: The clot develops into a scab and the epithelial cells begin to bridge the wound. The clearance of dead cells and devitalized tissue is started by the release of macrophages and fibroblasts. These are responsible for moving along the fibrin threads in the first process of repairing the wound.
- *Proliferative/epithelialization phase*: New blood vessels infiltrate the wound at this stage and epithelial cells beneath the scab are beginning to develop from the stratum germinativum (basal layer) of the skin. In superficial, uncomplicated 'sheer' type injuries, this process can take up to 24 hours.
- *Maturation phase*: This involves the reconstruction of a wound. New vessels are formed bringing oxygen and nutrients to the healing wound by a process known as neovascularization which can take up to 7 days post-injury. The scab then sloughs off and the scar tissue is formed.

When these phases are not allowed to progress naturally, assistance to heal the wound in the form of closure or repair is required. It is important to understand what stage the wound is at to determine the classification of the wound and how this may best be treated or repaired. Being aware of these categories identifies the time lapsed since the injury and how the wound will heal.

Categories of Wound Healing

Primary Healing

This type of wound should be repaired within 6–8 hours, healing by first intention. This is a primary wound for immediate closure and usually occurs from linear sheer injuries with minimal contamination and minimal tissue loss, and where end to end healing would occur.

Secondary Healing

This type of wound may have suffered large tissue loss and contamination. Granulation tissue develops in the base of the wound and scar tissue forms. This form can develop from wounds such as ulcers and abscesses. These wounds are described as healing by secondary intention. If large, many of these wounds require skin grafting at a later stage.

Tertiary Healing

These wounds usually develop from older injuries. They have suffered much tissue loss and contamination has set in. They may sometimes be closed with tapes or sutures and observed for 4–5 days.

The focus of this chapter will be on primary intention. This is the most common type of healing in wounds treated by nursing intervention. Depending on the anatomical site of the wound some may be sutured 24 hours post-injury, although the optimum time for wound closure is under 8 hours.

Reasons for Wound Closure within 12–24 Hours

- Granulocytes are at their peak within 12–24 hours. After this time bacteria may not be engulfed and the build-up of bacteria may break down the wound, increasing the risk of infection and delaying wound healing.

- The stratum germinativum (basal layer) is the parent layer for new cells to be produced. These new cells are responsible for epidermal formation during wound healing after injury. This process of producing new cells slows down after 12 hours.
- The stratum corneum is the keratinized layer that gives the skin a cosmetic finish.
- The corneum layer will become more bulky, adhering to scarring if wound edges are left unopposed after 12–24 hours.
- Macrophages engulf and destroy bacteria. They also stimulate fibroblasts that synthesize the protein collagen, allowing the third phase of wound healing to commence. These are large in number within 24 hours and reduce after this time. After 24 hours secondary/tertiary healing may develop making the wound difficult to close.
- Epithelialization promotes intact wound edges within 24 hours. Only lacerations by shearing forces with little epidermal damage may allow healing after 24 hours.

Primary Intention Wounds

To ensure that wound classification is correctly determined at the time of patient arrival, understanding the characteristics of wound appearance is necessary. The appearance of a primary wound that is suitable for primary wound closure is one with:

- fresh appearance;
- minimal bleeding;
- non-devitalized tissue;
- no visible contamination;
- no debris.

The wound must also be:

- aggressively cleaned;
- well irrigated;
- debrided.

All of these features make the wound suitable for repair by primary closure.

Cleansing of the Wound

Once it has been decided that treatment is to commence, the nurse's initial responsibility is to prevent any further contamination or infection. This is achieved by thorough cleaning of the wound to wash away any foreign bodies or debris. The wound should be cleansed using 0.9% normal saline because as well as cleansing the wound this may also cool the wound bed, therefore aiding the healing process (Doughty, 1992). If this is a deep wound it is advisable to administer a local anaesthetic prior to thorough wound cleansing and an aseptic technique should be maintained throughout to minimize the risk of infection and promote healing once the wound has been repaired.

Methods of Wound Cleaning

There are many methods of wound cleaning that may be considered, although in some cases, where wounds are heavily contaminated with dirt and bacteria, debridement may be necessary under general anaesthetic. However, less invasive measures of wound cleansing should also be considered.

Devitalized tissue is not difficult to identify as its appearance may be shredded, ischaemic, black or blue.

There are many different methods by which devitalized tissue can be removed. One way is by using a sterile swab moistened in 0.9% normal saline solution to sweep away superficial debris and blood. Further bleeding may be caused as a result of this, but by placing pressure on the margin the wound can be inspected to ensure that all material is removed. If the wound is deep, with dirt and grit embedded in the tissues, then deep cleansing may be required as leaving these foreign bodies in the wound not only contributes to infection but also to 'tattooing' (this is where debris penetrates beneath the skin and may cause pigmentation of the skin, leaving a tattoo effect).

Another way of cleaning dirt and foreign matter from the embedded tissues is to remove them using a sterile scrubbing brush. This is a very vigorous way to clean a wound and may be very painful. It is therefore advisable that the wound is well anaesthetized prior to carrying out the procedure. The method for cleaning in this way should involve a circular motion directed away from the wound. It is suggested that this should take 2–3 minutes, ensuring that all dried blood and foreign matter are removed. An alternative method of cleaning is by irrigating the wound with normal saline. The fluid should be introduced to the wound by forcing the saline through a syringe using high-pressure force. The syringe should be held 1–2 inches or 2.5–5cms above the wound and this procedure should continue until the wound is clean of dried blood and contaminants.

A more invasive way of cleaning the wound is by using forceps and scissors. This should not cause pain as the tissues have been severed during the injury and therefore the nerve endings are severed until repair. Smaller particles can actually be picked out from the wound using sterile forceps. In deeper wounds the subcutaneous fat can be excised using sterile scissors and forceps. As this is deeply embedded in the wound there is no concern over cosmetic results.

In preparation for the wound to be repaired with good cosmetic results and good apposition, the wound edges must be straight and linear. This can be achieved by using sterile scissors to trim any jagged wound edges. A wound that is not properly cleansed and debrided may give rise to infection and delayed wound healing, thus both must be completed prior to closure or repair.

Wound Closure

The purpose of primary closure of a wound is to approximate the wound edges correctly and there are different types of wound closure to be considered. The type of wound closure selected will very much be dependent on the depth and age of the wound, the appropriate training and skill of the practitioner to perform the procedure and the patient's tolerance.

The different types of wound closure discussed will be:

- suture material;
- skin staples;
- tissue adhesive;
- adhesive strips.

It is very important for the nurse to understand the reasons for, and advantages and disadvantages of suturing versus the other forms of wound closure as, once the wound is assessed, the rationale for selecting one form of wound closure over another will need to be given to the patient. This not only allows for full explanation of pending procedures to reassure the patient but also involves the patient in the plan of his/her care, therefore allowing verbal consent to be gained.

Wound Closure using Suture Technique

The healing of a wound is reliant on the practitioner's experience and skills in suturing. It is therefore important that the nurse has gained the necessary skills, involving both practical training and local competence assessments, prior to carrying out the task.

Selecting the Correct Sutures, Suture Materials and Instruments

Incorrect or inappropriate consideration of the suture material selected for wound closure may cause the wound to react to the suture, resulting in infection and wound breakdown. Considerations for selecting suture materials are based on the material being easy to handle, free from infection risk and well tested. It is also important that the suture material is strong and has good tensile strength to prevent breaking and unravelling.

Suture materials are divided into two types:

- absorbable sutures;
- non-absorbable sutures.

They are either monofilament (single thread) material or braided (twisted thread) materials.

Absorbable Sutures

These are often used to close deeper tissue injuries. They have the advantage that they will remove tension from the surface of the wound and close dead space. As they are embedded in the inner tissues there is a possibility that the tissues could react to the sutures, leading to infection. Also, they may not always be absorbed within the time duration expected.

Non-absorbable Sutures

These sutures are used on the outer surface of the skin to appose outer wound edges. They are the most common type of sutures used in superficial, uncomplicated wounds. They can guide the practitioner to the tension placed on the wound and they generally cause less irritability and are less likely to be rejected by the wound. However, the nurse should remain aware that their tensile strength might produce some inflammation around the wound site once closed.

There are different characteristics of suture materials that give the practitioner choice over what to use and why:

- *Monofilaments*: These sutures are single stranded fibres. They are more slippery than other suture materials, which is why they require secure knotting. As there is only one strand this material carries a low risk of infection, as there is nowhere for bacteria to get trapped. The material is strong yet pliable, and therefore offers very good security over joints and produces less inflammatory reactions.
- *Braided*: In these sutures, two strands of material are entwined. This has the advantage of requiring only minimal knotting to give a secure finish. However, the braided material can allow bacteria to be harboured between the fibres, leading to infection in the wound (Boriskin, 1994) and if infection becomes evident the sutures must be removed immediately.

The indication for suturing is for primary closure of a wound that is uncomplicated but may be too deep or bleeding too much to allow for any other form of wound closure.

Advantages of Suturing

- Effectively keeps the tissue edges of the wound together aiding natural healing, minimizing scarring and therefore obtaining a better cosmetic finish.
- Facilitates secure supportive movement of the laceration, particularly when over a joint.

Disadvantages of Suturing

- Can be painful despite local anaesthesia infiltration as the initial injection of lignocaine to the wound may cause discomfort.
- Time consuming.

There are also complications of suture insertion, which are usually related to the practitioner's experience. These include:

- fascia is not closed;
- subcutaneous sutures are too tight;

- angle of the needle at the entry and exit of the wound is incorrect and uneven, causing skin edge eversion;
- sutures are too far from wound edge making the wound gape;
- skin sutures may be either too tight or too loose.

Needles

The needles used for suturing vary in size and are measured in gauges dependent on the needle width and suture material thickness; the lower the gauge the more appropriate for thin and delicate skin.

Table 12.1 gives a general guide for the choice of suture needles. The needles for the suturing procedure are curved and are known as cutting needles. They are designed so that the outer edge is sharp for precise penetration of the skin whilst the inner portion is flattened so that the needle puncture mark is not enlarged.

Table 12.1 Choice of suture needles

Anatomical site	Suture needle size
Scalp	3/0 or 4/0
Face	6/0
Eyelid	6/0 or 7/0
Ear	4/0 or 5/0
Inside mouth	4/0 or 5/0
Arm	4/0 or 5/0
Leg	3/0 or 4/0
Foot or hand – dorsal	4/0 or 5/0
Foot or hand – palmar	3/0

Infiltrating Lignocaine to Wounds Prior to Closure

Lignocaine comes in different concentrations: 0.5%, 1% and 2% ampoules. It works by acting as an inhibitor to nerve impulses from sensory nerves by stabilizing the neuronal membrane. The choice lies in the strength of lignocaine. If 1% is used this will numb the wound, blocking pain stimuli and leaving touch and pressure intact. If 2% is used all stimuli are diminished, including both pressure and touch. A side-effect of lignocaine toxicity is a myocardial

inhibitory effect and therefore the doses have to be carefully monitored. It is advised that the maximum doses for adults of lignocaine
are:

1% lignocaine: 20 ml maximum;
2% lignocaine: 10 ml maximum.

Steps to Close the Wound using the Suturing Technique

Sutures may be applied using a variety of techniques: interrupted,
continuous, mattress, blanket or subcutaneous. For the purpose of
this chapter the interrupted technique will be discussed as this is the
most common form of suturing used within the A&E setting.

Once the wound is fully anaesthetized it is cleaned thoroughly,
trimming any excessive damaged tissue edges and removing debris
and devitalized soft tissue as required. This will aid optimum, uncomplicated healing and prevent the later appearance of tattooing. Suturing should then commence, aiming to distribute even tension
throughout the wound. The practitioner should aim to start suturing
somewhere near to the middle of the wound with an anchor stitch,
entering at a 90° angle. This helps to approximate the wound edges,
allowing even tension throughout the procedure.

It must be noted that this basic description is no substitute for
practical demonstration and supervised practice.

Wound Closure using Staples

Staples (also known as clips) are an alternative method of skin
closure. They nip the skin edges together but, unlike sutures, they
can only be inserted using the interrupted technique.

Indications for Use

Staples can only nip the skin together for superficial, linear and
uncomplicated lacerations. It is not advisable to use staples on lacerations to the hand as hand movements are inhibited. Also they
should be discouraged on facial lacerations, as meticulous skin apposition is essential for cosmetic purposes.

As they are a close alternative to sutures, the nurse must understand the rationale for selecting staples over sutures so that this

choice may be explained to the patient. This will involve the patient in his/her plan of care and give him/her a choice of wound closure. The patient's records should also reflect this.

The advantages of staples are that:

- staples are not as time-consuming to use as sutures because they are inserted quickly;
- staples may enhance the patient's acceptance and cooperation, as there is no needle involved in the procedure. Furthermore, no needle involvement means less opportunity for needle-stick injuries to the practitioner;
- staples are made of stainless steel and are therefore less likely to cause irritation or infection than sutures (Macgregor et al., 1989);
- staples are easily identified at time of removal.

The disadvantages of staples are that:

- staples are more expensive;
- patients are known to experience more discomfort on removal of staples than sutures;
- using staples may mean the practitioner is less inclined to explore the wound than if the wound is sutured.

Evaluation following Closure using Sutures/Staples

The wound must be evaluated post-closure (Table 12.2).

Procedure for Applying Tissue Adhesive to Close Wounds

Nurse Assessment

Tissue adhesive could be described as 'superglue for the skin' owing to its instant adherence to the skin, approximating wound edges. The wound must be fully assessed as described earlier prior to selecting a wound suitable for closure using tissue adhesive. As with all wounds, a primary laceration is the wound that is more likely to heal without complications using glue. To optimize wound healing with tissue adhesive a wound must be linear, superficial, non-bleeding and uncomplicated.

Table 12.2 Advice to patient following wound closure with sutures/staples

Action	Rationale
The neurovascular status of the wound must be checked	To ensure no neurological deficit has occurred following invasive repair of the wound (it should be noted that the effects of lignocaine will last for approximately 75 minutes but may last up to 2 hours). The patient must be informed that sensation in the sutured area may be reduced for this time
Note the wound edges for apposition, inflammation or further bleeding	For elimination of primary infection, breakdown of the wound or haematoma formation, which may be evidence of continued internal bleeding
Advise the patient to observe the wound for bleeding or oozing, inflammation, redness or pain. Patients should be advised to keep the dressing clean and dry for at least 5 days or until the sutures/staples are removed. Provide the patient with a wound care leaflet to reinforce verbal health advice	To detect early signs of secondary infection so that the patient may return to his/her GP. Also this will self-empower the patient to care for his/her wound, utilizing the principles of asepsis
Advise the patient of when to visit his/her health centre for removal of sutures/staples	To optimize wound healing and prevent infection from delayed wound closure material

Indications for using Tissue Adhesive

These are:

- small scalp wounds;
- superficial minor skin wounds, especially in children;
- wounds < 3 cm long which do not extend through the dermis (Pope, 1993; Bache et al., 1998);
- wounds that are not bleeding.

Advantages of using Tissue Adhesive

- Tissue adhesive is much quicker to apply than sutures or staples. It is also easier to apply, requiring less training.
- No equipment is necessary, making tissue adhesive more cost effective.

- It may be popular with many patients, particularly children, because no local anaesthesia is required prior to glue application.
- General practitioner visits are unnecessary as no sutures or staples need to be removed.

Disadvantages of using Tissue Adhesive

- Tissue adhesive should be applied only to wound edges. If it is applied into the wound it may be the focus of an infection.
- Some tissue adhesives generate heat on bonding and the initial exothermic reaction can cause patient discomfort and some tissue damage.
- Glue cannot be used close to blood vessels or wounds that are haemorrhaging as a thrombosis may originate from the exothermic polymerization not adhering to the skin edges.
- If tissue adhesive is used across moveable surfaces such as joints the wound will be more likely to split open.
- The tissue adhesive bonds very rapidly. This may be advantageous but also means that revision of the closure is precluded once the wound edges are opposed.

Tissue adhesive may be applied either by squeezing the ampoule to spread a fine line across the wound or by applying it in a series of dots across the wound.

Evaluation of Wound following Closure with Tissue Adhesive

The nurse must carry out a post-application check once the glue has been applied to the wound. The wound must be checked to note that:

- there is no further bleeding;
- the wound edges are approximated, the laceration is firmly closed and the glue is hardened and set.

The evaluation process also involves the advice given to the patient following the procedure to prevent any complications of wound closure (Table 12.3).

Wound Closure using Adhesive Strips

There are particular types of wounds that may be closed using adhesive strips. These are minor, uncomplicated, superficial wounds or

Table 12.3 Advice to patient following closure with wound adhesive

Action	Rationale
The patient should be advised to leave the wound uncovered (unless it is a child)	For glue to lift off naturally with the scab
The area should be kept clean and dry for 5 days, avoiding hair washing or combing over the area if applied to the scalp	This may cause the wound to re-open
Advise the patient not to pick at the wound	This may cause the wound to re-open and bleed
Inform the patient that the glue dissolves naturally, lifting off with the scab	To prevent premature concerns as to how glue is removed
Advise the patient to seek review if the wound begins to become painful, swollen, bleeds or discharges exudate	This may be the first sign of secondary infection

skin flaps. The wound must therefore be examined fully to ensure that there is no damage to inner structures, which would exclude using adhesive strips for wound closure.

Planning for Wound Closure using Strips

Indications for using adhesive strips are:

- for flap and pretibial lacerations where the flap edge can be pulled together;
- superficial linear lacerations that are under little tension;
- patients on steroids who may have fragile skin, because adhesive strips are non-invasive and therefore prevent further trauma;
- lacerations with a greater than usual potential for infection (e.g. dog bites) because sutures and staples may act as a foreign body in an infected wound and may therefore be rejected, causing the wound to break down;
- adhesive strips may be used in addition to sutures or staples for gaping areas following closure;
- following suture removal to offer support to the wound.

Advantages of using Adhesive Tapes

- No residual marks are left, unlike the case of sutures or staples.
- They are cheap, quick and easy to apply with no need for invasive removal.
- Tapes are painless because they do not require local anaesthetic infiltration.
- They have a greater resistance to wound infection than sutures.
- They allow an even distribution of tension across the wound.

Disadvantages of using Adhesive Tapes

- They cannot be used on sweaty, oily, hairy or scaly skin as they will not adhere.
- They may be inappropriately used as a quick alternative option to suturing.
- They cannot be used on wounds that need to be kept dry and immobile such as wounds over joints, the palmar surface of the hands or feet, or deep wounds involving inner structures or irregular wounds.
- They are difficult to use on young or uncooperative children.
- They may cause gaping wounds under tension.

Strips must never be applied circumferentially around a digit as this may result in a constricting band.

Evaluation

Once the strips have been applied it is important to check wound apposition using gentle movements and the patient should be able to demonstrate that he/she has a full range of movements before he/she is discharged home. The advice to be given to the patient is listed in Table 12.4.

Summary

This section has outlined the most common methods of wound closure used within the accident and emergency setting. The role of the A&E nurse is key in assessing all wounds; this will subsequently determine which type of wound closure method is most appropriate. Knowledge of the physiological processes of wound healing is therefore very important as this will help determine the current stage of wound healing. A subsequent understanding of the wound, healing process and advice on

Table 12.4 Advice to patient following wound closure with adhesive tapes

Action	Rationale
Advise patient to keep the wound covered with a non-adhesive dry dressing which applies slight pressure	This allows the wound to heal with no further bleeding
Advise patients to seek review if the wound bleeds through the dressing, becomes painful, discharges exudate or the tapes come away	These may be the first signs of secondary infection
Advise the patient to initiate passive exercises to the limb	To promote wound healing

discharge will allow the patient to understand the importance of caring for his/her wound at home, preventing complications of wound infection and empowering the patient to optimize wound healing.

Soft Tissue Injuries and Support Strapping Techniques

Many injuries that occur to upper and lower limbs are the result of minor trauma. This section covers the assessment process that the nurse may use for injured limbs following minor trauma, and how these injuries can best be managed. The main injuries discussed are sprains and strains. Although these injuries are considered to be minor it is important to note that prompt management may also be limb saving, reducing the risk of any subsequent disabilities.

- A strain is a weakening or stretching of a muscle at the tendon attachment.
- A sprain is a ligament or muscle associated with a joint that has been stretched and partially or completely torn.

Assessment of an Injured Limb

Limbs are comprised of many structures and it is important that the nurse understands these structures, their position and their function in order to allow a thorough assessment to take place:

- *Bones*: These protect organs and serve as levers for movement.
- *Ligaments*: These are fibrous connective tissues connecting bone to bone.

- *Tendons*: These are fibrous tissues connecting muscle to bone.
- *Cartilage*: This is dense connective tissue that has no neurovascular supply.
- *Joints*: These connect two bones to allow mobility and stability providing flexion, extension, medial and lateral rotation, adduction and abduction movements.
- *Blood vessels and nerves:* There is a large network of blood vessels and nerves in the lower limbs which can be affected when an injury occurs. They must be assessed for damage during examination.

When the patient arrives in A&E the nurse must not assume that a single limb complaint is the sole injury as a history of falls, contact trauma or assault may mean that there are concomitant injuries to exclude. During the assessment it is important for the nurse to establish certain factors about how the injury occurred. These include:

- identifying the mechanism of injury. This determines how the injury occurred, assessing whether the sprain/strain is mild, moderate or severe, which will allow for a subsequent plan of action to be devised;
- establishing the time elapsed since the injury to help assess the extent of internal soft tissue damage;
- establishing the neurovascular status of the limb. This will involve checking pulses distal to the limb involved in the trauma. Checking the colour for pallor or blanching may further determine any neurovascular compromise or damage of peripheral nerves. The temperature of the limb should be checked by touching the limb and any reduced or raised temperature should be noted. Localized redness and increased temperature in a limb may indicate underlying infection;
- performing a capillary refill test to determine the flow of oxygenated blood to the injured limb. This is performed by applying pressing to the finger/toe nail and then quickly releasing the pressure. This should be applied for 5 seconds and capillary refill should return in 2 seconds;
- removing all jewellery because a constricting band may cause restriction in the flow of blood to the limb as a result of associated swelling;

- ensuring normal function and movements of the upper and lower limbs to determine which part of the ligaments, tendons or muscles has been affected;
- determining the dominant hand for upper limb injuries so that consideration may be given to the most appropriate treatment, which will minimize limb immobilization.

Management of Upper Limb Soft Tissues Injuries

Shoulder Injuries

The shoulder is a ball and socket joint supported by strong muscles and ligaments. Any soft tissue injury here may result in the shoulder becoming very stiff or cause clicking within the shoulder joint which may indicate that the cartilage or joint capsule in the shoulder are injured. The movement which determines any injury in the shoulder is the abduction movement. The range of this movement is 0° to 180° and any restriction in the movement would identify an injury in the shoulder ligament or muscle.

The muscle which initiates abduction is the supraspinatus muscle. Whilst this muscle is moving the deltoid and other rotational cuff muscles abduct to 90°, then the scapula begins to rotate. The practitioner must be aware that difficulty in initiating the abduction movement may indicate partial or complete rupture of the supraspinatus tendon or acute or chronic inflammation of the supraspinatus tendon (this is normally a condition known as acute or chronic supraspinatus tendonitis). Stiffness of the shoulder may indicate an injury to the rotator cuff and scapula muscles or strain and sprain of the acromioclavicular joint. These injuries are very common in the elderly and specific management and advice about exercises for these injuries is very important.

Nursing Intervention and Management of the Shoulder Injury

The patient should be advised to carry out passive exercises to gently strengthen the shoulder ligaments and aid full movement. If inflammation of the joint or ligaments is noted, the patient may recover with non-steroidal anti-inflammatory drugs, absent any underlying contraindications to such medication. Resting the shoulder is an important part of the healing process and a broad arm sling should be applied. Gentle shoulder and neck exercises should be advised to regain normal movement at 90° and to prevent frozen shoulder.

Hand Injuries

In the hand, soft tissue injuries can affect the flexor tendons, extensor tendons or the intrinsic muscles. Tendons in the hand may be assessed by extending the fingers. Normal tendon function is then identified through extension and flexion of the fingers under passive movements. Any restriction in these movements means that the tendon may be injured. Other movements that may detect a soft tissue injury in the hand are flexion, extension, adduction and abduction of the wrist, fingers or thumb. Restriction of movements must be reported as poor management of this may lead to permanent disability of the upper limb.

A rupture of the terminal extensor tendon, known as mallet finger, leaves the distal interphalangeal joint with an inability to get extension. Nursing intervention for this type of injury is by applying a mallet splint to the finger, straightening the terminal joint and avoiding any flexion or extension. Elastic adhesive tape is applied to the splint to keep it secure in an extended position.

Other common soft tissue injuries of the hand are tenosynovitis (inflammation of the sheath in which the tendon runs), collateral ligament injuries, repetitive strain injury and swelling and bruising of the soft tissues.

Nursing Intervention and Management of Hand Injuries

As with the shoulder, the patient must be encouraged to regain full mobility of his/her hand through passive exercises. Any inflammation of the hand that is not red or hot indicating signs of infection may be treated with anti-inflammatory medication. To reduce swelling and bruising the patient should be advised to adhere to the following non-invasive treatments:

- *rest*: other than passive exercises;
- *ice*: ice packs will help to reduce swelling;
- *compression*: using appropriate supportive strapping;
- *elevation*: by raising the limb to reduce swelling.

There are a number of bandaging techniques that may be used to support and aid healing of the injured hand and the choice will depend on local protocols. A common type of simple wrist strapping may be achieved using elasticated tubular bandaging. This is applied just below the elbow to the metacarpo-phalangeal heads of the hand, allowing movements of the joint. The patient should avoid creating creases in the bandage and folding the bandage over, which will result in uneven pressure on some limb parts. This type of support strapping may also be used for soft tissue injuries to the upper and lower forearm and the elbow region. If the injury is due to tenosynovitis or a repetitive strain injury to the tendons and ligaments, a simple wrist brace with support backing will aid support, allowing the hand to rest.

For soft tissue injuries to the fingers or thumbs, individual strapping devices may be used. If a finger is injured, advice to rest the finger with support against a neighbouring finger will aid healing by allowing for gentle exercises of the fingers. Similar support may be given for the injured thumb by applying a thumb spica (a figure-of-eight elasticated strapping).

Advice on Discharge

It is important to advise the patient of symptoms that may indicate reduced circulation due to restriction of blood flow by the splint or bandaging, and all proximal phalanges of the hand must be checked for movement, colour, warmth and sensation following application of strapping and splints. Any decrease or alteration in these must result in removal of the strapping and review/reapplication as appropriate. All patients must be given an indication of how long the injured limb takes to heal, as many people will be keen to recommence their normal activities. This will vary dependent on the extent of the injury and loss of function involved. It is important that all of this advice is given to patients verbally and then reinforced by appropriate injury advice sheets. This will subsequently promote faster healing of the injury by empowering the patient to best manage his/her care at home.

Management of Lower Limb Injuries

Ankle Injuries

Sprains or strains to the ankle are commonly divided into mild, moderate or severe:

- Mild strain:
  - local tenderness;
  - spasm.

- Moderate strain: as above but also:
  - swelling;
  - discoloration;
  - short-term loss of function.
- Severe strain: as above but also:
  - snapping noise at time of injury.

The three levels of sprains are listed below:

- Mild sprain:
  - slight pain;
  - slight swelling.
- Moderate sprain: as above but also:
  - tenderness on palpation;
  - short-term loss of function.
- Severe sprain: as above but also:
  - discoloration.

Assessment of Lower Limb Injuries

To assess the level of sprain or strain a neurovascular assessment must first be performed as the peripheral nerves in the lower limb may be affected by soft tissue trauma. As with upper limb injuries colour, warmth and sensation checks of the injured limb must also be assessed on patient arrival. To assess the nerve functions, the peroneal and sciatic or tibial nerves must be checked. To test the peroneal nerve the nurse should instruct the patient to extend either the great toe or the foot as inability to do this may indicate nerve damage. The sciatic and tibial nerves may be tested by localizing sensation of pain and touch by identifying sensation to the sole of the foot. The pedis pulse in the lower leg should be palpated, noting its presence or absence and whether it is weak or strong. Any decrease in circulation, nerve loss or absence of the pulse must be documented and reported to a medical colleague immediately to prevent permanent neurovascular damage.

Nursing Intervention and Management of Ankle Injuries

How the patient with an injured ankle should be treated is dependent upon the level of sprain or strain. Mild to moderate sprains and strains should follow the RICE mnemonic (see page 335), with advice to bear slight weight on the injured limb. This treatment is also advised for severe sprains and strains with the additional advice to use crutches and remain non-weight bearing for approximately 3 days, with gentle passive exercise and physiotherapy as indicated. It is also advisable for patients with moderate to severe sprains and strains to take non-steroidal anti-inflammatory drugs.

The most common below-knee support strappings for such injuries are listed below, although these may vary dependent on local protocols:

- *Elasticated tubular support bandage*: These are often applied for effusions and sprains/strains or general soft tissue injuries. The patent's leg width around the calf is measured and the appropriate size tubular bandaging is then applied using an applicator. The bandaging should cover the lower leg from just below the knee, over the ankle and ending at the metatarsal head joints of the foot. This is to allow for passive exercises to be performed. The patient must be advised to remove the support bandage at night-time to allow for adequate circulation to occur.
- *Wool and crepe bandage*: This is useful for sprains/strains where severe swelling and loss of function has occurred. Cotton-wool roll is applied from the knee down to the foot at right angles (following a figure-of-eight pattern). The crepe bandage is then applied in a similar fashion.

Injuries to the Toes

Non-bony injuries of the toes may be treated in the same way as injuries to the fingers and thumb. A sprain or bruising to the big toe may be treated with a toe spica to allow support and comfort. Injuries involving the other toes may be treated with neighbour strapping to add support and comfort. The importance of pain relief and passive exercises also applies to toe injuries in order for the patient to regain normal function and ability within a short period post-injury.

Other Lower Limb Injuries

Another injury that requires treatment is a rupture of the Achilles tendon. The Achilles tendon is situated at the back of the leg, below the calf and just above the calcaneum bone. Patients presenting with this injury are usually athletic and commonly give a history of running downhill, moving on their toes during uphill running, stop-and-start games such as tennis or wearing incorrect running shoes. The person complains of a 'snapping' sound or sensation and acute pain above the heel. The diagnosis of this injury can be determined by a positive Simmond's Test. The patient is asked to lie on his/her front with the injured leg extended and foot over the couch. The calf muscle is then squeezed. A test is positive when no heel pull or upward movement is seen and the foot remains still. The treatment for Achilles tendon rupture is initial immobilization, often with plaster of Paris application. Such ruptures often require surgical repair and are therefore referred to the orthopaedic team.

Another foot problem is plantar fasciitis, which is a soft tissue condition affecting the heel region. It is an inflammatory condition of the plantar aponeurosis, which is fascia in the sole of the foot. The patient often gives a history of constant walking or running. The treatment for this is with below-knee strapping or heel pads, passive exercises, RICE advice and non-steroidal anti-inflammatory medication.

Advice on Discharge

The general advice for patients in respect of compression strapping is as for upper limb injuries. However, it is more important for patients with lower limb injuries to be advised to carry out passive exercises frequently soon after the injury as long-term stiffness of a lower limb joint may result in a longer rehabilitation programme. Assistance of mobility with the use of walking aids should be encouraged as a minimum requirement only, and patients must be discouraged as soon as pain allows from relying on additional aids to help regain independence.

Conclusion

This chapter has summarized the basic pathophysiology of wound healing and soft tissue injuries to allow the nurse to determine which inner structures may have been damaged following injury, therefore enabling him/her to prioritize care accordingly. It is apparent that the assessment skills of an A&E nurse are a fundamental part of the management of such injuries as prompt and accurate assessment can determine the immediacy of treatment for the injury, ensuring that normal function is regained quickly by allowing the healing process to take place.

Suggested Further Reading

Apley GA, Solomon L (1993) Apley's system of orthopaedics and fractures, 7th Edn. Oxford: Butterworth-Heinemann Ltd.
Bache JB, Armitt CR, Tobiss JR (1998) A Colour Atlas of Nursing Procedures in Accident and Emergency. London: Wolfe Medical Publications.
British Medical Association (1999) Advanced Paediatric Life Support: The Practical Approach, 2nd Edn. London: Latimer Trend & Company Ltd UK
Trott AF (1991) Wounds and Lacerations: Emergency Care and Closure. St Louis, MO: Mosby Year Book.

References

Bache JB, Armitt CR, Tobiss JR (1998) A Colour Atlas of Nursing Procedures in Accident and Emergency. London: Wolfe Medical Publications.
Boriskin MI (1994) Primary care and management of wounds: cleaning, suturing and infection control. Nurse Practitioner 19(11): 38–55.
Doughty D (1992) In Bryant RA, Acute and Chronic Wounds: Nursing Management. St Louis, MO: Mosby Year Book.
Macgregor F, McCombe A, Macleod D (1989) Skin stapling of wounds in the accident and emergency department. Injury 20: 347–8.
Morison M (1992) A Colour Guide to the Management of Wounds. London: Wolfe Medical Publications.
Pope S (1993) The use of histoacryl tissue adhesive in children's A&E. Paediatric Nursing 5(2).
Tortora GJ, Anagnostakos NP (1990) Principles of Anatomy and Physiology. New York: Harper & Row.
Trott AT (1991) Wounds and Lacerations: Emergency Care and Closure. St Louis, MO: Mosby Year Book.

Chapter 13
Ophthalmic Injuries

LYNN BEUN

Introduction

Eye injuries are a frequent cause of attendance at the accident and emergency (A&E) department. The international incidence of eye trauma is difficult to identify as reporting methods are not complete (McGrory, 1997). A study in an English A&E department demonstrated that 6.1% of patients had an ophthalmic problem (Edwards, 1987). It is important to remember that such injuries require skilled nursing and a sympathetic and caring approach to the patient. Any eye problem that causes visual disturbance can lead to fears and anxiety that permanent visual loss may occur.

Some patients may also express an anxiety about having the eyes touched and this can be similar in nature to a phobia. This can make first aid treatment difficult, so it is important to acknowledge these fears and talk to the patient about them rather than being dismissive. This anxiety in the population about eye problems is reflected by health care staff who frequently express concerns about treating patients with ophthalmic conditions and who lack confidence in doing so.

This chapter aims to provide the reader with a basic knowledge of the eye injuries most frequently encountered within the A&E department and enable the nurse to provide appropriate nursing care for the patient.

Anatomy and Physiology

In order to gain understanding about eye injuries and how they affect the patient, it is essential to first have a basic knowledge of the anatomy and physiology of the eye.

Despite their perceived vulnerability, the eyes are surrounded by structures that form some protection from injury. They are placed within the bony orbit of the skull, which affords some security from blunt injury. Eyebrows and eyelashes protect the eyes from foreign particles and perspiration.

The eyelids protect the eyes from excessive light/foreign bodies and provide a protective seal during normal sleep.

Small sebaceous glands known as Meibomian glands are situated within the eyelids. There are approximately 30 in the upper eyelid and 20 in the lower lid (Snell and Lemp, 1989). Their function is to produce an oily secretion which makes the closed lids airtight and which forms part of the tear film. Tears are produced in the lacrimal gland and flow onto the eye from small ducts in the upper lid. Tears keep the eye moist and clean and also contain an enzyme called lysozome that is bactericidal. Injury or irritation to the eye results in the eye watering, which is a protective mechanism and an attempt by the body to rid itself of the foreign particle or substance. This is why the patient complains of watering eyes when he/she has had a chemical injury or foreign body in the eye.

Tears are then drained away through the lacrimal punctae into the lacrimal sac and then into the nasal cavity. Dacryocystitis is a painful infection and blockage of the lacrimal sac. The conjunctiva is a loose mucous membrane that lines the inside of the eyelids and anterior surface of the eyeball. The blood vessels become inflamed or injected when infection or irritation is present and makes the eye appear red.

The sclera is the white fibrous coat of the eye that comprises strong connective tissue which gives shape to the eye. The cornea is a clear, sensitive and non-vascular structure that enables light to pass through into the eye. Sensory nerve fibres supply the cornea from the trigeminal (V cranial) nerve. If the cornea is damaged, this results in a particularly acute pain, which is sharp and stabbing in nature (Cheng et al., 1997).

The iris consists of pigmented muscle fibres that control the size of the pupil. The nerve supply is from the sympathetic and parasympathetic nervous systems. In conditions of poor lighting, the pupil enlarges to allow in more light to enable us to see. The pupil also dilates when the sympathetic nervous system is stimulated (e.g. in fright). In bright light the pupil constricts. Drugs may also affect the size of the pupils, for example atropine dilates the pupils whilst opiates cause constriction. When comparing the size of the pupils, it is worth remembering that it has been estimated that approximately 25% of people have pupils that are slightly unequal in size (Snell and Lemp, 1989); this is known as physiological anisocoria. The patient and his/her family or friends may be aware of this and this fact, if known, should be documented. In anisocoria the pupillary reflexes are normal. If in any doubt, the nurse should report all suspected pupillary abnormalities to the medical staff for further investigation.

The lens is a crystalline avascular structure that refracts the light onto the retina. The retina is a layer of specialized nerve cells that are sensitive to light. When the image is focused onto the retina, it is inverted due to the refractive properties of the cornea and lens.

The choroid is the vascular layer between the sclera and retina. The function of the choroid is to provide a blood supply to part of the retina. The light impulses pass from the retina to the optic nerve (second cranial nerve) and through a complex pathway to the visual cortex area of the brain, which interprets the messages received by the eyes. Because the visual pathway through the brain is long and complex, head injuries and neurological problems can result in visual disturbances and loss of visual field. Movement of the eyes is effected by the extra-ocular muscles via specific cranial nerves. Damage to the pathways of these cranial nerves (e.g. from trauma, disease or aneurysm) will result in muscle paralysis and the patient will complain of double vision which is relieved by covering one eye.

Nursing Care

The nurse's involvement with the patient's care may begin before the patient arrives in the department, if the patient or their representative telephones for advice. Recent research has shown that large numbers of patients seek advice to enable them to make empowered decisions about their eye problems (Rendell, 1997). The advice required varies from first aid to health education.

History

On arrival in the department, a careful history should be taken, which will enable the nurse to obtain an accurate assessment of the urgency of the eye problem. Pain is not always a good indicator of the seriousness of an eye condition and nurses should be wary of the fact that a vision-threatening perforating injury may be almost painless (Marsden, 1996). A patient presenting with a history of hammering metal or using a hammer and chisel may have an intra-ocular foreign body (Owen et al., 1987). The nurse should also be aware that the abused child may present with eye injuries (Tongue, 1991) and be alert to that fact and observe the child for evidence of other injuries or behavioural indicators. First aid should be given promptly, especially if the patient has experienced a chemical injury to the eye. Any history of previous eye problems and any known family history of eye disorders, in particular glaucoma, should also be noted. As with all patients, details of general health, medications and known allergies are required prior to treatment.

Assessment

During the assessment stage, if the patient is experiencing severe pain, a local anaesthetic eyedrop may be instilled in order to examine the patient and facilitate first aid treatment. The patient should be warned that the effects are temporary and that it is not a form of treatment. The visual acuity should always be tested. This can be a useful medical indicator of the type of eye pathology and is a legal requirement. The most common eye-test chart in use is called the Snellen Chart. It should be well-illuminated and placed six metres from the patient. If the patient wears spectacles for distance vision, such as driving, the visual acuity should be tested with the patient wearing his/her spectacles. If the patient is wearing contact lenses, this should also be noted. Each eye should be tested separately and the result recorded in the patient's notes. When examining the patient, a pen torch may be used to obtain a preliminary assessment but a slit-lamp microscope is desirable for comprehensive examination of the patient.

Examination of the Patient

First, observe the patient to see how he/she appears. A pain scale may be used to identify the patient's level of pain. The nature of the pain can assist in identifying the diagnosis. For example, corneal abrasions have a characteristic sharp pain with foreign body sensation, which can give the patient pain at the back of the eye. When the general demeanour and pain level of the patient has been identified, the face should be examined. There may be signs of rash, redness or bruising, or, if the patient is burnt, blistering of the skin. Next, focus on the eyes. A skilled nurse can obtain an accurate assessment of the problem using a pen-torch. Observe whether the patient appears to be very sensitive to the torchlight. Look at the eyelids and then concentrate on the eye itself. Examine each structure in turn, relating your findings to the history and also checking for consistency between history and findings.

Eye Injuries

Blunt Injuries

A periorbital haematoma (commonly known as a 'black eye') is caused by blunt injury such as a fist or following sports injury. The tissues around the eye become very bruised and swollen and it may be difficult to visualize the patient's eye. An ice pack applied to the lids may help to reduce the pain and swelling. When the patient presents with bilateral periorbital haematoma following head injury, staff should be aware that this may be a sign of a fractured base of skull and should assess the patient carefully. Following blunt injury, the eye may appear red, due to sub-conjunctival haemorrhage. Examination of the fundus by an eye specialist is advisable as the patient may have bruising to the retina known as commotio retinae, and retinal detachment is known to be a complication of blunt injury (Johnston, 1991).

A blow-out fracture of the orbital floor may follow blunt injury and all patients with periorbital haematoma should be checked to exclude this diagnosis. The key signs and symptoms are:

- pain on ocular movement;
- double vision and restricted ocular movement;
- surgical emphysema;
- numbness of the lower lid.

These symptoms are caused when the impact causes a compression fracture of the orbital floor. The inferior rectus muscle then herniates into the fracture and becomes trapped, causing restriction of ocular movement and diplopia. Enophthalmos, or retraction of the globe, may be present, but this is often difficult to identify within the A&E department, particularly when the lids are bruised and swollen.

An orbital X-ray will provide evidence of fracture and the patient should be referred for ophthalmic assessment, as some fractures require surgery.

Following blunt injury, damage to the underlying blood vessels may lead to hyphaema, which is the presence of blood in the anterior chamber of the eye. The majority of patients may be treated as outpatients, by resting at home (Williams et al., 1993) but should always be referred for an ophthalmic opinion, as about 7% of patients with hyphaema have been shown to develop more serious eye pathology, including raised intra-ocular pressure and retinal tears (Ng et al., 1992).

Corneal Abrasion

Corneal abrasion is a common eye injury, which has been found to account for 12.5% of the total number of attenders at an ophthalmic A&E department (Knox and McIntee, 1995). A corneal abrasion occurs when there is damage to the corneal epithelium, which exposes the sensitive nerve fibres and the result is a superficial but very painful problem. Corneal abrasions may be caused by a variety of injuries. The following is a list of common causes:

- gardening injury (e.g. on plants or garden canes);
- use of contact lenses (e.g. insertion and removal);
- assault (e.g. rings on fists, deliberate scratching);
- craftwork injuries (e.g. on paper, card or pencils);
- sports injury (e.g. rugby, squash);
- animal scratches (e.g. cats and dogs).

In many departments simple corneal abrasions are now treated by nurse practitioners. Skill is required to treat this problem as the pain may be very severe and as a consequence the patient may have anxieties about the long-term visual outcome. Providing information about the condition can help the patient with pain control; for example giving reassurance that although the injury is painful, recovery will occur within a few days. It should also be carefully explained to the patient that although local anaesthetic eyedrops have been instilled, they cannot be given as a regular form of treatment as they can cause corneal damage (Bolijka et al., 1994). Medical treatment involves providing a topical prophylactic antibiotic ointment, such as chloramphenicol. The ointment also acts as a lubricant. Some concerns about topical chloramphenicol have recently been raised as it has been linked with bone marrow depression, mainly after long-term use (Doona and Walsh, 1995). However, it remains at present the treatment of choice and is believed to be relatively safe provided the patient uses it for no longer than 14 days (Diamond and Leeming, 1995).

Some of the pain of corneal abrasion may be relieved by dilating the patient's pupil using a cycloplegic eyedrop, which relieves some of the spasm that makes the pain even worse. Before instilling this drop the nurse should check with the patient to see if there is any known personal or family history of glaucoma as individuals with shallow anterior chambers may be predisposed to developing acute angle closure glaucoma and using a dilating eyedrop can precipitate this. Oral analgesics with a combination of paracetamol and codeine phosphate may be helpful for this type of pain. Occasionally, if the pain is intractable, intra-muscular analgesia may be required to control pain.

Eyepads

Previously it was thought that all patients with corneal abrasions should have their eye firmly patched for 24 hours. The rationale was that the eyelid acted as a splint and helped the cornea to heal evenly. However, there is a growing body of evidence which indicates that the use of eyepads is not required (Kirkpatrick et al., 1993) and may actually prevent healing (Kaiser, 1995). Experiments on subjects with healthy eyes demonstrated that patching caused blurring of vision and corneal damage (Frucht-Pery et al., 1993). A recent systematic review of randomised controlled trials has indicated that eye patches produced no significant difference in the rate of healing (Flynn et al., 1998).

Sometimes patients may request a patch, stating that they would feel more comfortable with one on. The author recommends that in these cases a patch may be applied, but it should be made clear to patients that it has no therapeutic use, it is for their comfort only and should be removed if they feel discomfort. The nurse should suggest use of dark glasses to relieve photophobia in preference to patching.

Long-term Problems

A long-term problem that may occur after corneal abrasion is known as recurrent corneal erosion. The patient typically complains of recurrent episodes of pain in the eye early in the morning with photophobia and watering. The symptoms are caused by a breakdown of the healed corneal epithelium. Various treatments have been tried (Hykin et al., 1994) but the most frequently used therapy is simple lubrication using paraffin ointment at bedtime to prevent further attacks. Acute episodes should be treated as a corneal abrasion. Referral to an ophthalmologist is desirable if problems persist.

Foreign Bodies

Superficial foreign bodies may easily be treated by the nurse within the A&E department.

Sub-tarsal

The patient may give a history of a foreign body entering the eye, especially on windy days when walking outside. On examination the eye is watering and the patient is in discomfort, complaining that it hurts more when he/she blinks. Often the patient is able to locate the foreign body him/herself underneath the upper lid.

Procedure

The nurse should explain that the foreign body may be located underneath the upper lid and that it may be removed by everting the upper lid. Local anaesthetic eyedrops may not be required if the practitioner is skilled and experienced. The patient should be seated in a chair or on a couch with the head supported. The nurse should then firmly grasp the lid margin with the thumb and forefinger and the lid should be gently flipped over using a glass rod or the wooden end of a cotton bud.

Using a cotton bud that has been moistened with saline, the conjuctival surface of the inner eyelid should then be gently wiped in order to remove any dust or foreign particles. The practitioner should always wipe the conjuctival surface, even if there is no obvious foreign body, as some small fragments and particles of wood may be similar in colour to the conjunctiva and are not always easily discernible. The eyelid should then be returned to its normal position and the patient evaluated. If the patient has not required local anaesthetic eyedrops, he/she will express almost immediate relief. If local anaesthetic eyedrops have been instilled in order to facilitate treatment, it is wise to wait 20 minutes prior to evaluation until the anaesthetic has worn off. Some discomfort will still be present, as the patient will have developed scratches on the cornea. These will heal in 24 hours. One stat dose of topical antibiotic will prevent infection from developing.

If the patient reports that the foreign body sensation persists after removal of a sub-tarsal foreign body, or that the discomfort has increased, referral to a medical officer may be required in order to exclude other eye pathology.

Corneal Foreign Body

A superficial corneal foreign body is a very common eye injury. A study in a district general hospital has indicated that 33% of the eye injuries presenting were for corneal foreign body (Edwards, 1987). Causes of corneal foreign bodies are grinding, hammering and drilling and so are often work related (Harker et al, 1991). The use of protective eyewear may reduce the risk of injury, and the Personal Protective Equipment at Work Regulations were introduced in 1993, placing responsibility on both employer and employee to conform. The nurse has a subsequent role to play in providing health promotion advice to patients on the use of protective eyewear.

Intra-ocular Foreign Bodies and Penetrating Eye Injury

These two types of injury will be considered together, as they may occur at the same time and also the management and care of the patient is similar. Both of these injuries are ocular emergencies and the patient may require urgent surgery to avoid further visual loss. Males of all ages have been identified as being more likely to have a serious eye injury requiring hospitalization and these injuries were found to occur predominantly in the home (Desai et al., 1996). In children, penetrating eye injuries most commonly occur during play, particularly in boys aged 4 to 7 years (LaRoche et al., 1988).

A penetrating eye injury may be defined as an injury that causes a full-thickness perforation of the cornea or sclera. Typical causes are:

- sharp trauma (e.g. pencil points, knives, glass, garden plants, toys needles, etc.);
- high-velocity particles;
- blunt injury (which can cause rupture of the globe of the eye).

An intra-ocular foreign body occurs when a foreign body penetrates the eye and is retained within the eye. This is an ocular emergency that requires prompt action. The patient may present with an obvious foreign body protruding from the eye and a distinct history of the event. If this is the case, the nurse should not attempt to examine the patient too vigorously, but should ensure speedy referral to an ophthalmologist. Any protruding foreign body should be left in place and no attempt should be made to remove it. Some patients with intra-ocular foreign bodies may be initially asymptomatic, particularly if the foreign body is a small particle that has penetrated at high velocity, a common cause of which is using a hammer and chisel or hammering nails. Patients who give this history may require an X-ray of the orbits to exclude this.

Common causes are:

- using a hammer and chisel/hammering nails;
- airgun pellets;
- explosions;
- debris from a penetrating injury source.

Patient Care

- Ask the patient to remain nil by mouth until further notice.
- Keep the patient as still as possible and avoid touching the eye.
- Leave any protruding foreign body in place.
- Cover the eye with an eye shield if possible. Do not apply an eyepad or apply any direct pressure to the eye or lids.
- Refer to an opthalmologist urgently.
- Check patient for shock/monitor of blood pressure and pulse.
- Identify patient's tetanus status.

The patient and his/her carers may be very distressed and concerned about the possible long-term visual outcome. If the patient is a child and the injury occurred during play, other children such as siblings may be very concerned and also require reassurance. Pain may or may not be present. The nurse should be aware that pain may not be a good indicator of the seriousness of the injury, as some patients with intra-ocular foreign bodies or penetrating injuries do not complain of severe pain.

Burns to the Eye

Chemical

Chemical injuries are one of the few true ophthalmic emergencies and prompt action can influence the outcome for the patient. Whilst both acid and alkali injuries should be treated seriously, generally acids do not cause the severe problems associated with alkalis. Alkali substances rapidly penetrate the tissues of the eye and can cause perforation of the cornea. Acids cause protein precipitation on the eye surface, which limits the penetration of the substance (Cheng et al., 1997). All chemical injuries, however, require prompt action.

Staff should also be aware that if the patient gives a history of handling plants, certain species such as euphorbia can cause pain and burning if the sap is rubbed into the eye (Kendra, 1991). Such cases should be treated as a chemical injury.

First Aid

The first treatment for almost all chemical injuries to the eye is to irrigate profusely with normal saline or water; the only exception to this is CS gas, which is discussed later. Within the A&E department, treatment may be facilitated by instilling local anaesthetic eyedrops to relieve pain. Even if the patient has received irrigation at home or by ambulance crews, it is important to repeat the washout at the hospital in order to remove particles and ensure a thorough irrigation.

The patient should be seated in a chair or laid on a couch with the head well supported. Their clothing should be protected with appropriate capes. The pH of the conjunctiva should then be assessed by using Universal paper. The conjuctiva should normally be of pH 7.5. Any alkali substance in the eye will register on the

Universal paper as pH 8 and upwards and an acid as pH 7 and below. If a sample of the substance is available, it is also useful to test that as well. The eye should then be irrigated with normal saline. A normal saline infusion administered through a giving set may be used to provide a steady flow of fluid although some practitioners prefer to use saline directly from an eyewash bottle. Either method is satisfactory.

During the irrigation the eyelid should be everted and irrigated and any cement or particles should be swept away using a moist cotton bud. The pH should be regularly tested and the irrigation continued until the pH is neutral. All patients with alkali injuries should have irrigation for at least 30 minutes and should be referred to an eye specialist for management.

CS Gas

CS gas may not be legally sold to the public in the UK, but it is known to be used in cases of assault (Morgan, 1997). The police force currently uses it to control riots and in some areas individual police officers carry it as a small aerosol. Unlike all other chemical injuries, irrigation of the eye with water or saline has been shown to prolong the burning sensation. The preferred treatment of CS gas injury is to place the patient in a well-ventilated room and direct an electric fan at the face. The passage of the air helps the gas to vaporize and rapidly relieves the irritation (Yih, 1995). This treatment is recommended only when the nurse is absolutely sure that the chemical substance that has been sprayed into the eyes is actually CS gas. Great care should be taken with victims of assault, as the substances used on the victim may be unknown and have been shown in the past to include ammonia and other strong alkalis, all of which require immediate irrigation. If there is any doubt about the nature of the chemical substance, the first aid treatment should be as for all other chemicals.

Ultra-violet

Ultra-violet light burns may be experienced by welders using a welding arc, careless use of sunlamps or occasionally after excessive sunbathing. The most common cause is from workmen welding and using inadequate eye protection. The patient complains of onset of pain, which occurs 4 to 6 hours after exposure to the UV light. On examination, the face of the patient may appear reddened. The corneal epithelium becomes damaged by the light and at first the patient develops a gritty feeling in the eye, which gradually intensifies and becomes severe. Staining with fluoroscein eyedrops reveals a punctate appearance. Treatment is similar to that for corneal abrasion: a topical antibiotic ointment, oral analgesia and cycloplegic eyedrops to reduce the ciliary spasm if required. The patient may be reassured that although the experience is painful and frightening, the eye will heal within 24 hours. The nurse should also ensure that the patient is provided with information about eye protection and welding, as persistent exposure to this problem has been shown to lead to long-term changes to the outer part of the eye (Norn and Franck, 1991).

Conclusion

This chapter has explored the care of patients presenting with some of the most common eye injuries that the nurse in A&E is likely to encounter. By taking a careful history, looking at the eye and measuring the visual acuity, the nurse should be able to identify the nature and extent of the injury and identify those that require prompt first aid or specialist referral. The reader who seeks more detailed information about injuries or ophthalmic medical problems should consult the textbooks indicated below in recommended further reading.

Recommended Further Reading

Cheng H, Burdon MA, Buckley SA, Moorman C (1997) Emergency Ophthalmology. London: BMJ Publishing Group.
Ragge NK, Easty DL (1990) Immediate Eye Care. London: Wolfe Publishing.

References

Bolijka M, Kolar G, Viden Sek J (1994) Toxic side effects of local anaesthetics on the human cornea. British Journal of Ophthalmology 78: 386–9
Cheng H, Burdon MA, Buckley SA, Moorman C (1997) Emergency Ophthalmology. London: BMJ Publishing Group.
Desai P, MacEwan CJ, Baines P, Minassian DC (1996) Incidence of cases of ocular trauma admitted to hospital and incidence of blinding outcome. British Journal of Ophthalmology 80: 592–6.
Diamond J, Leeming J (1995) Chloramphenicol eye drops: a dangerous drug? The Practitioner 239: 608–11.

Doona M, Walsh JB (1995) Use of chloramphenicol as topical eye medication: time to cry halt? British Medical Journal 310: 1217–18.

Edwards RS (1987) Ophthalmic emergencies in a district general hospital casualty department. British Journal of Ophthalmology 71: 938–42.

Flynn CA, D'Amico F, Smith G (1998) Should we patch corneal abrasions? A meta-analysis. Journal of Family Practice 47(4): 264–70.

Fox J (1988) Nursing care of patients with eye injuries in A&E. Nursing 3(31): 9–11.

Frucht-Pery J, Stiebel H, Hemo I, Ever-Hadani P (1993) Effect of eye patching on ocular surface. American Journal of Ophthalmology 115: 629–33.

Harker C, Matheson AB, Ross JA, Seaton A (1991) Accidents in the workplace. Journal of the Society of Occupational Medicine 41: 73–6.

Hykin PG, Foss AE, Pavesio C, Dart JKG (1994) The natural history and management of recurrent corneal erosion: a prospective randomised trial. Eye 8: 35–40.

Johnston PB (1991) Traumatic retinal detachment. British Journal of Ophthalmology 75: 18–21.

Kaiser P (1995) A comparison of pressure patching versus no patching for corneal abrasions due to trauma or foreign body removal. Ophthalmology 102(12): 1936–42.

Kendra J (1991) Horticulture's perennial health risk. Hospital Doctor 7 February: 41.

Kirkpatrick J, Hoh HB, Cook SD (1993) No eye pad for corneal abrasion. Eye 7: 468–71.

Knox KA, McIntee J (1995) Nurse management of corneal abrasion. British Journal of Nursing 4(8): 440–4.

LaRoche G, McIntyre L, Schertzer R (1988) Epidemiology of severe eye injuries in childhood. Ophthalmology 95(12): 1603–7.

Marsden J (1996) Ophthalmic trauma in accident and emergency. Accident and Emergency Nursing 4: 54–8.

McGrory A (1997) Eye injuries: a review of the literature with nursing implications. International Journal of Nursing Studies 34(2): 87–92.

Morgan SJ (1997) The management of chemical burns of the eye. Eyenews 4(3): 7–13

Ng CS, Sparrow JM, Strong NP, Rosenthal AR (1992) Factors related to the final visual outcome of 425 patients with traumatic hyphaema. Eye 6: 305–7.

Norn M, Franck C (1991) Long-term changes in the outer part of the eye in welders. Acta Ophthalmologica 69: 382–6.

Owen P, Keightley SJ, Elkington AR (1987) The hazards of hammers. Injury 18: 61–2.

Ragge NK, Easty DL (1990) Immediate Eye Care. London: Wolfe Publishing.

Rendell J (1997) Telephone triage in an ophthalmic accident and emergency department. Ophthalmic Nursing 1(3): 4–9.

Snell RS, Lemp MA (1989) Clinical Anatomy of the Eye. Oxford: Blackwell Scientific.

Tongue AC (1991) Editorial: The ophthalmologist's role in diagnosing child abuse. Ophthalmology 98(7): 1009–10.

Williams C, Laidlaw A, Diamond J, Pollock W, Bloom P (1993) Outpatient management of small traumatic hyphaemas: is it safe? Eye 7: 155–7.

Yih JP (1995) CS gas injury to the eye: blowing dry air onto the eye is preferable to irrigation. British Medical Journal 311: 276.

Chapter 14
Ear, Nose and Throat Emergencies

YVONNE WIMBLETON

Introduction

Patients presenting to the accident and emergency (A&E) department at St Mary's Hospital, London with ENT conditions accounted for about 7% of all attendances for one year up to April 1999. Approximately 8.5% of these patients were admitted and the degree of urgency of these cases is illustrated using the Manchester Triage categories (Mackway-Jones, 1997) (Table 14.1).

Table 14.1 Percentages of patients presenting to A&E with ENT conditions within each clinical priority

Triage priority	1	2	3	4 and 5
ENT patients presenting within category	0.3	2.5	22.3	74.9

Whilst it is acknowledged that many people attend A&E departments with ENT problems of a 'primary care' nature, this chapter seeks to address those conditions that constitute an accident or an emergency. Table 14.2 lists some common conditions seen which are deemed more appropriate for treatment by either self-care or GP intervention and will not be covered within this chapter.

355

Table 14.2 Primary care ENT conditions

Ear	Nose	Throat
External otitis	Rhinitis	Sore throat
Otitis externa	Sinusitis	Tonsillitis
Otitis media		Laryngitis
Mastoiditis		
Hearing loss (insidious onset or chronic)		
Ear wax		

Emergency Nose Conditions

Epistaxis

Common Causes and Incidence

Around 90% of all nosebleeds occur due to a ruptured vein at the front of the nasal septum, an area also known as the 'Little's area'. In older people the bleeding is usually arterial and from the posterior part of the nose. It has been estimated that at least one-seventh of the population will have at least one nosebleed in their life. There are thought to be two peaks in incidence: one peak between the ages of 2 to 10 years and another between the ages of 50 to 80 years. Most cases are minor and only 5–10% need urgent referral to the ENT team for management or admission.

It is often difficult to pinpoint the cause of an acute nosebleed as some are triggered by the most minimal trauma, including sneezing or blowing the nose. Other causes include nose picking, soft tissue or bony damage caused by trauma, local or systemic infections and, in elderly people, hypertension and degenerative arterial disease (Ludman, 1988; Lawrence and Watts, 1989; Lund and Howard, 1997; Widell, 1997).

Anatomy and Physiology

Anterior nosebleeds arise from an anastomotic network of blood vessels known as Kiesselbach's plexus (Little's area). Anterior bleeds are usually unilateral, with blood coming out of only one nostril, and the point of bleeding can usually be visualized unless bleeding is very severe.

Posterior nosebleeds occur behind the nasal septum. It is common for the blood to come out of both nostrils and for large clots to accumulate within the nasopharynx. It is also possible for these patients to present with blood trickling down the nasopharynx instead of through the nostrils. These patients are at the greatest risk of airway obstruction and re-bleeding as the source is usually arterial.

Signs, Symptoms and Potential Complications

Although visible bleeding is the most common sign, it is vital to assess the airway and breathing for signs of airway obstruction, and for an increased respiratory rate which may indicate cardiovascular compromise. The circulation should be assessed for signs of hypovolaemia, such as tachycardia or delayed capillary refill. These should be dealt with immediately if compromised.

Most commonly there will be bleeding of any degree from one or both nostrils. The patient may describe a trickling sensation down the back of the throat and blood will be visible in the oropharynx and mouth when inspected. If the patient has a posterior epistaxis, bleeding from the nostrils may be absent. Patients will often feel nauseous and may vomit, due in part to the emetic effect of swallowed blood within the stomach.

The airway may become obstructed, particularly if the bleeding is very heavy, contains clots or originates from the posterior part of the nose. As blood collects in the nasopharynx the patient may find it progressively more difficult to clear his/her airway. The patient may appear distressed and breathing may be noisy and laboured. The patient's ability to breathe may deteriorate and aspiration of blood into the lungs can result.

The most common complication is likely to be shock due to severe or prolonged bleeding. The patient may feel dizzy, nauseous, thirsty, weak or restless. He/she may present with pallor, have a thready tachycardia, be tachypnoeic and hypotensive. It is important to remember that the blood pressure may not start to fall until there has been a 30% blood volume loss. If the patient is hypertensive, taking anticoagulant medication or has a clotting disorder, response to treatment is likely to be slower and therefore the risks of shock and airway obstruction are greater.

Nursing Intervention in A&E

A rapid assessment of airway, breathing and circulation is essential in determining whether the patient requires resuscitation. A patient presenting with massive haemorrhage may need suction and emergency intubation in order to protect his/her airway and breathing. If the patient is tachycardic or pale, high flow oxygen should be administered via a non-rebreathing mask with reservoir, and venous access should be established promptly with subsequent IV fluid resuscitation. Blood samples should also be obtained for cross-match, full blood count, clotting screen and glucose. If the patient presents with a compromised airway, breathing or circulation then medical intervention should be requested and the ENT team informed.

First aid measures should be instigated immediately if bleeding is still occurring and should be continued until medical review. The patient should be nursed upright to reduce the venous pressure at the site of bleeding, unless signs of shock are evident. If bleeding persists or increases in severity the patient should be reassessed and appropriate intervention employed. The frequency for recording the pulse, respiratory rate and blood pressure should be based on the nursing assessment and documented accordingly.

It is more common, however, that patients will present in a stable condition with a mild to moderate epistaxis. The patient should be reassured, his/her physical condition assessed and a brief history taken to establish the cause, duration and severity of bleeding so that a clinical priority can be assigned.

The choices of treatment available in the A&E department include cautery, anterior packing and posterior packing dependent on the nature and extent of bleeding.

If the bleeding is minimal and an anterior site can be identified, cautery can be performed using a silver nitrate stick. The patient should be informed about the possibility of brief associated discomfort.

Typically the nose is first treated with a vasoconstrictor and anaesthetic. This may be a solution of cocaine or lignocaine with adrenaline applied topically. Packing materials for an anterior bleed include the use of half- to one-inch ribbon gauze (up to two metres per nostril) impregnated with Vaseline or a compressed sponge (or nasal tampon) such as Merocel (Hunt and Rothenhaus, 1996; Lund and Howard, 1997; Widell, 1997). If a post-nasal pack is to be used for posterior epistaxis, a Foley catheter (around 18 gauge) can be used, the balloon being inflated with either air or water. Following insertion of the nasal packs a bolster should be applied. It should be noted however, that Foley catheters are not licensed for this purpose.

All patients with nasal packing should be admitted for observation of their airway, breathing and vital signs. It is also suggested that patients who have had a posterior epistaxis be admitted because of the high risk of a re-bleed (Widell, 1997). Those who are not to be admitted should be given appropriate health education and follow-up arrangements explained prior to discharge.

First Aid / Health Education

Health education should begin at the point of first meeting the patient by reinforcing and praising appropriate home care and re-educating where interventions have been inappropriate.

The nurse should reiterate and explain the importance of pinching the soft part of the nostrils together as the main method of stopping bleeding (many people incorrectly think that they should be pinching the bridge of the nose). The patient should also be advised to tilt the head forwards, to breathe through the mouth and to avoid sniffing, picking or blowing the nose both during and after a bleeding episode. Lifting, bending forwards and drinking hot drinks should also be avoided as all these activities can produce vasodilation in the nose and may cause the bleeding to restart. The use of ice packs on the forehead or back of the neck to produce vasoconstriction has not been proved to have any beneficial effect (Lund and Howard, 1997). The patient should be advised that if bleeding occurs and does not stop following two 10-minute attempts at first aid, professional attention should be sought.

Nasal Injury and Fractures

Common Causes

The most common facial fracture is that of the nose, mainly due to its prominence (Lund and Howard, 1997), and a direct blow to the nose is the most likely cause of fractured nasal bones. It is relatively uncommon for a person to land on the face when he/she falls; consequently, most people presenting with nasal fractures have been assaulted or have more severe mid-facial trauma such as that suffered in a road traffic accident (Ludman, 1988; Lund and Howard, 1997).

Anatomy and Physiology

The nose is an organ of respiration. The irregularly shaped nasal cavity is divided equally by the nasal septum. This consists of hyaline cartilage anteriorly and posteriorly; the bony part is formed by the perpendicular plate of the ethmoid bone and the vomer. The nasal bones are two small oblong bones that are side by side, the junction of which forms the bridge of the nose.

Fractures to the nose may be linear or comminuted 'smash' fractures. Fractures to the nasal bones are often accompanied by a C-shaped fracture of the nasal septum, when there may also be displacement of the upper lateral cartilages. The external appearance of the tip of the nose and columella (the visible exterior skin that separates the nostrils) can be affected even when it is only the septum that is injured. Nasal fractures are usually closed but occasionally are open when the nasal bones are exposed by facial lacerations or abrasions.

Signs, Symptoms and Potential Complications

Patients attending A&E with nasal trauma will usually have pain to the bridge of the nose with bruising and swelling. The main distinguishing feature of a fractured nose as opposed to soft tissue injury is that the nose may be deformed as a result of lateral dislocation of the nasal bones or the septum (the nose being displaced sideways) or depression of the bridge. This is often accompanied by nasal obstruction and epistaxis. The fractured nose will be acutely tender on palpation and there may be crepitus and abnormal mobility of the external part of the nose.

The most serious immediate complication is the potential for airway obstruction, the risk of which is increased if epistaxis is present or if there is a septal haematoma. These two conditions need to be treated within A&E to ensure the safety of the patient's airway and breathing and to stabilize the circulation in a person with severe haemorrhage. Another serious and potentially life-threatening complication which is indicated by the presence of CSF rhinorrhoea (a leak of cerebrospinal fluid through the nose), is a fracture to the roof of the ethmoid labyrinth into the anterior cranial fossa. The result of this may be that the dura of the brain is interrupted, thus allowing the passage of bacteria that may cause meningitis. A septal haematoma, unless treated soon after injury, will lead to necrosis of septal cartilage. It is easily recognized by the presence of gross swelling to both sides of the septum that is visible from the front of the nose. This complication will result in the collapse of the nasal septum and an unsightly deformity due to the retraction of the columella; this should not be confused with a deviated septum, which gives an apparent unilateral swelling.

Following the acute phase of the injury, the complication that patients are usually most concerned about is the deformity that they may be left with and/or the sensation of having a blocked nose. The treatment for these conditions is always delayed until the swelling has subsided.

Nursing Intervention in A&E

A rapid assessment of the airway and breathing is essential in determining whether the patient requires emergency intervention and any bleeding should be treated before assessing for signs of underlying fractures. If a septal haematoma or CSF rhinorrhoea is present, as indicated by the presence of glucose, then urgent medical intervention is required in order to prevent serious complications. A subsequent ENT opinion should be obtained. A patient with CSF rhinorrhoea should be instructed not to blow his/her nose and should be nursed upright to avoid forcing air-carrying bacteria through the fracture site or causing a surgical emphysema by inducing positive pressure within the nose. The patient may subsequently be referred to a neurosurgical unit for closure of defects in the dura.

In the absence of bleeding, analgesia should be given and an ice pack applied in order to relieve pain and slow the development of swelling. Wounds will require thorough cleaning and debridement and lacerations will need to be closed by primary intention. Broad-spectrum antibiotics are indicated for the treatment of open fractures, with the nurse's aim being to promote the patient's compliance with treatment by giving thorough advice and explanations of potential complications.

First Aid/Health Education

First aid for nasal injuries is primarily aimed at controlling bleeding, pain and swelling. Advice regarding epistaxis should be given where appropriate. Otherwise patients should be advised how to administer ice packs and to avoid activities that increase the pain. The patient should also be advised regarding appropriate over-the-counter analgesia.

Many patients who attend A&E with nasal injuries expect to be X-rayed and the majority are keen to know whether their nose is broken or not. Radiography of the nose soon after injury is not helpful because the amount of swelling usually masks the presence of deformity and/or fractures (Lund and Howard, 1997). In the majority of cases, therefore, the main role of the nurse is to provide health education advice regarding the condition, the potential complications and the reasons as to why definitive investigations and treatment are delayed.

The patient should be advised that once the swelling subsides, usually about five to seven days from the time of injury, that he/she should inspect his/her nose for deformity and ensure that he/she can breathe through both nostrils as freely as he/she could prior to the injury. As nasal bones will set within about three weeks of the injury, the patient should see his/her GP no more than one week following injury if he/she has identified that he/she needs treatment or has further concerns.

Patients who have suffered an open fracture, have had CSF rhinorrhoea and those who have had a septal haematoma drained will be discharged with antibiotics. Patients are more likely to comply with treatment if they understand why they are taking them and it is also essential that they understand the signs and symptoms of an impending infection and when to seek subsequent medical attention.

Foreign Bodies in the Nose

Common Causes and Incidence

Most nasal foreign bodies are found in childrens' noses and are usually inserted on purpose. Anything smaller than the diameter of the nostril may become a nasal foreign body.

Anatomy and Physiology

Many children are brought to A&E soon after insertion of a foreign body and it can be easily visualized within the nostril. If the foreign body is organic in nature, or has been *in situ* for some time, an inflammatory response may occur in the nasal mucosa. This may result in swelling and a foul-smelling, purulent discharge that may then obscure the view of the nasal cavity and foreign body. Foreign bodies are easily trapped in the nose, partly due to the irregular shape of the three turbinates which can also make visualization difficult (Hunt and Ellison, 1996).

Signs, Symptoms and Potential Complications

More often than not the history is the most significant indicator that a foreign body is present. The object may also be visible on inspection of the nasal cavity, either unaided or by using a nasal speculum and a bright light. The patient may present as asymptomatic, may be experiencing some discomfort or may even be in pain.

Serious complications include transfer of the foreign body into the upper airway, which could lead to partial or even total obstruction. This may result from the object being forced into the nasopharynx during attempts at removal, particularly if the object is shiny and round (e.g. a bead or a sweet). The risk may also be increased by causing distress to the child, who may then inhale the object. Other complications are infection and inflammation, which could both lead to pain and systemic illness.

Nursing Intervention in A&E

A rapid assessment of the airway and breathing should be performed and immediate medical and/or ENT intervention sought if either is compromised.

A history should be taken to establish the type of foreign body and the duration of its placement. Unless the child is distressed or too young to understand, the nurse should try to get the child to blow his/her nose in order to expel the object. This can be easily and quickly achieved at the time of assessment and, if successful, may in the absence of complications avoid the need for a lengthy wait to see a doctor.

If a child is distressed, time and energy should be devoted to calming the child down by using play therapy and distraction techniques. Depending on the response, a mild sedative may be considered. Help should be given in assisting the carer to immobilize small children for a short time to enable swift removal of the foreign body and the avoidance of complications. This can be achieved through strategic positioning of limbs and a secure embrace.

Methods for removal of nasal foreign bodies include applying suction via a catheter which has had its tip cut flat, gently grasping the object with a pair of Tilley's forceps, rolling the object along the floor of the nose using a hook and using a solution of cocaine to shrink the nasal mucosa, which would then facilitate expulsion when the patient blows his/her nose (Ludman, 1988; Hunt and Ellison, 1996; Widell, 1997). If the patient is uncooperative or the object cannot be removed easily a general anaesthetic will be necessary in order to protect the airway during exploration and removal. X-rays are of no value unless the object is known to be radio-opaque. Experience in foreign body removal, or close supervision, on the part of the doctor or nurse is essential since the situation can so very easily be made worse with apparently little intervention.

First Aid / Health Education

Because of the risks associated with pushing nasal foreign bodies into the nasopharynx, the only first aid that can be advocated is that a cooperative child can be encouraged to blow his/her nose. If there is a lack of understanding or cooperation, there is a risk that the child may sniff instead. Carers should be advised that if this fails, they should seek medical attention for removal of the foreign body.

The Ear

The ear is divided into three main parts: the external ear, the middle ear and the inner ear. The external, visible part consists of the pinna (also known as the auricle) with the opening of the external acoustic meatus.

Foreign Bodies in the Ear

Common Causes and Incidence

Similar to foreign bodies inserted into the nose, a foreign body in the ear is also primarily a childhood condition. However, adults may also present with objects in their ears, most commonly insects and the tips of cotton buds.

Anatomy and Physiology

Unless there is a perforated tympanic membrane, the only place a foreign body can be trapped is in the external acoustic meatus. The meatus extends for about 2.5 cm from the opening to the tympanic membrane. Since it is slightly 'S' shaped it can be difficult to visualize a foreign body unless the pinna is tugged in a postero-superior direction in order to straighten the canal. In addition to the curved shaped of the canal, the presence of cerumen (wax) and hair helps to prevent foreign objects from reaching the tympanic membrane.

Signs, Symptoms and Complications

Most often, a patient will present to A&E with a clear history of a foreign body in the ear, which can usually be visualized by using an auroscope. Live insects within the canal can cause discomfort or even pain and great anxiety. These need to be removed urgently before further damage is caused to the ear. Other signs may include bleeding and hearing loss. If the foreign body has been present for a relatively long time the patient may present with signs of otitis externa. These include inflammation and a purulent discharge from the ear. Children will often fail to admit to inserting an object into the ear for fear of being punished and so diagnosis may be difficult (Hunt and Ellison, 1996; Widell, 1997).

Complications include infection, and damage to the tympanic membrane and middle ear may also result if the foreign body is pushed further into the canal during attempts at removal. Patient cooperation is essential to reduce the risks of complication and a short general anaesthetic may be indicated.

Nursing Intervention in A&E

The patient should be assessed by taking a history and assessing the level of pain or discomfort suffered. Analgesia should be offered accordingly. Extreme discomfort and anxiety are likely if there is a live insect in the ear and so stilling or removal of the insect should be attempted without delay.

Methods for removal of foreign bodies include extraction with forceps, extraction by using a wax hook placed beyond the object, suction, gentle syringing with water warmed to 37°C or use of oil (such as olive or arachis) to float insects out. All these techniques should be used with extreme care and techniques that involve instilling fluids into the ear must be avoided if there is any risk that the tympanic membrane is disrupted. It has been suggested that a solution of 2% lignocaine instilled into the ear will quickly kill or paralyse insects, although cockroaches are best killed with oil (Hunt and Ellison, 1996).

If attempts to remove the foreign body are unsuccessful in the A&E department the patient will need to be referred to the ENT team. This consultation should be within 12 to 24 hours so that the risk of infection is reduced.

Prior to discharge, the patient's external acoustic meatus should be examined for retained pieces of foreign body as well as abrasions, lacerations and infection. It may be necessary for the patient to be discharged with antibiotic eardrops that also contain a steroid in order to prevent infection and inflammation.

First Aid / Health Education

When patients present to A&E it is important to reinforce correct first aid already given or to re-instruct as necessary. If a foreign object is lodged in the ear, it is important that lay attempts at removal are discouraged because impaction and further injury may result. However, advice may be given regarding first aid treatment for insects in the ear as these may be removed easily by gentle flooding of the ear with tepid water to float the insect out (Webb et al., 1997).

For patients who are treated in the A&E department, health education will include an explanation about the signs and symptoms of infection. For patients discharged home with antibiotics or eardrops, advice should be given as to how and when to take the medication with any special instructions reiterated.

Advice should also be given to avoid a repeat episode of the presenting injury, as many presentations of foreign bodies in the ear relate to cotton buds; an explanation of why the ear should not be cleaned using these may be appropriate.

Injury to the Pinna (Auricle)

Common Causes and Incidence

Blunt trauma to the external ear may cause a haematoma or lacerations to the pinna, whilst assaults and bites may result in avulsion injuries.

Anatomy and Physiology

The pinna is made up of deeply grooved fibroelastic cartilage covered with skin. The external prominent rim is the helix. The lobule is well supplied with blood capillaries and consists of tough areolar and fatty tissue. It is supplied by the posterior auricular artery, which arises from the external carotid artery, and anastamoses with the anterior auricular artery. As there is a good blood supply to the pinna, blunt trauma can cause a haematoma, which is very painful and can displace the pinna. Significant deformities can result from untreated haematomas, which can cause destruction of the cartilage – a condition known as 'cauliflower ear'.

Lacerations are repairable by suturing, and even when there is tissue loss of up to 2 cm of the helix the edges can be brought together, although may require additional wedge resection of the pinna. Reconstruction of the ear following avulsion can usually be carried out if the time between injury and surgery is kept short.

Signs, Symptoms and Complications

Patients presenting with trauma to the pinna of the ear may be in a great deal of pain. There may be a laceration, part of the ear may be missing or there may be the redness and swelling of a haematoma.

Unless treatment is carried out early it will not be possible to reattach avulsed parts of the pinna owing to a failing blood supply. The ear may then be permanently misshapen. Cauliflower ear is the complication of an untreated haematoma between the perichondrium and the cartilage, which again needs early treatment to avoid destruction of the cartilage.

Nursing Intervention in A&E

Following the triage assessment, first aid should be administered as required. A pressure dressing should be applied to control any bleeding and ice can be used to slow the development of any swelling. The patient's level of pain should be assessed, and analgesia given as indicated and as soon as is practicable. Before any surgical procedures are carried out, the nurse should ensure that the patient understands what is going to happen and that he/she is given the opportunity to have any questions answered. The nurse will need to be resourceful in creating a suitable dressing that will apply some pressure by conforming to the shape of the ear following any procedures.

First Aid / Health Education

Because of the risks of permanent damage to the pinna, it is important that patients who sustain injuries resulting in haematoma formation, lacerations or avulsions should seek medical attention as soon after the injury as possible. Pressure should be advocated to control any bleeding. By advising early application of ice to the ear following blunt trauma, the extent of haematoma formation may be drastically reduced, and this in turn will help to control the amount of pain experienced and lessen the risk of subsequent complications.

Patients who are discharged following any invasive procedures such as suturing or haematoma evacuation should be advised as to the signs and symptoms of wound infection. Patients who have had evacuation of a haematoma are likely to be discharged with a course of broad-spectrum antibiotics, and the nurse should emphasize the importance of completing the course as a means of preventing infection and reiterate any special instructions for the particular antibiotic prescribed.

Vertigo

Common Causes and Incidence

Vertigo refers to the hallucination of motion, either of the person or of the environment. Vertigo is always associated with imbalance; however, imbalance is not always due to vertigo. It is a symptom rather than a disease and may relate to a vestibular system lesion in the brain stem, in the eighth cranial nerve or of the inner ear, specifically the labyrinth (Ludman, 1988; Herr and Alvord, 1996; Lund and Howard, 1997).

There are two types of vertigo. About 85% of people presenting with the complaint are suffering from peripheral vertigo. These patients are suffering from rotational vertigo, nausea or vomiting with no signs of a brainstem deficit. Cochlear symptoms such as tinnitus or hearing loss may also be present. Peripheral vertigo tends to recur and although it can be very debilitating it tends to reduce in frequency and severity over time. Most young people presenting with vertigo are suffering from a peripheral cause. Central vertigo tends to have a slower onset and is often accompanied by neurological symptoms as it is caused by a lesion of the central nervous system (Herr and Alvord, 1996). Some of the conditions causing vertigo are given in Table 14.3. Other causes include motion sickness, impending faint and hyperventilation syndrome.

Anatomy and Physiology

The organs of balance are contained in the inner ear and are made up of two parts: the bony labyrinth and the membranous labyrinth. The bony labyrinth forms a cavity with the temporal bone and consists of the vestibule, the cochlea and three semicircular canals. The membranous labyrinth is the same shape and fits inside the bony labyrinth. The nerve fibres contained within the membranous

Table 14.3 Causes of vertigo

Peripheral vertigo	Central vertigo
Benign paroxysmal positional vertigo	Concussion
Acute labyrinthitis	Cerebellar tumours
Vestibular neuronitis	Acoustic neuroma
Menière's disease	Cerebellar infarction
Concussion	Cerebellar haemorrhage
Cholesteatoma	Intoxication with alcohol
Ototoxic drugs	Drugs
Rupture of the round window	Hypertensive dizziness
Impaction of ear wax	Complex partial seizure
Rupture of the tympanic membrane	Vertebrobasilar insufficiency

Source: Herr and Alvord (1996).

labyrinth combine to form the auditory part of the eighth cranial nerve. This travels through a foramen in the temporal bone to the hearing area in the temporal lobe of the cerebrum. The semicircular canals are the organs associated with the sense of position and balance. These canals lie in each of the three planes of space. Any change of position causes movement of the endolymph and peri-lymph, which are fluids within the semicircular canals. This in turn stimulates the nerve endings and hair cells in the utricle, saccule and ampullae. The resultant nerve impulses are transmitted to the cere-bellum via the vestibular nerve, which becomes the vestibulo-cochlear nerve once it joins the cochlear nerve. Vertigo occurs when the information from vestibular sources differs from that of other sensory systems such as the eyes, muscles and joints, as it is the coor-dination of all these senses that gives people their sense of balance.

Signs, Symptoms and Complications

Vertigo refers to the abnormal feeling of movement as opposed to feeling unsteady or light-headed, and is a symptom of other disease. The patient with vertigo may suffer from nausea or vomiting and be so unsteady that he/she is unable to stand up.

A thorough medical examination is required in order to establish the cause of the vertigo and to rule out any serious pathology, the complications of which may be life-threatening. Complications of vertigo include falls, especially in the elderly, and dehydration in a person with prolonged vomiting.

Nursing Intervention in A&E

The main objective of care in the A&E department is to control the patient's symptoms. The patient should be helped into whatever position is most comfortable for him/her and all unnecessary movements should be avoided. Adult patients need to have cardiac causes excluded and until this happens the patient should receive high flow oxygen, have an intravenous cannula inserted, have an ECG performed and be monitored for cardiac arrhythmias.

Medications such as diazepam or prochlorperazine may be effective in reducing the dizziness, nausea and vomiting and the earlier these can be given the sooner the patient can start to improve. Intravenous fluids may be given to patients with severe vomiting to prevent or treat dehydration, and blood should be taken for urea and electrolyte analysis as they can be affected by prolonged vomiting.

Patients presenting with vertigo will be very unsteady, so patient safety is a priority. Trolley sides should be elevated at all times and the patient should be escorted should he/she need to get off the trolley whilst symptomatic.

Whilst in A&E the patient may undergo various investigations, and treatment may be instigated for any causes found. The patient may be admitted if the symptoms do not subside or the cause needs inpatient assessment and treatment such as for cardiac or central nervous system abnormalities.

First Aid / Health Education

Patients who are discharged should be advised to rest and this may involve the need to take time off work until a full recovery is made. Until symptoms have completely resolved the patient should be advised against driving, operating machinery and working at heights.

Patients who have suffered from peripheral vertigo should be advised that there is a strong likelihood of the symptoms recurring.

The Throat

Foreign Bodies in the Throat

Common Causes and Incidence

It is quite common for patients to present to A&E with a foreign body stuck in the throat. The presentation may vary, with choking being the most serious and life-threatening presentation. Foreign bodies stuck in the oesophagus or oropharynx are usually painful but rarely life-threatening.

Foreign body airway obstruction is most commonly seen in children, with the highest mortality rate being among those of pre-school age (Hunt and Ellison, 1996; Advanced Life Support Group, 1997). The items inhaled are usually non-ingestible objects such as small toys and household items or anything that is small enough for a child to put into his/her mouth. Adults who present with foreign body airway obstruction usually present with lumps of food stuck in the larynx.

Adults most commonly present with foreign bodies of the oropharynx and oesophagus, the highest number of presentations being due to retained fish bones and chicken bones (Ludman, 1988; Hunt and Ellison, 1996). Although many adults presenting to A&E are able to point to the location of their discomfort, it is very common for the foreign body to be absent. This is often seen in patients who have eaten fish, who feel a sharp scratching sensation in their throat and who after full investigation have no retained foreign body. Indeed, a study cited by Hunt and Ellison (1996) concurred that only 31% of patients referred to an ENT clinic for pharyngeal foreign bodies were found to have one after full investigation.

Anatomy and Physiology

Small sharp foreign bodies often impact in the lower pole of the tonsils, and these are usually visible on examination with a good light source. Beyond this, ingested foreign bodies may get stuck at any part of the oesophagus but most often at the upper end of the oesophagus just below the cricopharyngeal sphincter, which is a band of pharyngeal muscle. Inhaled foreign bodies will usually impact in the narrowest part of the airway, which is the larynx in adults and the cricoid ring in children.

Signs, Symptoms and Potential Complications

Foreign Bodies in the Airway

Partial obstruction of the airway is indicated by coughing, choking, stridor (inspiratory respiratory noises indicative of upper airway obstruction) and difficulty with breathing. The patient will probably be unable to speak and will be distressed. In the acutely distressed patient facial colouring may be bright red during the period of distress and choking but subsequently he/she will become pale or cyanosed as respiratory efforts fail to supply enough oxygen and to expel carbon dioxide. A patient who has completely obstructed his/her airway and still has respiratory effort will present with exaggerated, paradoxical movements of the chest and abdomen. These patients will soon become pale, cyanosed and suffer respiratory arrest due to profound hypoxia.

Foreign Bodies in the Alimentary Tract

It is not always easy to confirm or refute the patient's belief that he/she has an oesophageal foreign body. Usually the symptoms develop whilst eating and are quite localized, with the patient able to point to the area where the damage has occurred. Symptoms which should cause suspicion of a retained foreign body include sharp pain on swallowing (especially if it radiates to the ear), difficulty swallowing saliva, tenderness of the neck, dysphagia and otalgia (Ludman, 1988; Hunt and Ellison, 1996).

Complications of inhaled foreign bodies include both partial and complete obstruction of the airway. An untreated partial obstruction can turn into a complete obstruction with the onset of spasm and oedema. A completely obstructed airway will soon lead to hypoxia, coma and death.

Pharyngeal and oesophageal foreign bodies can lead to abscess formation, necrosis of the lining of the oesophagus with bleeding and even oesophageal perforation if the foreign body is sharp or has been lodged for a prolonged period of time.

Nursing Intervention in A&E

An immediate assessment must be made of the airway, breathing and circulation. If there is a foreign body in the airway this will be either partially or completely obstructed and breathing is likely to be compromised or absent. In such cases medical attention must be obtained without delay and basic/advanced life support commenced for the apnoeic patient with subsequent attempts to clear the airway.

If first aid attempts to clear the airway are unsuccessful, laryngoscopic visualization of the larynx may reveal a foreign body that can then be removed with a pair of Tilley's forceps. In very rare cases and when attempts to clear the airway are unsuccessful, it may be necessary to perform an emergency tracheostomy or cricothyroidotomy.

A foreign body of the oropharynx is often easy to visualize and if the patient can cooperate it may easily be removed with a pair of forceps. Typically such foreign bodies are fish bones that have partly embedded themselves in a tonsil. It may then be safe for the patient to be discharged with advice on observing for any evidence of infection.

If the patient is symptomatic, suggestive of a foreign body further down the throat, referral to the ENT team is usual for endoscopic examination of the oesophagus. If the foreign body is radio-opaque this would usually follow an X-ray of the soft tissues of the throat.

First Aid / Health Education

Airway obstruction is a life-threatening problem that needs to be treated as soon as it happens. Five firm, sharp backslaps should be given between the shoulder blades to adults who are conscious and any child or infant (conscious or not). If unsuccessful in adults, these should be followed by five abdominal thrusts (the Heimlich manoeuvre). In children the first set of five backslaps is followed by five chest thrusts. Chest thrusts are carried out by pressing sharply against the same part of the sternum used for chest compressions during resuscitation (this being dependent upon age and size). Five more backslaps are then given if the airway is still obstructed, followed by five abdominal thrusts. Abdominal thrusts are given by applying a sharp inward and upward movement in the centre of the abdomen just below the diaphragm. In infants (children less than one year old) the rescuer alternates between five backslaps and five chest thrusts as the abdominal organs and viscera are too delicate to withstand abdominal thrusts. The aim of any first aid intervention is to expel the object from the trachea by forcing air from the lungs. Gravity will also aid expulsion, so all manoeuvres should be carried out with the patient's head as low as possible. In the unconscious patient the patient should be lying on his/her side for the backslaps or on his/her back for the abdominal thrusts.

Infections causing Emergencies of the Throat

Epiglottitis

Common Causes and Incidence

Epiglottitis is a serious and often fatal infection that is most common amongst children between the ages of 3 and 6 years. It has been identified as affecting about 1:100,000 adults per year (Murphy and Armstrong, 1996). *Haemophilus influenzae* type B is the main cause of the illness in both adults and children, with *Streptococcus pneumoniae* being the infection most associated with causing epiglotittis in immunocompromised patients. However, the condition is becoming much rarer since the introduction of the HIB immunisation. Rarely, epiglottitis may be thermally induced, such as following ingestion of hot fluids (Peters, 1993).

Anatomy and Physiology

Inflammatory disorders of the laryngeal region that affect the epiglottis and the aryepiglottic folds and the false cords are known as epiglottitis. The physiology of the illness can vary from slight erythema and oedema of an isolated region, to involvement of the whole area with gross oedema, inflammation and complete obstruction of the airway. Factors thought to be involved in obstructing the airway include mucosal oedema, aspiration of secretions, laryngospasm and fatigue.

Signs, Symptoms and Potential Complications

The presentation of epiglottitis in children is usually much more dramatic than that in adults. In children the illness usually has a very sudden and rapid onset with increasing difficulty in breathing over a period of about 3 to 6 hours (Advanced Life Support Group, 1997). The sick child will usually be sitting very still with the neck extended and chin forwards (a posture known as the 'tripod' position) and probably be unable to speak as the throat is so painful. The mouth will normally be slightly open and he/she will be drooling as such patients are unable to swallow their saliva owing to the severity of the sore throat. Stridor, if present at all, will be soft and coughing is usually absent. The child will usually have a pyrexia of 39° C or higher, be tachycardic and will look toxic with signs of poor peripheral circulation due to septicaemia. Subcostal, sternal and intercostal recession will also be present in the child with airway obstruction due to the use of the accessory muscles of ventilation. The child will not tolerate being laid flat and attempts to do so may result in total airway obstruction and death.

The onset of epiglottitis in adults is often slower and the presentation is characterized by a sore throat that is disproportionate to the physical findings (Murphy and Armstrong, 1996). If the patient is able to speak, the voice associated with supraglottic swelling is muffled and thick. All the symptoms of childhood epiglottitis may also feature in adults.

Epiglottitis is a life-threatening condition. Deterioration may be rapid with the patient's airway suddenly becoming totally obstructed. Death may result unless immediate action is taken to secure both the airway and breathing.

Nursing Intervention in A&E

The key to preventing total airway obstruction and death is by prompt medical/nursing management of the airway. In caring for any drooling, toxic-looking child it is essential to consider epiglottitis early on and to treat the situation in a calm and quick manner. No interventions which could distress the child should be carried out by anyone; this especially includes trying to look inside the child's mouth as respiratory collapse may ensue (Lawrence and Watts, 1989; Murphy and Armstrong, 1996; Advanced Life Support Group, 1997; Lund and Howard, 1997). A patient who has signs and symptoms of epiglottitis should be prioritized for immediate medical management and should be cared for in the resuscitation room. A calm, quiet atmosphere is essential and it is preferable that the parents are encouraged to stay with the child. Attention should be sought from a senior doctor, preferably an ENT specialist and an anaesthetist. The child will need to be anaesthetized in order to allow laryngoscopy and intubation, which are both likely to be difficult because of the extent of the swelling and inflammation of the epiglottis.

For A&E nurses it is essential to be able to recognize the cardinal signs of epiglottitis and to be able to react with certainty and confidence whilst providing a reassuring and supportive role to the patient and parents. The parents of a sick child are unlikely to realize the severity of the situation and it will be distressing for them to see their child being intubated and treated so aggressively. The nurse will have a major part to play in ensuring that the parents understand the situation and the significance of all interventions.

Once the airway is secure, intravenous access is the next priority in order to correct circulatory deficit and to obtain essential blood samples for culture in order that antibiotic therapy can begin. Early administration of antibiotics is also key to the survival of the patient and treatment may begin with cefuroxime, cefotaxime, ceftriaxone or chloramphenicol. Opinions differ as to whether these patients will benefit from treatment with steroids, although it is suggested that they may be lifesaving in the case of angioedema (Murphy and Armstrong, 1996; Lund and Howard, 1997).

The patient with epiglottitis should be monitored very closely with frequent documentation of vital signs and urgent attention being paid to deficits of the airway, breathing or circulation. He/she should be cared for in an intensive care unit, whether intubated or not, and once the patient's condition is stabilized transfer should be arranged at the earliest opportunity. Children treated for epiglottitis are often extubated after about 24–36 hours and will have made a full recovery within 3 to 5 days.

Quinsy

Common Causes and Incidence

Quinsy, also known as peritonsillar abscess, is a complication of tonsillitis. It is usually seen in teenagers and young adults and is seen most often in patients who do not have a long-standing history of recurrent tonsillitis (Picken, 1996; Lund and Howard, 1997). Quinsy results when an abscess forms in the space between the tonsil and the tonsillar bed. It is usually unilateral and accompanied by a mild tonsillitis on the opposite side. Patients presenting to A&E with an apparent quinsy will often be at the stage of cellulitis, which occurs prior to the localization of pus.

Quinsies are usually polymicrobial abscesses, with cultures often showing both aerobes (such as group A beta-haemolytic streptococci, pneumococcus, *H. influenzae* and staphylococcus), and anaerobes (particularly Bacteroides). Quinsy may follow infectious mononucleosis (glandular fever) which is an acute virus caused by the Epstein-Barr virus (EBV). It is transmitted by droplet infection and is characterized by pyrexia, sore throat and swollen lymph glands.

Anatomy and Physiology

The tonsils consist of lymphatic tissue located between the mouth and the oropharynx. At the place where the soft palate and the lateral walls of the pharynx blend, there are two folds on each side of the throat and it is between these folds that the tonsils are located. The tonsillar tissue is known as mucosa-associated lymph tissue (MALT) and is involved in the development of immunity. The tonsils are strategically positioned to protect the respiratory tract from microbes.

The illness usually begins with a simple tonsillitis. The patient may present to A&E at this stage with a peritonsillar cellulitis and have a mild inflammation characterized by unilateral erythema extending to the soft palate or oedema. There is little or no bulging of the soft palate, no displacement of the uvula and little or no trismus (spasm of the muscles of the jaw).

When the patient presents with quinsy, examination of the oropharynx is difficult as the patient will find it hard to open his/her mouth owing to the trismus. The view of the affected tonsil will be obscured as the soft palate on the side of the quinsy will be very erythematous, bulging forwards and medially, and also the tonsil will be displaced medially and backwards. Because of the expanding collection of pus, the uvula will be displaced across the midline and will be swollen and oedematous. There will usually be a mild tonsillitis on the opposite side and the cervical lymph glands will be enlarged and tender.

Signs, Symptoms and Potential Complications

Patients presenting to A&E with quinsy are often generally unwell. They will probably have had a sore throat for two or more days. The pain usually increases in severity and becomes unilateral on the affected side. They will have severe dysphagia and will even be unable to swallow saliva and so may be drooling. Trismus will often develop with pain radiating to the ear and consequently the patient will find it very difficult to open his/her mouth. The patient will also be pyrexial, tachycardic and may be showing signs of dehydration if the symptoms have been prolonged.

Complications of quinsy can be life-threatening. Airway obstruction is the most immediate and sudden complication and can result from delayed treatment due to misdiagnosis. Rarely, the infection can extend into contiguous neck spaces (those next to the affected area) leading to deep neck abscesses which may then lead to erosion of the carotid artery or septic thrombosis of the internal jugular vein.

Nursing Intervention in A&E

A prompt assessment of the patient's airway, breathing and circulation should be undertaken. Any patient who is drooling with swollen structures in the oropharynx should be prioritized for immediate medical intervention (Mackway-Jones, 1997). It is vital that the A&E nurse recognizes the clinical presentation of quinsy and is respectful of the potential complication of airway obstruction. The patient should be cared for in the resuscitation room with equipment for advanced management of the airway immediately available. The patient should receive a high concentration of oxygen via a non-rebreathing mask with reservoir and early cannulation of a large peripheral vein should be achieved.

Early intervention by the ENT team may involve either conservative management with intravenous antibiotics and fluid replacement, drainage via needle aspiration, or incision and drainage under local anaesthetic. The latter procedures are usually carried out with the patient sitting up and the head tilted forwards. If the airway is compromised an emergency tonsillectomy may be performed. The nurse will need to ensure that the patient is prepared promptly for the procedure and that the patient has an adequate understanding of what is going to happen.

Once the quinsy is treated the patient may be offered a tonsillectomy, particularly if there is more than one episode.

Ludwig's Angina

Common Causes and Incidence

Ludwig's angina is a rare but life-threatening illness. Patients present with an acute cellulitis or localized abscess of the floor of the mouth. It usually occurs following dental infections, particularly of the second and third lower molars. It is often caused by streptococcus and may occur following trauma.

Signs, Symptoms and Potential Complications

Patients with Ludwig's angina may have a history of dental pain and infection. There will be inflammation and obvious swelling within the mouth and there may even be abscesses. The condition will be painful and cause dysphagia. The patient is likely to be drooling due to the inability to swallow saliva. He/she will also be pyrexial and tachycardic.

Hypoxia will result if the swelling obstructs the airway but the potential exists for rapid, complete obstruction of the airway leading to respiratory arrest. Other complications include septicaemia, empyema, pneumonia and mediastinitis (Fritsch and Klein, 1992).

Nursing Intervention in A&E

An assessment should be carried out to evaluate the airway, breathing and circulation. If there is any airway deficit or if the patient is drooling he/she should be prioritized for immediate medical intervention and cared for in the resuscitation room. Continuous monitoring of vital signs should be carried out and documented accordingly.

If the airway becomes so obstructed as to cause difficulty with breathing a nasopharyngeal airway may be inserted as this is usually well tolerated in a patient who is still conscious. Oxygen should also be administered via a non-rebreathing mask with reservoir in order to ensure a high percentage. Complete obstruction of the airway will necessitate intubation but, if unsuccessful, then tracheostomy or cricothyroidotomy will be required. Early cannulation of a large peripheral vein is essential in order to replace fluids and for administration of antibiotics.

The patient is likely to feel very anxious and it is important for the nurse to be prepared for emergency airway management whist maintaining a calming and reassuring approach to the patient. It is important that the patient has an understanding of the likely course of events so that he/she is not unduly alarmed by the urgency of his/her treatment.

Other Emergencies of the Throat

Two other conditions resulting in emergency situations involving the throat are inhalation injury causing burns that will lead to oedema and obstruction of the airway, and strangulation injury resulting in compression of the trachea and obstruction of the airway. Like the previous conditions discussed, priority should be given to the prompt assessment of the airway, breathing and circulation. Resuscitative measures should be carried out if there is any deficit to these vital functions, the key to survival being in the maintenance of an adequate airway and in ensuring the patient is ventilated with high concentrations of oxygen. It is absolutely vital to have a high index of suspicion when caring for patients with these injuries. The seriousness of the patient's condition may not be obvious on arrival in the department. However, facial burns, sooty nostrils, carbonaceous sputum, difficulty in swallowing and voice changes should alert staff to the high likelihood of airway burns. Early consultation with a senior doctor and the ENT team is also advocated in order that definitive treatment can be given for the underlying condition.

Conclusion

This chapter has given an overview of common ENT conditions that may present within the A&E department and it is apparent that an accurate and informed nursing assessment can achieve early recognition and intervention for potentially life-threatening conditions within this patient group.

Suggested Further Reading

Bull PD (1991) Lecture Notes on Diseases of the Ear, Nose and Throat, 7th edn. Oxford: Blackwell Scientific.
Coleman BH (1992) Hall and Coleman's Diseases of the Nose, Throat and Ear, and Head and Neck, 14th edn. Edinburgh: Churchill Livingstone.

References

Advanced Life Support Group (1997) Advanced Paediatric Life Support: The Practical Approach, 2nd edn. London: BMJ Publishing Group.
Fritsch DE, Klein DG (1992) Ludwig's angina. Heart and Lung 21(1): 39–47.
Herr RD, Alvord SL (1996) Vertigo and labyrinthine disorders. In Harwood-Nuss AL, Linden CH, Luten RC, Moore-Shepherd S, Wolfson AB, The Clinical Practice of Emergency Medicine, 2nd edn. Philadelphia: Lippincott-Raven, pp 105–9.
Hunt M, Ellison J (1996) Foreign bodies in the ear, nose, and throat in children and adults. In Harwood-Nuss AL, Linden CH, Luten RC, Moore-Shepherd S, Wolfson AB, The Clinical Practice of Emergency Medicine, 2nd edn. Philadelphia: Lippincott-Raven, pp 97–100.
Lawrence N, Watts J (1989) Handbook of Emergencies in General Practice. Oxford: Oxford University Press.
Ludman H (1988) ABC of Ear Nose and Throat. London: BMJ Publishing Group.
Lund VJ, Howard DJ (1997) Ear, nose and throat emergencies. In Skinner D, Swain A, Peyton R, Robertson C (Ed) Cambridge Textbook of Accident and Emergency Medicine. Cambridge: Cambridge University Press, pp 481–97.

Mackway-Jones K (Ed) (1997) Emergency Triage: Manchester Triage Group. London: BMJ Publishing.

Murphy MF, Armstrong PMJ (1996) Adult epiglottitis. In Harwood-Nuss AL, Linden CH, Luten RC, Moore-Shepherd S, Wolfson AB, The Clinical Practice of Emergency Medicine, 2nd edn. Philadelphia: Lippincott-Raven, pp 77–80.

Peters SJ (1993) Commentary on thermal epiglottitis after swallowing hot tea. ENA's Nursing Scan in Emergency Care 3(3): 8.

Picken CA (1996) Acute infections of the adult pharynx. In Harwood-Nuss AL, Linden CH, Luten RC, Moore-Shepherd S, Wolfson AB, The Clinical Practice of Emergency Medicine, 2nd edn. Philadelphia: Lippincott-Raven, pp 80–4.

Webb M, Scott R, Beale P (1997) First Aid Manual, 7th edn. London: Dorling Kindersley.

Widell T (1997) Eye, ear, nose, throat and dental emergencies. In Plantz SH, Adler JN (Eds) Emergency Medicine. Philadelphia: Williams & Wilkins, pp 355–94.

Wilson KJW, Waugh A (1996) Ross and Wilson Anatomy and Physiology in Health and Illness, 8th edn. Edinburgh: Churchill Livingstone.

Chapter 15
The Role of the Triage Nurse

JANET PARKER

Introduction

Determining precedence for patients who have an urgent condition, establishing rational and consistent assessments for lesser injured patients and creating an environment conducive to high standards of patient care has always been a pre-eminent role of the accident and emergency (A&E) nurse. Until recently, however, this role was *ad hoc*, unpredictable and without structure. A contemporary method of patient assessment had to be developed to provide an effective and safe environment for A&E patients; this process is known as triage.

Historical Perspective

Triage has its origins in military history. In the early 1700s, Baron Dominique Jean Larre, a surgeon in the Napoleonic army, adopted the principles of modern triage by developing a system under which soldiers requiring the most urgent care were attended to promptly. The term 'Triage' is derived from the French 'trier' meaning to sort, classify or choose, and this is the principle upon which the current triage system is founded. The strategy, as we now recognize triage, was initiated in the United States in a New York hospital in 1964, becoming more widely used in the United Kingdom by the 1980s. The need for a patient assessment system was initially recognized by the Royal College of Nursing (1984) when only three hospitals in the United Kingdom were using a triage system.

One of the main objectives of establishing the Royal College of Nursing Accident and Emergency Nursing Association in 1990 was the advancement of triage in A&E departments. Gorton (1993) subsequently reported that very few United Kingdom A&E departments used such an assessment tool.

Rationale

Triage establishes a patient management system and through this system identifies any problems and appraises relative priorities of patients. The general principle is to take the patient through all the decision-making processes involved in his/her assessment at the triage point, to identify at the earliest opportunity those patients who are more seriously injured and to determine the urgency of their condition. It is not the purpose of triage to diagnose the patient's condition.

The rationale for introducing such a system and taking this course of action evolved from increasing workload demand, greater expectations from the public, and the necessity to conform to the Patient's Charter. Parmer and Hewitt (1985) argued that the increasing number of patients in A&E departments posed the threat that acutely ill or injured patients would go unrecognized if they were not initially assessed through a triage system.

It became clear that local guidelines and protocols were necessary to ensure that a safe and accurate service was offered, the implication being that the less time taken to perform triage, the less accurate the subsequent assessment and therefore the less precise the prioritization of patient care.

With the arrival of clinical governance, it is crucial to provide a safe quality service in the correct place and at the correct time, consequently developing a proactive rather than reactive practice.

This chapter will now discuss the concept of triage, variations in training, accountability issues, legal issues, the role and responsibility of the triage nurse and the necessity of evaluation for such a system.

Concept

The principles upon which triage is founded are those which will provide a safe environment for the patient attending the A&E department, to enable the effective screening of patients and the provision of first aid, and to categorize patients to reflect the severity of their condition. Mackway-Jones (1996) identified that it is essential for there to be a system in place to ensure that patients are seen in order of clinical need rather than in order of attendance. Hendricks and Harris (1996) suggested that this interpretation of the patient's needs resulted from nursing intuition, knowledge and experience.

The triage system has several distinct features but continues to be complex and varies remarkably between departments. The principal aim is the provision of a quality service that offers appropriate care at an appropriate time, interpreting and synthesizing the information obtained from patients.

Training and Development

The triage nurse is required to adopt a tactful, approachable and non-judgemental manner, demonstrating the ability to assess the total situation immediately. In the chaotic environment of a busy waiting room this can help reduce friction and verbal aggression from patients and relatives. To develop this ability, triage nurses require competence, knowledge, skill and to be able to apply such knowledge and skills to an established standard of performance.

There appears to be no consensus on training and development programmes that can be adopted nationally and that are suitable to every A&E department. The diversity is illustrated through the following authors. An observation approach was recognized by Nuttall (1986), York and Proud (1990) advocated the use of seminars and lectures, Gray (1991) favoured a three-day study programme. Rock and Pledge (1991) further argued that the triage nurse role should be performed by a Registered General Nurse with a minimum of two years' A&E experience but did not advocate the need for special training, although a period of preceptorship was recognized as beneficial. Crouch (1994) also suggested a nationally recognized course for triage. The diversity of workloads within A&E departments and the continuous succession of healthcare delivery means that training in the triage system is modified considerably and is often initiated appropriate to local needs.

If larger departments have separate 'resuscitation', 'major' and 'minor' treatment areas, their use of the triage system will be very different from a smaller department where the triage nurse role may integrate assessing patients from all these areas of work. Therefore, in the absence of national training for triage nurses, a clear educational process for individual departments needs to be facilitated at the local level to fit in with local standards, protocols and patient demand. It is the responsibility of each department to define clear guidelines and policies that will allow nurses to practise with confidence.

An understanding of the expectations of role definition will help outline how triage nurses view their role. With recent debate regarding multi-skilling and boundaries between the doctor/nurse role frequently being moved, a clear definition is needed. A distinct philosophy, criteria, protocols, provision of substantial resources, staff appraisal and monitoring of the effectiveness of the system are imperative to the success of the triage system. Minimum standards of experience before consideration for accreditation in the role of triage need to be included in the criteria. Experience of the A&E nurse role is almost a prerequisite to becoming a triage nurse, the optimal functioning of the triage nurse being dependent upon the aforementioned knowledge, intuition, experience and also formal education. It is generally acknowledged that to perform a high level of skilled assessment requires a person adept at excellent communication and interpersonal skills.

National Triage Classifications

Implementation of a triage methodology in an approved and standard format and following comprehensive training has long been awaited. The British Association for Accident and Emergency Medicine (1996) and the Royal College of Nursing (1984) recognized that a standard scale for triage needed to be adopted and after widespread debate developed new national categories incorporating the triage scale and target times (Table 15.1). They recognized that comparison of the patterns of work and demands on A&E services between different departments would be more meaningful if there were a standard way of talking about urgency. The intention was that the five-point scale would become the standard scale by which patients are categorized according to their priority for treatment when they arrive in an A&E department.

This scale has been adapted throughout the country and ranges from the use of a colour-coded system, a 1-5 numbered system or the use of a five-point definition system ranging from immediate to

Table 15.1 Triage scale and target times

Number	Name	Colour	Target time
1	Immediate	Red	0
2	Very urgent	Orange	10
3	Urgent	Yellow	60
4	Standard	Green	120
5	Non-urgent	Blue	240

non-urgent. However, all of these are interchangeable and identify the same priorities. The percentage of patients seen within target times incorporated into the scale is stipulated locally and managers will need to scrutinize accurate and organized information on clinical activity to determine the effectiveness of the system within individual departments.

Manchester Innovation

The Manchester Triage Group, established in 1994, developed a methodology to allow practitioners of triage to work to a set standard when applying the national triage scale. The design adopted a systematic approach to triage through the use of algorithms and offered a patient management system modifiable to most A&E departments. Through the use of decision-making strategies and general discriminators the aim is to provide a standard triage method. With a combination of the British Association for Accident and Emergency Medicine and Royal College of Nursing national triage scale and structured techniques such as those developed by the Manchester Triage Group, analysis of national standards of triage and subsequent actions of triage personnel should be more rational and logical.

The New NHS

The New NHS (DoH, 1997) has established a National Institute for Clinical Excellence to ensure that standards are met and cost effectiveness is achieved. The Government proclaimed that nationally this means consistent access to services across the country. Locally, clinical governance will mean NHS Trusts ensuring clinical standards are achieved, whilst a Commission of Health Improvement will oversee the quality of services and intervene directly when a problem arises. If effective, this should go some way toward monitoring a national standard of triage including issues such as assuring quality, good practice and maintenance of performance standards.

O'Dowd (1998) expressed concern that there had been no mention of membership for the United Kingdom Central Council within the National Institute for Clinical Excellence. The author echoes this concern and believes that modification to practice cannot take place effectively without consultation with members of all multidisciplinary teams involved in assuring that quality and standards are met.

The Patient's Charter

With raised expectations on the part of health service consumers and the publishing of the Department of Health *Patient's Charter* document (1992), nurses and managers are aware of the need to conform to national and local Charter standards. The document coerced A&E departments into providing a formal triage assessment by inclusion of Standard Five, which guaranteed patients an immediate clinical assessment to determine their need for treatment. This was undoubtedly effective in ensuring a reduction of possible detrimental effects of delays in the waiting room for seriously ill or injured patients. However, the fluctuating workload within A&E departments made the provision of immediate assessment unrealistic within most departments, even after the introduction of a formal triage system. This resulted in brief encounters, which denied patients an effective, safe and accurate assessment and failed to give those involved time to develop patient/nurse relationships. Structured local protocols have now ensued and most A&E departments have established their own Charter guidelines detailing standards and waiting times. Difficulties and differences in opinion still occur but these protocols have helped resolve many problems.

Local Charter guidelines offer a longer period of time for triage assessment, allowing a higher and safer level of assessment with improved standards of care for all categories of patients. Local NHS Trusts have concentrated their efforts on adapting and implementing guidelines in priority clinical areas to suit local needs.

An effective triage system and patient reception combine detailed nurse assessment with a definitive approach. Careful consideration should be given to observations, intuitive reactions and concise but accurate documentation. Priorities are then established effectively and the information can be interpreted and synthesized to enhance and balance patient care.

Priorities and Responsibilities

When making an assessment the triage nurse must remain aware of his/her priorities, conscious that the main objective is the rapid assessment of whether the patient has an obvious need for resuscitation indicated by impairment or potential impairment to his/her airway, breathing or circulation. The provision of first aid measures and then immediate delegation of care for priority patients to other team members must take precedence unless triage responsibilities have been allocated to individuals.

Ensuring that priorities are met is a responsibility of the triage nurse but this does not mean that he/she necessarily has to perform these tasks him/herself as acknowledging limitations, acting as mediator and delegating these tasks is essential for the triage system to function effectively. Once patients with immediate needs have received attention, those patients who do not need urgent assistance and can wait for further assessment or treatments are prioritized.

Having ascertained that the patient is a designated non-urgent category, the triage nurse has to decide whether it is appropriate to continue with a fuller assessment. This is not appropriate if there is an excess of patients or if the next patient has been waiting longer than agreed local Charter times for assessment. The triage nurse's responsibility is to perform only mandatory investigations for the safe assessment of patients and return to patients for a more thorough investigation when time allows. If it is not appropriate to proceed with a full assessment and the delay may be detrimental to the patient, the triage nurse should delegate this care. The role of the triage nurse involves provision of care for patients in the waiting room, the continual reassessment of waiting patients, and appropriate communication and actions.

Patient Charter Standard 8 (DoH, 1992) can be related to triage as the named nurse is a possible focus for the development of the relationship between patient and triage nurse. A named nurse is a qualified nurse allocated to a patient and therefore the triage nurse can be the named nurse for patients in the waiting room, with subsequent responsibility for providing care and monitoring reassessment. The working of most A&E departments does not allow the same nurse to provide all care to the patient and communication between nursing colleagues with appropriate delegation of responsibilities is essential.

During the initial assessment, ensuring patient privacy by avoiding interruption and by using a dedicated triage facility will help to develop an understanding and tactful approach. The triage nurse should offer credible explanations for his/her actions and triage decisions made, remaining observant of issues such as parental consent and special needs of the patient. This can be a complex and extended process and should not affect patient assessment times. The triage nurse should identify practices that cause delay in triage assessment such as extensive waits for patient registration or multiple telephone enquiries and subsequently rectify these problems before they affect the assessment times. He/she must remain aware of the department and personal workloads, so that information can be given accordingly as to the effects on waiting times. To offer a supportive and attentive approach to patients can limit the degree of isolation they feel at being asked to wait, and maintaining open communication links between triage nurse and patient reassures them and reduces the risk of physical or verbal aggression.

No categorization made by the triage nurse should be final and priorities may be changed taking into consideration additional information or changes in patient condition.

Health Promotion and Health Education

If workload allows, another role of the triage nurse can be to advocate appropriate health promotion and health education. The triage nurse role is now well established and the general public will readily accept advice from a nurse. In this advantageous position the nurse must consider his/her responsibility toward health promotion and health education and incorporate these issues into the role.

Walsh (1985) claimed that A&E nurses should use opportunities that present themselves daily to practise health education as patients will tend to be motivated by the fact that they have just had a first-hand experience of illness or trauma and are therefore more receptive to health advice. There will, however, be times when distressed carers or relatives are not receptive to advice and recognizing these times is essential.

Advocacy and Empowerment

The triage nurse should encourage patients to become active participants in the decision-making process, empowering them in a positive and supportive manner and so providing a holistic, individualistic approach to care. UKCC *Ethical Guidelines* (1996) Clause 21 emphasized this point by stating that if possible the patient or client should be able to make a choice about his or her care even if this means that he/she may refuse care. A state of ignorance regarding their healthcare can be highly stressful and anxiety-provoking for patients and access to a triage nurse, although minimal, may help to allay these concerns. To enable individuals to take a proactive role in their choice of healthcare the triage nurse can empower them by developing their ability to make the right decision. The triage nurse can make accessible any relevant information and resources, giving patients the opportunity to discuss issues of their choice. The importance of clinical judgement and involving the patient in arriving at clinical decisions was stressed by Sackett et al. (1996).

When making decisions for the subsequent care of patients, the triage nurse must be aware of many factors including his/her own professional Code of Conduct, the practicality of the decision, the legal implications, religious beliefs, moral obligations and aesthetics. Nurses should assume this role of advocate only according to the extent of their knowledge, skill, and ethical and legal maturity (Cahill, 1994).

There are inherent benefits to this proactive approach, such as patient satisfaction and decreased waiting times. Devlin (1998) stated that patient satisfaction will become the vital domain of healthcare assessment with the new NHS charter addressing the principles relating to standards of treatment and care and informing patients of what they can expect (DoH, 1997). Nuttall (1986), Grose (1988) and Mallett and Woolwich (1990), all claimed that triage subsequently results in an overall reduction in waiting times. However, we must also recognize the capacity for problems if not implemented carefully.

Accountability

The triage nurse should be aware of the consequences of any actions and recognize that A&E nursing is an area where scope of professional practice underpins the development of nursing practice (Autar, 1996). The *Scope of Professional Practice* document (UKCC, 1992b) stated that nurses should acknowledge any limitations in their knowledge and competence and decline any duties or responsibilities unless able to undertake them in a safe and skilled manner. Using acquired knowledge should help the triage nurse to develop an appreciation and thorough understanding of his/her decisions and help to solve problems, foresee results and develop self-reliance.

Throughout any aspects of triage assessment, the nurse continues to have professional responsibility for his/her practice and must retain awareness of his/her accountability. The *Scope of Professional Practice* (UKCC, 1992b) supported the *Code of Conduct* (UKCC, 1992a) and clarified that all nurses and other healthcare workers are accountable for their practice, including the giving and receiving of delegated tasks.

The triage nurse must also remain aware of confidentiality, ethical underpinnings, moral obligations and legal considerations and recognize his/her own accountability for actions and non-actions in respect of these issues. Awareness of his/her responsibility to the UKCC, to employers, to him/herself and to the patients allows the triage nurse to balance these issues.

Potential Problems

It would be contentious to conclude this discussion regarding the role of the triage nurse without highlighting the potential pitfalls of such a role. Triage decision-makers should be able to deviate from guidelines if dilemmas occur, taking into account variables such as the cultural, legal and ethical implications. Nevertheless, triage nurses should avoid making purely emotional responses and abstain from lengthy deliberation on these aspects by retaining the ability to reason, with the intention of improving patient care and attempting to avert problems by risk reduction. It is impossible to evaluate every situation as similar and each episode needs independent assessment to prevent difficulties from occurring.

Problems may develop when there are no written protocols from local Trusts, or when there is minimal liaison regarding protocols with outside agencies such as general practitioners. Medical restrictions such as the reluctance of general practitioners, practice nurses and other hospital specialities to accept referrals from triage nurses can also impede the system.

Concise and accurate documentation of triage assessment is essential for clinical and legal reasons. The *Guidelines for Records and Record Keeping* document (UKCC, 1998) stated that the purpose of the records is to provide clear evidence of the care planned, the decisions made and to provide current information on the condition of the patient. This is of particular benefit for A&E patients allocated to the waiting room because, if the notes are precise, the triage nurse can identify from previous documentation whether reassessment of the patient or a change in patient categorization is indicated.

If inadequate note-taking is allowed, this can be detrimental to patients and to the triage nurse taking over responsibility for the waiting patients. If there is no mention of special circumstances of certain patients or those patients requiring reassessment then the nurse taking over the role of triage has no basic information to enable adequate continuation of care. If he/she feels that there is a lack of information in the patient records further assessment may be needed, thereby increasing the demand on the nurse's already over-stretched time.

Environmental factors also need to be taken into consideration to avoid problems. Not having access to suitable triage facilities to enable patient privacy is detrimental as the amount of information the patient may offer at this point may be restricted. A noisy and overcrowded waiting room is not conducive to patient assessment, particularly when there are constant interruptions from patients, relatives and reception staff. Increased demand on the triage nurse role, such as integrating the role with that of the emergency nurse practitioner or with added responsibility for giving telephone advice to callers, adds considerable duress to the expectations made of the triage nurse and is not advocated.

In A&E departments where triage nurses are expected to assess ambulance patients as well as walking wounded patients, answer telephone enquiries and perform reception and porters' duties the potential for the system to fail is high because the priorities and functions of the triage nurse become indistinct.

If in extreme circumstances triage is not performed, the reasons should be documented as this acknowledges the periods when the work environment is chaotic and when additional provision of staff is needed, and offers reasons as to why Charter standards have not been achieved when audit is performed.

Evaluation/Audit

Read et al. (1992) advised that continual monitoring and evaluation of triage is necessary to identify training needs and service improvement. Evaluation should include the identification of realistic goals, collection of data and the use of measurable indicators of goal achievement. These can be performed by a systematic activity analysis of the triage nurse resource, retrospectively, by a doctor's assessment, clinical audit and audit of triage notes. The NHS Management Executive (1993) recommended that clinical audit should be professionally led and, once established, should become part of routine practice in guideline implementation.

Conclusion

The author believes that the practice of nurse triage is essential to ensure safe and effective positive care for all patients. Expert triage nurses effortlessly fulfil the expectations of their role by delivering appropriate care, and are skilled to a level of professional expertise far beyond that provided by courses or training. They excel by interpreting and optimizing care and through taking a proactive approach by demonstration of innovative and challenging practice. To integrate the triage nurse service and to adequately prepare triage nurses to meet the needs of the public, individual Trusts must recognize that training is needed. Such training can subsequently help the triage nurse become efficient and productive, with the ability to identify high-risk situations and contend with complex and challenging dilemmas.

The implications for the future role of the triage nurse are continuing extensive responsibilities encompassing new technology, patient-centred care pathways and development of their multi-skilled ability. The triage nurse must practise within local guidelines, and essential to this role is to have an awareness of hospital and Trust policies, current research and up-to-date nursing practice. To be credible and acceptable as an expert triage nurse the nurse must take initiative, delegate responsibilities efficiently and develop analytical and problem-solving approaches to patient assessment. The future role of the triage nurse is determined by the development of these professional and autonomous decisions.

References

Autar R (1996) The scope of professional practice in specialist practice. British Journal of Nursing 5(16): 984–90.

British Association for Accident and Emergency Medicine and The Royal College of Nursing (1996) Priorities for Accidents and Emergencies: A Standard Scale of Triage. London: BAEM and RCN.

Cahill J (1994) Are you prepared to be their advocate? Issues in patient advocacy. Professional Nurse 9(6): 371–5.

Crouch R (1994) Triage, past, present and future. Emergency Nurse 2(1): 4–6.

Department of Health (1992) The Patient's Charter. London: HMSO.

Department of Health (1997) The New NHS: Modern, Dependable. London: HMSO.

Devlin HB (1998) Clinical governance: another stick to beat managers with? British Journal of Health Care Management 4(7): 318–19.

Gorton B (1993) The Patient's Charter and the Accident and Emergency Department. Report of evaluative research to the Department of Health. London: DoH.

Gray R (1991) Introducing triage to a new department. Nursing Standard 5(30): 25–7.

Grose A (1988) Triage in accident and emergency. Professional Nurse 3(10): 400–2.

Hendricks J, Harris J (1996) The lifeline of triage. Accident and Emergency Nursing 4(2): 82–7.

Mackway-Jones K (1996) Emergency Triage. Manchester Triage Group. London: British Medical Journal.

Mallett J, Woolwich C (1990) Triage in accident and emergency departments. Journal of Advanced Nursing 15: 1443–51.

National Health Service Management Executive (1993) Achieving an Organisation-wide Approach to Quality. Leeds: NHSME.

Nuttall M (1986) The chaos controller. Nursing Times 82(20): 66–8.

O'Dowd A (1998) Report on UKCC open session. Nursing Times 94(36): 8.

Parmer M, Hewitt E (1985) Triage on trial. Senior Nurse 2(5): 21–2.

Read S, George S, Westlake L, Williams B, Glasgow J, Potter T (1992) Piloting an evaluation of triage. International Journal of Nursing Studies 29(3): 275–88.

Rock D, Pledge M (1991) Priorities of care for the walking wounded. Professional Nurse 6(8): 463–5.

Royal College of Nursing (1984) Cited in Blythin P (1988) Triage in the UK. Nursing 3(31): 16–20.

Sackett DL, Rosenburg WMC, Gray JAM (1996) Evidence based medicine. What it is and what it isn't. British Medical Journal 312: 71–2.

United Kingdom Central Council for Nursing, Midwifery and Health Visiting (1992a) Code of Professional Conduct. London: UKCC.

United Kingdom Central Council for Nursing, Midwifery and Health Visiting (1992b) The Scope of Professional Practice. London: UKCC.

United Kingdom Central Council for Nursing, Midwifery and Health Visiting (1996) Ethical Guidelines. London: UKCC.

United Kingdom Central Council for Nursing, Midwifery and Health Visiting (1998) Guidelines for Records and Record Keeping. London: UKCC.

Walsh M (1985) Accident and Emergency Nursing: A New Approach, 3rd edn. London: Heinemann.

York S, Proud G (1990) Ophthalmic triage. Nursing Times 86(8): 40–2.

Chapter 16
The Role of the Emergency Nurse Practitioner

ELLEN TURNER

Introduction

This chapter has been written to give an insight into the development of the nurse practitioner (NP) role and how the role has expanded to include emergency nurse practitioners (ENP) working in minor injury units and accident and emergency (A&E) departments across the UK. It highlights the ENP role within major A&E departments and the subsequent advantages. Legal aspects of the role and the importance of suitable training are also discussed.

The Nurse Practitioner: Background

A programme was commenced in the early 1970s in North Carolina and other American states to train NPs to work in rural areas where access to physicians was limited (Stilwell, 1982).

In the late 1960s and early 1970s the expectations of the American public for its healthcare system grew considerably. The public demanded a system that was available, accessible and comprehensive (Geolot et al., 1977). The American Academy of Nurse Practitioners estimates that 32,000 NPs work in clinics, nursing homes, hospitals or their own offices. Most specialize in adult, family or paediatric healthcare. According to the American Nurses Association there is currently one NP available for every seven open positions (Curry, 1994).

In the UK the role of accident and emergency (A&E) nurses was greatly limited in 1968 by a DHSS circular on A&E services which prevented nurses treating any patient unless seen by a doctor first (DHSS, 1968). In the first half of the twentieth century, the role of the nurse was seen as subservient to the more powerful medical profession. However, the nursing profession has attempted to break away from perceived medical domination in the last twenty years (Brooking, 1991). The doctor/nurse relationship has changed dramatically since the late 1970s owing to the increasing knowledge base of the nursing profession. Guidelines issued in 1977 by the DHSS on the 'extended role of the nurse' allowed the delegation of tasks from a doctor to a nurse, providing training had been received (DHSS, 1977). This allowed extension of the role of the A&E nurse within local guidelines (Davis, 1992). Although nurses were seen to be competent in carrying out extended roles such as suturing, application of plaster of Paris (POP) or gastric lavage, they had no control over diagnosis or prescriptions (Potter, 1990).

The role of the NP was not developed in the UK until the mid-1980s and arose from inadequacies in the provision of medical care. This has occurred for three main reasons:

- a lack of appropriately qualified medical practitioners;
- patient dissatisfaction with the quality of care, including consultation time and choice of treatment;
- difficulty in access to primary healthcare.

In the UK the role of the NP has therefore developed in areas where resources are under scrutiny, where patients are able to express (and have expressed) dissatisfaction, where they can be offered choices and where nurses can be the primary point of access for patients (Fawcett-Henesy, 1990).

A&E staff have recognized for many years that a significant proportion of patients attending A&E departments do not necessarily require the services of a medical practitioner (Jones, 1986; Yates, 1987). The development of the emergency nurse practitioner (ENP) role in A&E departments has confirmed this observation.

The development of the NP role in the UK has been slow and restricted. In 1987 Yates conducted a research study of 230 A&E department consultants in the UK to seek their opinion regarding the development of the ENP role. The results showed that only a minority of the consultants supported the nurse practitioner concept, and 103 respondents (66%) thought that the nurse practitioner concept would increase medico-legal consequences. The majority of doctors maintained that nurses should not step outside their traditional role.

James and Pyrgos (1989) stated that nurses in GP surgeries and industry treat patients, therefore it seemed logical that they do so in A&E departments. They conducted a comparative study to assess whether the investigations and treatments suggested by experienced nurses and doctors were the same. The study was carried out using four nursing sisters who had over 5 years' A&E nursing experience. For the duration of the study the nurses saw 332 patients and recorded their findings and theoretical management plan. They did not institute any treatment. A middle-grade doctor subsequently examined and treated the patients without being aware of the nurse's findings. The patients were seen by the doctor at their original position in the patient queue in order to assess any potential saving in waiting times. After assessment they were asked if they would be happy to be seen and treated by a nurse if he or she were appropriately trained. The patients seen by the nurses were limited to the walking wounded over the age of 5 years who did not have any significant head, eye, chest or abdominal complaints apart from superficial wounds to the skin.

The results showed that of the 332 patients seen, there were 150 patients for whom both the nurse and the doctor thought an X-ray was required. The nurse's requests differed from the doctor's in 18 patients. There were 22 patients for whom the nurse would have requested an X-ray but were not sent for X-ray by the doctor. During the period of the study, the nurses performed well in treating most of the patients. They were assessed against experienced doctors and had no specific training for the role. The nurses' examination techniques, however, relied more on experience and intuition than on method. Of those patients deemed suitable to be treated by the nurse, 94% stated that if a nurse practitioner system were introduced they would agree to use it. This study highlighted the fact that, with appropriate training, nurses are able to care for patients with minor injuries and that the public will accept the concept of the ENP role.

The A&E department at Oldchurch Hospital, Essex, was the first to establish ENP services in the UK in 1986. Following a trial period of 10 weeks, where an ENP saw the majority of the minor-injured patients, a clinical audit of 50 patients' notes showed that 44 had been appropriately managed by the ENP. Although six patients had been mismanaged, they would not have suffered any adverse effects as a consequence (Morris and Head, 1989). During the trial period the Essex Community Health Council sampled the response of the general public to the nurse practitioners, questioning 124 consecutive patients. They found that 91% were satisfied with the treatment they had received and 86% felt it was a great improvement to the department. As the trial demonstrated that an ENP would be viewed as a positive addition to the department, a full-time ENP post was established utilizing existing senior nurses in the department. The scheme was subsequently given the Royal Institute of Public Administration (RIPA) award.

A study was undertaken by Read et al. in 1992 to determine the distribution and scope of ENP schemes in England and Wales. From the 465 departments surveyed only 27 (6%) had an official NP scheme. In contrast, unofficial NP schemes were reported in 159 departments, more commonly in specialist departments and minor injury units and less frequently in major A&E departments. Three main conclusions emerged from this study:

- Official NP schemes were rare and most commonly occurred in specialized A&E departments (particularly ophthalmology) where many nurses had relevant postgraduate qualifications and many years of specialized clinical experience.
- Differences between the work of official and unofficial NPs in equivalent departments were relatively minor.
- The range and volume of NP work in major general departments was small, reflected in the estimated small numbers of patients treated by NPs nationwide.

The researchers indicated that the presenting problems of patients attending major general or minor A&E departments were broadly similar, despite the wide discrepancy in the proportion of patients managed by doctors and NPs in the two types of department. They recommended that if the role of the NP in A&E departments was to become more clearly defined rather than to continue to develop sporadically and largely unofficially, four issues must be considered:

- Where official NP schemes are in place staffing arrangements must ensure that the ENP can actually practise and not be diverted to other tasks.
- Clear protocols should be drawn up and properly constituted audit arrangements made to monitor the outcome of an increased volume of treatment by NPs.
- As well as establishing the degree of conformity to present standards, auditing arrangements should compare the management of similar cases by NPs and junior doctors for both process and outcome.

Finally, national training and accreditation for NPs should be discussed in the context of the moves to extend the role of the nurse (Read et al., 1992).

The ENP role has been well established in the A&E department at Southend Healthcare Trust in Essex. The ENPs there are able to order and review X-rays, organize analgesia, cannulate patients and admit to a ward (Dillner, 1995). Southend Healthcare Trust is one of the main hospitals to offer a nationally recognized ENP training course.

Woolwich (1992) described the ENP concept as an exciting and innovative role for the A&E nurse seeking to extend the boundaries of practice within the clinical area and also his or her own expertise. Woolwich developed the ENP role in the A&E department of St Mary's Hospital, London. A pilot study was designed to highlight any unforeseen problems that may have hindered the NP role. The issues of requesting and interpreting X-rays, the availability of senior medical staff to discuss patient referral and the range of patients that could be seen by the ENPs were problems identified by the pilot study. These issues were addressed and guidelines implemented. The ENP role has now been successfully set up in the department.

Role of the Emergency Nurse Practitioner in A&E Departments: Definition of an Emergency Nurse Practitioner

The ENP is an experienced nurse who is able to make a detailed physical, social and psychological assessment before providing care and treatment and arranging appropriate referral and follow-up care. In A&E departments, the ENP may act as an alternative professional and first point of contact for those with minor injuries. The role of the ENP encompasses the principles of both care and cure and enables the nurse to provide an autonomous holistic approach to care (Potter, 1990).

ENPs are totally accountable for their actions. Walsh (1989) stated that the development of the ENP role should not be seen as being that of assistant to the A&E doctor. Rather, the ENP should be viewed as someone with much more to offer such as time, understanding and a listening ear. He argues that the role of the ENP in A&E departments should include providing health education and a holistic approach to care.

Potter (1990) advocated that the development of the ENP role offered real scope for improvement in A&E services. His research study on the potential role of NPs highlighted that the use of NPs in A&E departments significantly reduced waiting times, not only for those patients seen by the NP but for those seen by medical officers as they were relinquished to more appropriate patients. The author concluded that the introduction of NPs undoubtedly improves patient services within A&E departments and offers patients an alternative and efficient system of care.

The UKCC *Scope and Extended Practice of Nursing* document (UKCC, 1992c) is governed by the principles outlined in the UKCC *Code of Professional Conduct* (UKCC, 1992a), which places particular emphasis on knowledge, skill, responsibility and accountability. The code therefore provides a firm framework within which decisions about adjustments to the scope of professional practice can be made. The practice of nursing requires the application of knowledge and simultaneous exercise of judgement and skill.

Practice must therefore be sensitive, relevant and responsive to the needs of individual patients and clients and have the capacity to adjust where and when appropriate to changing circumstances. The values that underpin nursing practice and thus the role and function of the professional nurse are set out within the *Strategy for Nursing, Midwifery and Health Visiting* (DoH, 1989). Similarly, principles and values for good practice are documented in *The Patient's Charter* (DoH, 1991). These are:

• an understanding and appreciation of each patient or client as a whole person;

- a fundamental respect for the individual, acknowledging that
  each person is unique and has the basic human right to be treated
  as such;
- respect for the integrity of the person and his/her right to expect
  honesty, respect and the preservation of dignity.

These principles and values apply to every nurse but are of paramount importance in the role of the ENP, who has the responsibility
and autonomy for the total care of individual patients.

Rationale for the Emergency Nurse Practitioner Role in Accident and Emergency Departments

The continuing rise in attendances at A&E departments has resulted
in increased waiting times, particularly for the patient with a minor
injury. There is an increasing demand for healthcare facilities and
the public in many areas has come to regard the A&E department as
an alternative to the GP for minor injuries, ailments and non-urgent
conditions.

A&E departments have to deal with an uncontrolled fluctuating
workload involving a wide range of conditions from the acutely ill
and severely injured to the relatively minor injury/ailment which
does not require the full facilities of an A&E department. The ENP
can contribute by safely treating many patients and by educating
them on the appropriate use of both A&E and GP services. In light
of changes in the NHS in recent years and in the future with respect
to the Community Care Bill 1989, the Patient's Charter 1991,
Health of the Nation 1993 and the Audit Commission 1996, health
authorities have addressed, or will be required to, the issue of
ENPs. Shortage of doctors and the reduction of doctors' hours are
additional issues.

There is no legal requirement for patients to be seen by a doctor
merely because they present to A&E departments (Yates, 1987) and
research has shown that where an ENP is employed, conditions for
both the patients and the A&E department as a whole have
improved (Potter, 1990). These include:

- waiting times reduced;
- abuse and aggression reduced;

- staff morale improved;
- better use of medical time;
- better use of nursing time;
- reduction of departmental misuse;
- a good 'patient focus' system is demonstrated.

Training

The ENP role enables the experienced A&E nurse to use his/her skills to the full whilst the role is continually expanding and the protocols and parameters of practice extending. James and Pyrgos (1989) advocated that the ENP must have at least three years' A&E experience in a senior position and that appropriate training must be given. The role demands skills not taught during the RGN training and therefore requires post-basic training combined with experience. The RCN (1990) recommended that the ENP be given training that will develop the knowledge and skills to carry out the role. Such training should enable the ENP to make a clinical assessment and diagnosis based on the history and examination of the minor illness or injury attendee. The ENP is then able to draw up a logical plan of care to manage the patient's health problems, and make arrangements for appropriate follow up. Training should include:

(1) Assessment and diagnosis:
  - to enable the ENP to recognize signs and symptoms of minor trauma and to distinguish between the normal and abnormal;
  - to make an accurate assessment and diagnosis of patients;
  - to undertake defined diagnostic tests related to the presenting condition and interpret and evaluate the results.
(2) Treatment and prescribing:
  - to enable the ENP to select appropriate treatment based on an accurate diagnosis;
  - to prescribe and implement a programme of care and refer to appropriate agencies to continue care.
(3) Communication skills:
  - to improve public relations skills and develop productive relationships with outside agencies;
  - to develop skills for documenting accurately patient history, diagnosis and treatment;

- to ensure that documentation is concise and relevant, written in a manner acceptable in medical practice, legally sound and in accordance with the policies of the department in which practice is taking place.

(4) Health behaviour and the prevention of illness:
  - to enable the ENP to demonstrate knowledge, skills and attitudes to the main health problems in the community, providing health promotion, preventive, curative and rehabilitative care;
  - to understand the contributory factors in health and illness including social, ethnic and occupational factors;
  - to be able to recognize the relationships between life behaviour and health and illness.

The role of the ENP is wide and varied and continually developing. Whilst it is assumed an experienced A&E nurse will already have the necessary knowledge to deal with the majority of minor injuries referred to him/her, specific tutorials are necessary to ensure that knowledge is complete.

The ENP must keep updated on the changes that occur in the treatment of the minor injury/ailment patient to ensure the best possible care for the patient. Limited prescribing of dressings and medications is still the subject of debate at government level. The first Crown Report in 1989 led to legislation in 1994 that saw the creation of nurse prescribing in pilot studies. This is currently being extended throughout the UK with a £12 million government-backed campaign (Waters, 1999).

The educational requirements of the ENP role have also been the subject of much debate (RCN, 1992; Cooper, 1996; Bland, 1997; Walsh, 1997). There are various university-accredited courses, although Walsh (1997) argued that anything less than the RCN two-year diploma for NPs may be inadequate.

Legal Implications and Accountability

The legal implications for the ENP role are covered in the DHSS Health Circular *The Extended Role of the Clinical Nurse* (1997).

This guidance makes the employing authority liable for the extension of the nurse's role. The nurse must have been specifically and adequately trained for the role, which must be one that can be properly delegated to the nurse and has been recognized by the professions and by the employing authority. An acceptable training programme must be offered and appropriate refresher courses provided.

Consultations with all disciplines involved in patient care must take place and it is essential that the health authority take full responsibility for the action of its nurses. It is important for all current and future practising ENPs to note that the *Code of Conduct* (UKCC, 1992a) makes nurses vulnerable when they take on new roles without adequate preparation and training (Mitchinson, 1996). The RCN Accident and Emergency Nursing Forum recommends that the ENP should be able to prescribe simple analgesia, tetanus vaccinations and over-the-counter medicines. It is hoped that this may be extended in the future. Section 58 (2) of the Medicines Act (1968), which underpins the legal position regarding nurses giving to patients medicines that have not been prescribed by a doctor, stated that requests for 'prescription only medicines' should be given only by a doctor, dentist, veterinary surgeon or a person acting in accordance with the direction of an appropriate practitioner. It has been suggested that protocols may constitute such directions (Marshall, 1997).

It is recognized that the ENP belongs to a professional organization providing indemnity insurance. Young (1989) stated that a nurse practitioner employed in the health authority is legally the employee of the health authority, and where this relationship exists the employer is vicariously liable for the tasks of the employee during the course of his/her employment. This liability exists whether the acts were authorized or not, unless the act was solely for the employee's own purpose.

Walsh (1989) stated that NPs are totally accountable for their own actions. Indeed, no nurse should carry out a procedure he/she does not feel confident in doing or has not received appropriate training to do. Whilst the ENP is accountable for his/her own actions, the UKCC *Scope and Extended Practice of Nursing* (UKCC 1992c) document is governed by the principles outlined in the UKCC *Code of Professional Conduct* (UKCC, 1992a), which places particular emphasis on knowledge, skill, responsibility and accountability. Derrick (1989) stated that nurses extending their role, although trained for practice, may not fully appreciate the legal issues surrounding it. Primary liability is held by the individual nurse for his or her own actions. Rea (1987) stated that negligence is divided into three main components:

- *The duty of care*: The legal duty of care encompasses the professional, moral, ethical and sociological duties of care within which nurses operate. It is what the nurse is required to do under the terms of his/her contract of employment. Deviation from this in any way is 'negligence'.
- *The breach of the duty*: This is the alleged wrongdoing.
- *The resultant damage*: The damage to the patient must be the result of the breach of the duty of care.

The law relating to negligence principally seeks to identify conduct that does not reach an acceptable professional standard. If injury results from such conduct, the possibility of an action for damages arises (Rea, 1987). As each registered nurse is accountable for his or her practice, it should also be every nurse's individual responsibility to understand the legal implications underlying that accountability. It is therefore essential that individual health Trusts promote interest in and provide knowledge of the legal side of nursing, particularly in respect of the extended role in nursing and the development of ENPs.

The Way Forward

Public expectations of the health care system in the UK are growing. The public demands a system that is available, accessible and comprehensive (Geolot et al., 1977). This is now being recognized by the Government with its current proposal to open twenty 'walk-in' health centres in shopping precincts in the next three years.

Minor Injury Units (MIUs) have already been set up in many areas where smaller A&E departments have been closed. There are now more than 300 MIUs across the UK (Dolan 1999). These have proved invaluable to the public and have allowed experienced nurses to fully utilize their skills as ENPs. At many of these MIUs, ENPs are trained not only to request but also to interpret X-rays (Freij et al., 1996), and have limited powers of prescribing. The Audit Commission (1996) produced a report dealing mainly with the running of A&E departments. It identified the steps needed to improve the provision of care to all who are currently examined or treated in A&E departments, and how these requirements may change as alternative settings for the provision of care develop. Some of the recommendations included the role of ENPs:

- There should be more effective use of ENPs, and courses specifically for NPs working in A&E departments should be offered, with a common core content and accredited by the English and Welsh National Boards.
- There are currently wide differences in agreed local protocols. Some ENPs are allowed to treat children aged over 12 months, at other hospitals the minimum age is 5 years. Comparative information on current practice and specimen protocols should be made available to guide these local decisions.
- Experienced ENPs should have the same access to senior medical advice as A&E doctors and should not be supervised by junior doctors.
- All ENPs need to rotate to other roles to avoid losing their broader skills. This report demonstrated that there is significant scope to improve services provided by many A&E facilities without the need for increased funding.
- Rostering can often be improved so that there is a better match between staff availability and patient demand.
- The scope of nursing practice can be expanded and procedures modified to treat and discharge some patients more quickly.

Conclusion

From the many research studies carried out it is acknowledged that the majority of the public accept an ENP service. The ENP role in A&E departments is therefore set to expand and widen its horizons. The continued rise in new A&E attendances, on average 2% per year since 1981 (Audit Commission, 1996), has helped A&E consultants to accept the contribution of the ENP. However, managers still need to address the issues surrounding the role, including the availability of adequate nursing staff to match expected workload and other appropriate resources. There must also be courses specifically for NPs working in A&E departments, with a common core content and accredited by the National Boards, to standardize the variations in local protocols. In this way, a high standard of holistic care will benefit both patient and staff and the ENP will be regarded as a safe, autonomous professional.

Suggested Further Reading

Guly HR (1996) History Taking, Examination, Record Keeping. Oxford: Oxford University Press.
Ewles L, Simnett I (1995) Promoting Health: A Practical Guide, 3rd edn. London: Scutari Press.
Raby N, Berman L, de Lacey G (1995) Accident and Emergency Radiology: A Survival Guide. London: WB Saunders.

References

Audit Commission (1996) By Accident or Design: Improving A&E Services in England and Wales. London: HMSO.
Bland A (1997) Developing the ENP role in accident and emergency. Accident and Emergency Nursing 5: 42–7.
Brooking J (1991) Doctors and nurses: a personal view. Nursing Standard 6(12): 24–8.
Cooper M (1996) A literature review. Emergency Nurse 4(2): 19–22.
Curry JL (1994) Nurse practitioners in the A&E department: current issues. Journal of Emergency Nursing 20(3): 207–12.
Davis J (1992) Expanding horizons. Nursing Times 88(47): 37–9.
Department of Health (1989) Health Circular, HC, CMO (MH) 9 & CMO/CNO Letter, PL/CMO (89) 7, 20 September.
Department of Health (1991) The Patient's Charter. London: DoH
Department of Health (1993) Health of the Nation. London: DoH.
Derrick S (1989) Legal implications of extended roles. The Professional Nurse (April).
DHSS (1968) Accident and Emergency Services, HM (68) 82. London: HMSO.
DHSS (1997) The Extended Role of the Clinical Nurse: Legal Implications and Training Guidelines. London: HMSO.
DHSS (1989) Health Circular, HC, CMO (MH) 9 and CMO/CNO letter, PL/CMO (89) 7, 20 September.
Dillner L (1995) A matter of chance. Nursing Times 91(7): 14–15.
Dolan B (1999) MIUs help to revolutionise A&E care, report from RCN ENP Conference. Nursing Standard 13(31).
Fawcett-Henesy A (1990) Setting the scene for revolution. Nursing Standard 4(21): 35–9.
Freij RM, Duffy T, Hackett D (1996) Radiographic interpretation by NPs in a MIU. Journal of Accident and Emergency Medicine 13: 41–3.
Geolot D, Alongi S, Edich RF (1977) Emergency nurse practitioner: an answer to an emergency care crisis in rural hospitals. Journal of the American College of Emergency Physicians 6(8): 355–7.
HMSO (1993) Health of the Nation. London: HMSO.
House of Commons (1989) National Health Service and Community Care Bill, November. London: House of Commons.

James MR, Pyrgos N (1989) Nurse practitioner in the A&E department. Archives of Emergency Medicine 6: 241–6.

Jones G (1986) The waiting game. Nursing Times (October): 28–33.

Marshall J et al. (1997) Administration of medicine by emergency nurse practitioners according to protocols in an A&E department. Journal of A&E Medicine 14: 233–7.

Mitchinson S (1996) Are nurses independent and autonomous practitioners? Nursing Standard 10(34): 34–8.

Morris F, Head S (1989) The nurse practitioner: help in clarifying clinical and educational activities in A&E departments. Health Trends 21: 124–6.

Potter T (1989) Potential role of the nurse practitioner in A&E. Emergency Nurse 4(1): 2.

Potter T (1990) A real way forward in A&E: developing the nurse practitioner role. Professional Nurse (August): 586–8.

Rea K (1987) Negligence. Nursing 3: 533.

Read SM, Jones NB, Williams BT (1992) Nurse practitioners in A&E departments: what do they do? British Medical Journal 305: 1466–9.

Rees C (1990) The questionnaire in research. Nursing Standard 4(42): 34–5.

Royal College of Nursing (1990) A&E Nursing Forum, ENPs: Guidelines. London: RCN.

Royal College of Nursing (1992) Emergency Nurse Practitioners: Guidance from the Royal College of Nursing. London: RCN Accident and Emergency Nursing Forum.

Sheehan J (1985) Selecting the right method. Nursing Mirror 160(20): 19–20.

Stilwell B (1982) The nurse practitioner at work. Nursing Times (3 November): 1859–60.

United Kingdom Central Council for Nursing, Midwifery and Health Visiting (1992a) Code of Professional Conduct. London: UKCC.

United Kingdom Central Council for Nursing, Midwifery and Health Visiting (1992b) The Scope of Professional Practice. London: UKCC.

United Kingdom Central Council for Nursing, Midwifery and Health Visiting (1992c) Scope and Extended Practice of Nursing. London: UKCC.

Walsh M (1989) The A&E department and the nurse practitioner. Nursing Standard 4(11): 34–5.

Walsh M (1993) A&E or the GP: how patients decide. Nursing Standard 7(25): 36–8.

Walsh M (1997) Commentary: Nurse practitioner roles should be explicitly defined. Nursing Standard 11(17): 36–7.

Waters A (1999) Playing the waiting game. Nursing Standard 13(26): 12–13.

Woolwich C (1992) A wider frame of reference. Nursing Times 88(46): 34–36.

Yates DW (1987) Nurse practitioners for A&E? British Journal of Accident and Emergency Medicine (March): 10–11.

Young AP (1989) Legal Problems in Nursing Practice, 2nd edn. London: Harper & Row.

Chapter 17
Telephone Triage

Stuart Toulson

Introduction

> Imparting information over the telephone is analogous to nursing with your
> eyes closed and your hands tied behind your back. (Glasper, 1993a, p. 34)

Much has been written about the ever-expanding role of the qualified nurse, and the ensuing debate regarding what used to be termed
extended roles has been heightened by the recent drive to decrease
junior doctors' hours. There has been subsequent discussion about
what nursing actually is and what is therefore unique about the role
of a qualified nurse compared with that of a healthcare assistant.
The whole issue centres around the term 'professionalism' and the
continued drive by nurses to break away from the passive hand-
maiden image of the Nightingale era to become receptive to the
changing needs of their client group.

This chapter will discuss one such nursing initiative: the use of the
telephone to assess and advise patients regarding their healthcare
needs and how to access the most appropriate level of care. The implications of telephone advice both within the primary care and the accident and emergency (A&E) setting will be discussed. The current and
proposed development of NHS Direct will also be examined, highlighting why the need for such services exists and the underlying
professional and legal considerations for safe service implementation.

Telephone Advice within the Primary Care Setting

Hallam (1989) reviewed the use of telephone advice services and
concluded that it was far less common for the telephone to be a

vehicle for consultation in primary medical care in Great Britain than in the United States or Scandinavia. McCarthy and Bollam (1990) concurred that the use of telephone consultation in primary care had not been extensively studied in the United Kingdom, which appeared to lag behind other developed countries in the use of the telephone for consultation purposes (Virji, 1992).

Marsh et al. (1987) analysed all out-of-hours calls to a British GP practice during a one-year period, concluding that the commonest calls were from patients already diagnosed and under treatment; 20% were suffering from a chronic ailment and 16% from an acute condition which had been seen and treated previously. The commonest advice given was merely to enhance any existing treatments. Of the new ailments, upper respiratory tract infections and gastrointestinal problems (especially diarrhoea) were the most common and both were considered to be treatable without direct patient contact. The authors concluded that there was evidence that many of the calls received were for minor and/or self-limiting conditions. The findings are summarized in Table 17.1.

Of all patients who were given telephone advice, 45% did not consult again within a week and 35% of those invited for follow-up at surgery did not attend. Some 25% of those patients seen by a GP were also considered to be suffering from minor ailments that did not justify an out-of-hours visit.

The percentage of households in this country with access to a telephone had risen from 42% in 1972 to approximately 91% in 1992 (Oftel, 1992) and this figure has certainly increased as a result

Table 17.1 Summary of calls received and outcome

Problem	% of calls	% managed by phone	% managed by GP visit
Chronic (on treatment)	19.8	48.1	51.9
Acute (on treatment)	16.1	70.0	30.0
Upper respiratory tract	17.6	70.4	29.6
Acute gastric upset	11.7	69.5	30.5
Pain	11.6	50.0	50.0
Bleeding	04.0	57.1	42.9
Earache	03.5	57.1	42.9
Chest infection	03.3	00.0	100
Miscellaneous	12.4	54.5	45.5

Souce: Marsh et al. (1987).

of the current trend for mobile phone possession. Access to a doctor by telephone, reported as the most important improvement to general practice services desired by patients (Allen and Marks 1988), has also increased following the trend towards GP out-of-hours cooperatives. Lattimer et al. (1995) concluded that telephone communication had the potential not only for information giving but also for the assessment and management of patients. It is clear, therefore, that any telephone advice service made available to patients within the community has the potential to directly influence the access of the public to a healthcare professional.

Telephone Advice within Accident and Emergency

The A&E department has been described as the shop-front of a hospital and patients will often use it as a source of telephone advice on a wide range of medical problems (American Emergency Nurse's Association, 1991; Kunkler and Mitchell, 1994). The majority of these problems, however, tend to be minor and Verdile et al. (1989) estimated that only 1% of calls are of a true emergency nature. The practice of giving advice over the telephone has subsequently been encouraged by the National Audit Office (1992) to provide easy access to a professional, ranging from seeking urgent medical assessment to basic first-aid/self-care information.

Singh et al. (1991) demonstrated the perception of the general public that A&E was the most logical place to contact, with only 30% of patients attempting to seek advice from their GP. Egleston et al. (1994) reported a 'public demand' for medical advice by telephone, concluding that such services provided low-cost and safe access to health information. Knowles and Cummins (1984) also described a 'genuine community need' for service implementation. Glasper (1993b) concurred that telephone advice lines had 'genuine appeal' and provided an extra quality service analogous to the healthcare demands of many client groups. With growing demands for healthcare services to become more cost effective and responsive to consumer needs, consideration of telephone consultation has therefore become increasingly important (Dale et al., 1995).

A study within a Toronto children's hospital demonstrated that nurses could capably give medical advice over the telephone with subsequent reduction in emergency department attendance (Wilkins, 1993). Knowles and Cummins (1984) later studied callers to a major American Emergency Department (ER). The authors presented the results found among their 547 respondents, categorizing the main concern of the caller, and these are given in Table 17.2.

Table 17.2 Main concern of callers to an emergency department

Problem	Percentage of all cases
Gastrointestinal	14
Respiratory	12
Obstetrics/Gynaecology	10
Trauma	8
Orthopaedics (non-trauma)	6
Medications	5
Urinary tract	4
Ophthalmology	4
Emotional problems	4
Dermatology	4
Cardiac	4
Sexually transmitted disease	3
Neurology	3
Laboratory results	2
Allergy	2
Social work issues	2
Other (administrative)	13

Source: Knowles and Cummins (1984).

Singh et al. (1991) surveyed 155 calls to A&E for medical advice. Of these, 35 (23%) had previously consulted their GP and 15 (10%) had attempted to do so but were unsuccessful. The survey concluded that 67% of callers thought it necessary to contact only A&E, that problems were less than 24 hours old in 88 (57%) cases and that 63 callers described a complaint of between 48 hours and one month in duration. The nature of enquiries is categorized in Table 17.3.

The authors also categorized the advice given to callers (Table 17.4).

The Nurse as Service Provider

People will often call A&E to seek medical advice and these calls are usually answered by nursing staff (Dale et al., 1995). Kunkler and

Table 17.3 Nature of telephone enquiries to A&E

Problem	No.	%
Accidents and trauma	41	26
Medical	33	21
Parasuicide	21	14
Surgical	14	9
Dental	11	7
Stings and bites	6	4
Orthopaedic	5	3
Obstetrics and gynaecology	5	3
Psychiatric	3	2
Assault	3	2
Miscellaneous	13	9

Source: Singh et al. (1991).

Table 17.4 Advice given to callers by A&E

Advice	No.	%
Attend A&E	48	33
Urgent GP consult	27	18
Routine GP consult	16	11
Referral to dentist	10	7
Referral to speciality	5	3
Reassurance	41	28

Source: Singh et al. (1991).

Mitchell (1994) contacted 75 A&E departments within the United Kingdom, resulting in 93% of advice calls being answered by nursing staff. Of concern were the findings that 7% of calls were answered by reception staff and that requests to speak to a doctor were granted in only one case. No reasons were identified for this latter finding although the authors gave the following possible rationale:

(1) medical staff were busy with the immediate management of patients;
(2) the higher ratio of nursing to medical staff made it easier for a nurse to answer the telephone;

(3) nursing staff were more experienced at assessing patients and were able to give advice by telephone more readily.

Verdile et al. (1989) performed a similar study within the USA with comparable results: 4% of departments permitted consultation with a doctor, 9% of calls were answered by reception staff and 87% of calls were answered by nursing staff. Wheeler (1989) asked nurses to describe their most unusual telephone advice calls – the 'frightening, humorous, unexpected and bizarre'. Obscene calls were excluded from the study and the findings are given in Table 17.5.

Table 17.5 Nature of telephone advice calls

Complaint	Frequency
Ingestion/accidental overdose	23
CPR/respiratory arrest	14
Suicide in progress	7
Suicide threats	6
Chest pain	4
Homicidal threats	4
Labour/pregnancy complications	3
Homicide in progress	2
Bomb threats	2
Neuro/trauma	1
Unconsciousness	1
Seizures	1
Child abuse	1
Self-mutilation (orchidectomy)	1
Request for castration	1
Bee sting	1
Snake bite	1
Abdominal pain	1
Vaginal bleeding	2
Broken bones/lacerations	3
Sexually transmitted diseases	17
Bedroom full of bees	1
Psychiatric problems	3
Pranksters	4
Pet resuscitation/first aid	5
Non-urgent problems	30

Source: Wheeler (1989).

Advice Compliance

Toulson (1996) conducted a comparative survey of random A&E attendees, concluding that 85% of patients would use a telephone advice line if available and that 87% would be prepared to accept any subsequent advice. McGear and Sims (1988) earlier stated that cooperation was best achieved when both nurse and caller understood their roles and were able to contribute to the decision-making process. They stressed that the nurse was not responsible for the caller's feelings, subsequent actions or for guessing what the caller wanted. The following responsibilities of both nurse and caller were outlined:

- Nurse's responsibility:
  (1) being able to listen and gather information;
  (2) being knowledgeable about health and illness;
  (3) asking questions to gain relevant information;
  (4) giving information relevant to the problem in question or symptom described;
  (5) asking the caller to decide what he or she will do about the problem based on the exchange of information;
  (6) giving advice based on sound principles and stating when he or she does not agree with the caller;
  (7) documenting both the nursing assessment and the agreed plan for future action;
  (8) telephoning the caller back if the nurse is uncomfortable about the outcome of the communication.
- Caller's responsibility:
  (1) calling when he or she has a problem with, or a question about, his or her health;
  (2) giving accurate information about the problem;
  (3) being willing and prepared to answer any questions the nurse needs to ask in order to better assess particular needs;
  (4) listening to the information/advice provided by the nurse and asking questions if it is not understood;
  (5) deciding upon a course of action based on the information received and discussing this with the nurse;
  (6) contacting the service again if there is any change in symptoms or if there are further questions or problems.

Egleston et al. (1994) surveyed 145 calls to A&E with 104 respondents completing a follow-up questionnaire. Fifteen callers were advised to attend their GP with 12 complying, 67 were advised to attend A&E with 65 complying and 22 were given other advice with which they all complied. In total 95% of callers complied with advice given (in 78 [75%] cases by a nurse and in 26 [25%] by a doctor). The advice was deemed to be appropriate in 102 (98%) of cases.

Service Times

Knowles and Cummins (1984) concluded that most ER calls occurred during the late morning, that a typical call lasted 5.1 minutes, that the number of calls received was equally distributed between days of the week and that 49% of callers were regular attendees at the department. The timing of calls received is presented in Table 17.6.

Table 17.6 Timing of calls made to A&E

Time	%	Time	%
00.00–02.00	06.6%	12.00–14.00	09.7%
02.00–04.00	03.9%	14.00–16.00	06.9%
04.00–06.00	04.4%	16.00–18.00	07.3%
06.00–08.00	04.7%	18.00–20.00	08.2%
08.00–10.00	11.0%	20.00–22.00	10.2%
10.00–12.00	17.2%	22.00–24.00	09.9%

Source: Knowles and Cummins (1984).

Communication Considerations

Individuals will generally experience an interaction with a healthcare professional as an event of primary importance and will seek an understanding of the situation with a view to attaining control whilst making an assessment of a professional's social skills and responding accordingly. He/she may also try to extract from the professional the meaning of his/her remarks, whether these are questions or instructions, and to act when it is believed these questions and instructions have value. Where there are difficulties in extracting such meaning individuals may seek to act within some meaning which was not present in the original encounter and may well negotiate within themselves and act accordingly (Newell, 1994).

It should be remembered that, when giving telephone advice, the nurse must exercise a greater proficiency of interpersonal skills because the non-verbal cues of the patient will be less apparent. Patients may also call A&E with problems of every degree of severity, from the inconsequential to the life-threatening. Yet even a relatively minor problem can be experienced as severe by a patient. In such cases the tendency to 'catastrophize', to judge a situation to be more severe than it actually is, itself becomes an important part of the problem situation (Egan, 1994). Any communication skill employed by the nurse should therefore aim to help the patient to put his/her problem into perspective, to teach the distinction between differing degrees of problem severity and to advise accordingly.

Nurses all too often fall into the trap of assuming either that their health values are generally held or that, at the very least, lay people will acknowledge them as the right values since they are based on professional knowledge and expertise (Coutts and Hardy, 1985). Clearly professionals have no automatic right to expect the public to place their trust in them; instead it has to be earned and nurses are no different from any other professionals in this respect (Chadwick and Tadd, 1992). There is further danger that when an individual becomes a patient the healthcare team feel they 'possess' that individual and that as a patient the individual concerned has to surrender all 'rights' to them. This is clearly not so because the patient must retain the right to information regarding treatment and care and to be made aware of any alternative strategies that may be available (Burnard and Chapman, 1994). Smith (1980) earlier warned that a nurse must subsequently recognize that the patient carries the ultimate responsibility for determining his/her needs and what is in his/her own best interests.

Legal Considerations

Telephone advice is based on the quality of information provided by the caller, which can and may be deficient, and is given without any direct observation or tactile skills in symptom assessment (Glasper, 1993a; Henry, 1994). The current legal position is that although questioning a caller about a problem is acceptable, once telephone advice is given the individual becomes liable for the patient's well-being. Edwards (1994) examined the components of reasoning utilized by A&E nurses regarding telephone advice, concluding that a key consideration shown in decision-making was an awareness of professional vulnerability and the feeling that patients were putting the onus on them. Advice was altered in light of both professional and personal responsibilities felt towards callers, and nurses expressed a personal anxiety at the responsibility they felt for potential outcomes over which they had limited control.

Hospitals have no legal duty to provide telephone advice and nurses have no legal duty to impart advice over the telephone (Dunn, 1985). It may be argued, therefore, that the best rule for responding to a telephone request for medical advice is to advise the caller to come to the hospital for assessment because of the difficulty in diagnosing over the telephone (American Emergency Nurse's Association, 1991; Rich, 1993). Stell et al. (1996) advocated that telephone advice within A&E should not be promoted as such cautionary anxiety may create rather than reduce the demand for medical attention.

Much of the reluctance to use this medium is based on the premise that the practice is potentially hazardous in that no safe determination of a caller's condition can be made (Edwards, 1994). Declining to answer simple enquiries, however, may result in increased public frustration whereas an efficient response to a telephone enquiry may greatly increase the usefulness of A&E departments to surrounding communities. The British Association for Accident and Emergency Medicine (1992) stressed that, in such instances, the enquirer must always be reminded that he/she is the one directly aware of the severity and acuteness of the problem and that the final decision regarding when and where to seek help is ultimately his/hers.

Henry (1994) warned that a key element in defending any claim involving telephone advice would be the presence or absence of documentation. Dunn (1985) stated that there had been no recorded case of successful legal action against a hospital as a result of telephone advice, concluding 'let's keep it that way'. There are clear legal implications underpinning the use of the telephone as a medium for giving medical advice and the importance of keeping caller records is well documented (Verdile et al., 1989; Wheeler, 1989; Rich, 1993). Of concern is the *ad hoc* practice of giving telephone advice without any form of documentation. With the introduction of NHS indemnity, where hospital Trusts have to meet the financial consequences of negligence, it is clear that some form of documentation must become standardized practice. This is an era in which nursing is challenging itself and the other health professions to look carefully at fundamental issues and it is inevitable that this period of re-examination may result in uncertainty about the extent of the provider's legal and moral responsibilities (Murphy and Hunter, 1983).

NHS Direct

In December 1997 the Government published its commitment to NHS Direct, the 24-hour nurse-run telephone advice service, in the White Paper *The New NHS: Modern, Dependable* (Department of Health, 1997). The principle behind the initiative was to provide members of the public with easy and rapid advice/information regarding health, illness and the NHS so that they would be better able to care for themselves and their family.

The objectives of the service were:

- to provide a confidential and consistent source of professional advice on healthcare so that members of the public could manage many of their problems at home or be informed how best to access more appropriate care;
- to provide simple and speedy access to a comprehensive and up-to-date range of health-related information;
- to help improve quality, increase cost-effectiveness and reduce unnecessary demands on other NHS services;
- to allow professionals to develop their role in enabling patients to be partners in self-care and help them focus on those patients for whom their skills are most needed.

The service became available in November 2000 and, whilst still undergoing formal analysis, early results are encouraging with caller satisfaction high and service use increasing. Current patterns of use suggest that the service is especially used out of hours (evenings/weekends) and that the service appears to have been of great benefit to parents, with about one in four calls relating to children aged 5 years and under. Subsequent impact on A&E/GP workloads is still being debated, but a reduction in out-of-hours GP visits has been demonstrated (University of Sheffield, 1999).

Whilst the 24-hour medical advice line is the main component of NHS Direct, there is also wide support for a range of other current and proposed services (Kennelly and Dale, 1998). These include:

- NHS Direct integrated access – aiming to ensure effective nurse referral to the most appropriate out-of-hours agencies (GP, social services, mental health etc);
- NHS Direct outreach – involving nurses proactively calling patients at home who may need help and advice (e.g. those recently discharged from hospital);
- NHS Direct online – aiming to provide the public with easy access to health information via PCs and digital television;
- NHS Direct information points – providing public access points to NHS Direct in areas such as GP surgeries, A&E departments, libraries, post offices, pharmacies, shopping centres, deprived areas, etc.;
- NHS Direct healthcare guide – involving the publication and distribution of a guide covering common ailments, this is available free to the public and is included in 'bounty packs' for new parents;
- NHS Direct healthcare programme – planning to use the above guide to provide the basis for training the public on basic health care issues;
- Access to NHS Direct Services via e-mail and text;
- Referrals.

Some have compared NHS Direct with the current trend in telephone banking in which no face-to-face contact is required (Shamash, 1998) whilst some GPs have called for such 'airhead' nurse-led services to be scrapped (*Nursing Times*, 1999a, 1999b). However, many view the service as the way forward for the NHS and as a life-saving initiative (Metha, 1998; Slaughter, 1998; White, 1998).

In summary, the vision of NHS Direct is to provide one point of contact that will provide a single gateway to healthcare, ultimately giving patients more choice when accessing NHS services, as promised in The NHS Plan (2000), 'the front line of healthcare in the home'. The NHS subsequently aims to become a resource which people routinely use to help themselves, with the NHS telephone number becoming as well known as '999'.

Whatever the individual view, NHS Direct will certainly have a significant impact on A&E departments, primary care practitioners and health care delivery in general over the next decade. Therefore, whilst it is accepted that change is a threatening concept, such an initiative must be viewed as a much needed service of benefit to both patient and healthcare provider alike. What is important, however, is that the service is monitored and quality assurance strategies put in place to identify and address any areas of concern. Effective communication links between all professionals involved/affected by NHS Direct must also be maintained.

Conclusion

As healthcare evolves and becomes more responsive to consumer needs the consideration of structured nurse-run telephone advice lines should be viewed as an increasingly important and viable resource. Healthcare consumers are more selective about healthcare providers and the services on offer. Increasingly they are involved in decisions about their own care and desire the knowledge and support necessary to stay healthy and to treat non-acute problems themselves (Salvage, 1985; McGear and Simms, 1988; Hancock, 1995). Under the auspices of the *Patient's Charter* (DoH, 1992), coupled with *Health for All by the Year 2000* (WHO, 1981) and *A Vision for the Future* (DoH, 1993), purchasers of healthcare are exploring new initiatives that promote client-oriented services. The A&E nurse's role is one that has been identified for change and such change should be both desired and initiated by the nurse in the interest of his/her patients (Robinson, 1993). Telephone advice services may subsequently represent an example of such an initiative aimed at enhancing patient care, choice and autonomy.

Suggested Further Reading

McGear R, Sims J (1988) Telephone Triage and Management: A Nursing Process Approach. Philadelphia: WB Saunders.

References

Allen D, Marks B (1988) Patient access and appointment systems. The Practitioner 232: 1380–2.
American Emergency Nurse's Association (1991) Emergency Nurse's Association Position Statement - Telephone Advice. Journal of Emergency Nursing 17(5): 52.

British Association for Accident and Emergency Medicine (1992) Guidelines on the Handling of Telephone Enquiries in Accident and Emergency Departments. London: Royal College of Surgeons.

Burnard P, Chapman CM (1994) Professional and Ethical Issues in Nursing: The Code of Professional Conduct, 2nd edn. London: Scutari Press.

Chadwick R, Tadd W (1992) Ethics and Nursing Practice: A Case Study Approach. London: Macmillan.

Coutts LC, Hardy LK (1985) Teaching for Health: The Nurse as Health Educator. London: Churchill Livingstone.

Dale J, Williams S, Crouch R (1995) Development of telephone advice in A&E: establishing the views of staff. Nursing Standard 9(21): 28–31.

Department of Health (1992) The Patient's Charter. London: HMSO.

Department of Health (1993) A Vision for the Future. London: HMSO.

Department of Health (1997) The New NHS: Modern, Dependable. London: HMSO.

Department of Health (2000) The NHS Plan. London: HMSO.

Dunn JM (1985) Warning: Giving telephone advice is hazardous to your professional health. Nursing (August): 40–1.

Edwards B (1994) Telephone triage: how experienced nurses reach decisions. Journal of Advanced Nursing 19: 717–24.

Egan G (1994) The Skilled Helper: A Problem-management Approach to Helping, 5th edn. California: Brooks/Cole.

Egleston CV, Kelly HC, Cope AR (1994) Use of a telephone advice line in an accident and emergency department. British Medical Journal 308: 31.

Glasper A (1993a) Telephone triage: a step forward for nursing practice. British Journal of Nursing 2(2): 108–9.

Glasper A (1993b) Telephone triage: extending practice. Nursing Standard 7(15): 34–6.

Hallam L (1989) You've got a lot to answer for Mr Bell: a review of the use of the telephone in primary care. Family Practice 16(1): 47–57.

Hancock C (1995) Care in the year 2000. In Jolly M, Brykczynska G (Eds) Nursing beyond Tradition and Conflict. London: Mosby.

Henry FH (1994) Legal principles in providing telephone advice. Nurse Practitioner Forum 5(3): 124–5.

Kennelly C, Dale J (1998) Direct enquiries. Health Service Journal (July) 24–5.

Kenny C, Gulland A (1998) Dial N for nurses. Nursing Times 94(12): 19.

Knowles PJ, Cummins RO (1984) ED medical advice telephone calls: who calls and why? Journal of Emergency Nursing 10(6): 283–6.

Kunkler R, Mitchell A (1994) Advice over the telephone. Nursing Times 90(46): 29–30.

Lattimer V, Glasper A, Smith H, George S (1995) Out-of-hours Primary Medical Care: The Views of General Practitioners in Wessex and the North East of England on Three Models of Service Provision, report to the Department of Health. Southampton: University of Southampton.

Marsh GN, Horne RA, Channing DM (1987) A study of telephone advice in managing out-of-hours calls. Journal of the Royal College of General Practitioners 37: 301–4.

McCarthy M, Bollam M (1990) Telephone advice for out of hours calls in general practice. British Journal of General Practice 40: 19–21.

McGear R, Sims J (1988) Telephone Triage and Management: A Nursing Process Approach. Philadelphia: WB Saunders.

Metha R (1998) NHS Direct helps saves lives. Emergency Nurse 6(4): 4.

Murphy CP, Hunter H (1983) Ethical Problems in the Nurse-Patient Relationship. Boston: Allyn & Bacon.

National Audit Office (1992) NHS Accident and Emergency Departments in England. London: HMSO.

Newell R (1994) Interviewing Skills for Nurses and Other Health Care Professionals: A Structured Approach. London: Routledge.

Nursing Times (1999a) This week: Forget the gripes, NHS Direct is cutting GP workloads. Nursing Times 95(24): 9.

Nursing Times (1999b) This week: Doctors blast 'airhead' nurse-led NHS schemes. Nursing Times 95(28): 10.

Oftel (1992). Annual Report. London: Oftel.

Rich J (1993) Caring for ED patients: 13 ways to protect your practice. Nursing (February): 60–1.

Robinson DK (1993) Nurse practitioner or mini doctor? Accident and Emergency Nursing 1(1): 53–5.

Salvage J (1985) The Politics of Nursing. Oxford: Butterworth-Heinemann.

Shamash J (1998) Between the lines. Nursing Standard 12(28): 22–3.

Singh G, Barton D, Bodiwala G (1991) Accident and emergency departments' responses to patients' enquiries by telephone. Journal of Royal Society of Medicine 84(6): 345–6.

Slaughter S (1998) Soon, an NHS lifeline for 19 million of us. Daily Telegraph (28 October).

Smith S (1980) Three models of the nurse-patient relationship. In Spicker SF, Gaddow S (Eds) Nursing Images and Ideals: Opening Dialogue with the Humanities. New York: Springer.

Stell IM, Jackson RE, Rudkin ADM, Watson DP (1996) Telephone advice in accident and emergency. Is it worth it and is it safe? London (unpublished).

Toulson SM (1996) Telephone advice in accident and emergency: patients' views. Unpublished dissertation, University of Brighton.

University of Sheffield (1999) Evaluation of NHS Direct First Wave Sites Interim Report, Executive Summary (unpublished).

Verdile VP, Paris PM, Stewart RD (1989) Emergency department telephone advice. Annals of Emergency Medicine 42: 179–80.

Virji AN (1992) Usefulness of telephone consultations in general practice. British Journal of General Practice 42: 179–80.

Wheeler SQ (1989) ED telephone triage: lessons learned from unusual calls. Journal of Emergency Nursing 15(6): 481–7.

White C (1998) Smooth operators. Nursing Times 94(41): 44–5.

Wilkins VC (1993) Paediatric hotline: meeting community needs while conserving healthcare dollars. Journal of Nursing Administration 23: 26–8.

World Health Organisation (1981) Health for All by the Year 2000. Geneva: WHO.

Chapter 18
Health Education in Accident and Emergency

HELEN MARKHAM

Introduction

Health education has become a focal point within the NHS in recent years. As the service comes under increasing pressure, government initiatives such as the Health of the Nation (WHO, 1991) have begun to emphasize the importance of the prevention of ill health and this in turn has emphasized the value of health education. Within this climate of change nurses too have begun to recognize the need to develop their role in health education. Accident and emergency departments by their very nature provide a major point of contact between the general public and health services. As a result the opportunity exists to provide a health promotion and education service, which can enhance programmes run within the community and address the specific needs of the individual patient

The aim of this chapter is to expand on the subject of health education within the speciality of accident and emergency (A&E) nursing. It will address the overall aims of health promotion by examining relevant government initiatives, the role of the A&E nurse in health promotion and the practicalities of carrying out health education. The latter will include the identification of the patient's learning needs, planning the learning process (including methods of teaching) and methods of evaluation. The chapter will subsequently discuss some definitions pertinent to the subject that the reader may find useful.

Definitions

Health

The definition of 'health' can vary tremendously depending on the source. The *New Oxford Dictionary of English* (1998) simply defines health as 'The state of being well and free from illness'. However, this definition does not lend itself to defining the concept of health pertinent to those who suffer with chronic illness or disability and who will never achieve a 'perfect' level of function. It may be more effective for the purposes of this chapter, therefore, to consider that the term 'health' refers to the optimum level of performance that can be achieved on a social, psychological, physical and spiritual level for the individual.

Health Promotion/Health Education

Within the relevant literature the terms 'health promotion' and 'health education' appear to be largely interchangeable. Latter et al. (1992) defined health promotion as 'any combination of education and related legal, fiscal, economic, environmental and organisational interventions designed to facilitate the achievement of health and the prevention of disease'. Watson and Royle (1991) focused more on the input of education in health promotion that is directed towards 'sustaining or increasing the level of well being, self actualisation and personal fulfilment of a given individual or group'. Given definitions of health education/promotion that utilize the concept of teaching, it is appropriate to define teaching itself in this setting. Lane and Beales (1998) cite Hubley, who in 1993 defined teaching in health promotion as increasing knowledge and disseminating information related to health, thereby creating the basis of knowledge to make informed decisions. Within this collaborative process of health education the aim is to increase patient understanding, reduce anxieties caused by ill health or injury and thereby alter healthcare habits, with the ultimate aim of preventing the incidence of further ill health, injury or disease.

The aims and objectives of health promotion will now be addressed in more detail from both an individual and a national perspective.

Aims and Objectives of Health Promotion

Health promotion can have varying aims. The World Health Authority (WHO) definition in 1996 described a 'process of enabling people to increase control over the detriments of health and thereby improve their health'. Patients present to A&E because their health is compromised by an illness or injury that is preventing them from functioning fully (McConnell, 1997). The A&E nurse, through health promotion, should aim to help the patient manage and improve the condition of his/her immediate injury or illness. He/she should also aim to educate the patient to improve his/her general health through lifestyle changes to try and reduce further incidences of injury or illness. Many accidents may be preventable, or at least the risk of re-occurrence may be significantly reduced, through health promotion and education. With each patient, therefore, there are both short- and long-term goals concerned with health education. Whilst most patients are willing to participate actively in education related to their immediate presenting condition, the nurse must judge whether education in respect of longer term goals of health is appropriate at that time.

Watson and Royle (1991) provided a concise summary of the aims of health education in terms of long-term goals from the perspective of the individual nurse and patient. The authors listed three overall aims for health education:

(1) Health promotion can be aimed at restoring health, focusing on helping individuals to positively change their behaviour and alter their lifestyle in order to improve health.
(2) Health promotion may be aimed at altering the individual's behaviour and lifestyle in order to prevent disease and maintain his/her stable store of health.
(3) Health promotion can be aimed at those with long-term health problems who may never feel well but through education can obtain the knowledge, skills and resources needed to improve their current state of health and ultimately achieve a level of functioning that is maximal for them.

The health education and promotion that may be recognized as actively occurring within the NHS today has developed along with and in response to changes in the social and political attitudes to health. Not only does health promotion have aims and objectives that concern the individual nurse and patient, but also there are national objectives now established for the promotion of health and reduction of illness, injury and disease. The publication of *The Health of the Nation* document in 1991 by the World Health Organisation (WHO) demonstrated the government's commitment to health promotion on a national scale. This government initiative stimulated extensive public debate, with apparent support for the need to concentrate as much on health promotion and the prevention of illness as on healthcare. In her introduction the then Secretary of State for Health (Virginia Bottomley) stated at the time of its launch that there was a commitment to the pursuit of health in its widest sense, both within the government and beyond. She also advocated that the objectives and targets within *The Health of the Nation* were not just for the government and the NHS but the nation as a whole to achieve, thereby encouraging people to take responsibility for their own health (WHO, 1991).

The White Paper was meant to symbolize the start of a continuing process. It contained health promotion objectives including targets concerned with eating and drinking that focused on the reduction of intake of saturated fats in the diet, the reduction of the incidence of obesity and the reduction of alcohol intake. It also addressed smoking with the aim of reducing both the number of people actually smoking and the number of people who start smoking. These two combined are interlinked with objectives for the reduction of deaths and incidences of ill health related to coronary heart disease (CHD).

The document also contained objectives concerned with accident prevention, as one of the targets of the Health of the Nation report was to reduce the incidence of disability and death resulting from accidents by 25% by the year 2000 (WHO, 1993). The report contained many wide-reaching objectives and targets, many of which affected the health promotion aims of the individual nurse and patient within A&E. It is beyond the remit of this chapter, however, to fully analyse and document the implications of the Health of the Nation targets and it is perhaps of more benefit to focus on an area most pertinent to A&E: the reduction of disability and death resulting from accidents.

The original Health of the Nation paper stated that accidents were the most common cause of death in people under thirty years of age. The paper proposed that many accidents were preventable by providing information and education. Accidents take a particularly heavy toll on the lives of children. Statistics released with the White Paper in 1991 stated that 543 children died as a result of accidents that year. The older adult was also statistically at higher risk.

The targets outlined by the White Paper in the area of accident reduction encompassed the WHO targets for the reduction of ill health, disability and death set at 25% by the year 2000. In the UK the government has set targets to reduce the death rate in children under 15 years of age by 33%, in young adults aged 15–24 years by 25% and in those aged 65 years and over by 33% by the year 2005.

When the Health of the Nation was launched it was proposed that the Health Education Authority's national health promotion remit should extend to addressing the harm caused by accidents. In concurrence with this it was proposed that the NHS emergency services, including A&E departments, were in a position to collect and use information about the causes and results of accidents to facilitate the production of prevention strategies. The targets set in 1991 were bold statements of the government's commitment to and hope for the Health of the Nation initiative. A&E staff can certainly contribute towards the effort to achieve those targets. The paper suggested that in many accidents alcohol consumption, drugs and heightened emotions are all significant contributory factors. In light of this, the provision of information and education in the form of health promotion may be beneficial in appropriate situations as lifestyle changes could have a positive benefit. Subsequent statistics produced in a review of these targets did show promise in the area of accident reduction one year after the launch of the initiative. *The Health of The Nation: One Year On* (WHO, 1993) specifically mentioned A&E services as having developed initiatives toward accident prevention in conjunction with their normal treatment service. It stated that a working group had been developed to explore how best to realize the potential of A&E departments to contribute towards the prevention of accidents, and that there were future plans to integrate accident prevention information and education alongside other relevant aspects of health promotion including the misuse of drugs and alcohol. It was also proposed that professionals including A&E staff, general practitioners, occupational therapists and environmental health officers needed to develop their potential together to create and contribute to local multi-agency accident prevention schemes. With such active initiatives, A&E staff are now becoming increasingly aware that there is much that can be achieved to combat premature death by a change in attitude to ill health and by focusing on prevention and not just care.

The Role of the A&E Nurse

Within this climate the A&E nurse must identify his/her role within health education and promotion, ensure that patients receive all the relevant information to manage their presenting condition and provide information on improving health within their lifestyle where appropriate. Watson and Royle (1991) stated that nursing today can be defined as more than the care and nurture of individuals when they are ill, proposing that the primary goal of nursing should be health promotion, which involves assisting individuals to achieve a positive state of health and well-being, and consequently a better quality of life. The incorporation of activities related to the promotion of health, the prevention of disease and utilizing an approach which encourages individuals to take responsibility for their own health is an essential part of professional practice and one of the main routes to professional excellence. This emphasis on the health-education potential of the nurse's role has arisen in recent years, and the main reason would appear to be the recognition of the fact that many causes of morbidity and mortality are lifestyle related and consequently preventable. It follows logically that because of a nurse's continuous contact with a patient and the overall numbers of nurses within the NHS, that they are in a key position to carry out such health education programmes (Latter et al., 1992).

Carrying out health education and promotion should be central to a nurse's role in caring for his/her patient because one of the aims of nursing is to encourage patients to be their own advocates and assume responsibility for their own health. The potential benefits of this include an increase in health knowledge on the part of the patient, involvement in decision-making and self-empowerment. All these may help the patient to adapt to the stress caused as a result of their current illness, to reduce their anxiety and via the provision of information may result in a reduction in the risk of re-occurrence of the illness or injury.

The role of the nurse as health promoter and educator in A&E can be interwoven throughout the patient's stay in the department but is perhaps most clearly defined when the nurse is involved in patient discharge. McConnell (1997) suggested that the main involvement in health promotion activity for the A&E nurse is primary health education related to accident prevention. Secondary health education involves first aid advice for the immediate management of the patient's presenting illness or injury and discharge advice for longer-term management during recovery. The need for A&E nurses to give first aid advice is documented by Walsh (1985, 1996) and Jones (1990). Many old wives' tales perpetuate ineffectual practices such as applying butter to burns, whilst appropriate first aid methods, such as running a burnt hand under cold water, are easy to understand and apply (McKenna, 1993). Discharge advice may be specific (e.g. how to exercise a sprained limb) or more general (e.g. dietary advice to promote wound healing). This is a focus on the short-term goals of health promotion and education in the management of the patient's immediate problem. However, it is important to remember that, where appropriate, long-term goals for health promotion and education should also be considered by the A&E nurse. Such long-term goals of improved health lifestyle, such as the promotion of immunization and screening programmes and accident prevention, can only be achieved through informed decisions on the patient's part. The A&E nurse can subsequently provide such information or direct the patient to more appropriate services in the community. Indeed, it is an important role of the nurse to be able to direct people to appropriate and available local healthcare resources (Farquhar, 1990).

Having considered the relevance of health education and promotion to the role of the A&E nurse, it is important to consider the associated nursing skills required to perform this role and hence to facilitate effective patient education.

Practical Skills for Patient Teaching

It should be acknowledged that factors such as time, privacy and the stressful environment of the A&E department raise questions about its suitability for meaningful individual health education. Yet health education and promotion are a central part of the A&E nurse's role in providing holistic care for the patient. While people have the right to health knowledge, it is difficult to present this in a value-free way, particularly to the carers of a child who has had an accident. The nurse does not want the provision of information to add to existing feelings of guilt or appear to be victim blaming. The nurse providing health promotion and education should therefore possess the necessary skills to ensure this is a positive, beneficial and therapeutic experience for the patient. Watson and Royle (1991) suggested that for effective patient education the nurse must posses excellent communication skills, an awareness of his/her own personal strengths and weaknesses, an ability to work collaboratively with others, knowledge of the principles of learning and methods of teaching, knowledge and skills in the area to be taught and an awareness of the responsibility for patient teaching.

For effective health education the patient should be an active participant because he/she is ultimately responsible for his/her health. Patient-centred teaching is an interactive process between patient and nurse. Involving the patient throughout the educational process increases the likelihood of successful learning, the development of skills necessary to adapt to future changes in health and less hesitancy on the part of the patient in seeking information and resources in the future. Patient assessment prior to health education is a key element to ensure the advice and information given is achievable and acceptable and hence successful. For effective health education, patient empowerment is essential.

The nurse should briefly assess several factors including the patient's attitude to his/her responsibility for his/her health, whether his/her locus of control is external (believing that health and accidents are a result of fate) or internal (believing that the individual can influence his/her own state of health). This locus of control can be influenced by age, sex, education, occupation, family background and socio-economic factors. The aim of the nurse is to encourage an internal locus of control. The patient's past experience with illness and how he/she coped, whether any changes in health habits and lifestyle resulted and how the patient felt about this should also be taken into account, thereby assessing his/her willingness to learn in their current situation. The patient's general feeling of well-being or illness at the time will also influence his/her capacity and readiness to learn. Each individual's intellectual ability to understand his/her condition and solve related problems will also be an influencing factor. Attention span, basic knowledge and fluency in the language being used should also be considerations for the nurse (Watson and Royle, 1991). Any barriers to learning such as sensory deficits, confusion, reduced motivation due to stress or anxiety should be identified so that they can be compensated for and thereby overcome.

Health education is complex and requires more effort than simply imparting information or knowledge. An essential ingredient in effective communication is patient participation, encouraging individuals to take control and assume responsibility for part of the learning process rather than the nurse assuming control by giving the patient instructions which he/she may not be able to comply with. These factors in assessment are important considerations for the nurse in judging whether health education is appropriate and the extent and type of goals to aim for at that time.

The next stage following assessment is the identification of the learning needs of the patient. Watson and Royle (1991) defined a learning need as the educational gap between the existing level of competence and the desired level. A learning need should be identified by the nurse and patient together, rather than being the subjective opinion of the nurse alone. Once learning needs have been mutually identified, a plan of action is required. The nurse and patient can address short-term goals for immediate learning needs (e.g. the management of a laceration following sutures) and begin to examine any long-term learning needs that may need to be followed in the community (for example the management of alcohol intake). The immediate learning needs are those most frequently addressed in A&E as part of primary and secondary health education, as covered earlier. The long-term learning needs, once identified with the patient, should then be discussed with a view to where and how learning can be continued within the community setting.

When planning the content for patient teaching it is important that the information is accurate and expressed in terms and language understandable to the learner and that any adaptations for age, cognitive ability, education and culture taken into consideration. Although, as previously mentioned, the A&E department is not particularly conducive to teaching and learning, the nurse should attempt to provide teaching uninterrupted and allow time for patients' questions and any correction and repetition that may be necessary. Teaching methods will vary depending on the topic being discussed. With practical procedures, it is usually easier for the patient to have the procedure broken down into logical steps and to carry out the procedure, as this is more likely to assist him/her in committing it to memory and understanding the rationale behind it. Information can obviously be given verbally, although most A&E

departments also provide leaflets that can be combined with teaching and tailored to individual patient requirements by the nurse. These are often useful for the patient to take away and refer to because information given to a patient in A&E is not always fully retained owing to anxiety caused by preceding events. If it does not compromise patient confidentiality, it is often advantageous to carry out teaching in the presence of a relative or friend, who again may be able to retain more information than the patient and consequently act as a resource.

On completion of the education process, the nurse should evaluate the learning achieved, as it is necessary to ascertain whether the patient has acquired the necessary knowledge and skills with regard to his/her ability to cope with the current injury or illness. Observation and feedback from the patient are the primary ways in which the nurse can evaluate the learning process. If appropriate, the nurse may wish to ask questions or if teaching a practical skill may ask the patient if he/she would like to run through the process while being supervised so that any extra questions or helpful tips can be covered. Watson and Royle (1991) proposed that one learning programme in one health-care setting is unlikely to provide the patient and his/her family with the necessary knowledge and skills to achieve fully the goals that they have identified. Learning new healthier lifestyle skills takes time, and application in the home and the community is very different from the hospital setting. In teaching patients the skills to manage their immediate presenting problem the A&E nurse should ensure that they feel confident enough to manage at home. For the longer term goals for health that may have been identified, the A&E nurse can only begin the learning process. It is helpful, therefore, to provide information about relevant self-help groups and organizations in the community that may be of benefit to the patient. Appropriate referral to other related community agencies should also be considered.

Conclusion

The overall aim of health education and promotion in the A&E department is to equip the patient with the necessary knowledge and skills to cope with his/her current situation and if possible initiate a programme of learning that will improve his/her health and quality of life. The A&E nurse must aim to be supportive and work in a collaborative manner with the patient to ensure that the learning experience is positive and beneficial and to encourage him/her to use healthcare resources as a source of health information in the future. It is hoped that this chapter has provided a summary of the relevant issues and factors concerned with health education and promotion. It is not an exhaustive account of the process, as there are many excellent articles and books that examine the issues in more detail. It has aimed, however, to provide an overview of the A&E nurse's role in health education and its importance, the practicalities of performing that role and how the process of health promotion is incorporated in the national strategies identified in *The Health of the Nation*.

Suggested Further Reading

Broomfield R (1998) More safe, Less sorry (potential for A&E nurses' contribution to health promotion by involvement with community initiatives). Nursing Times 94(46): 42–3.

Lane M (1998) Health promotion in relation to domestic violence: role of the A&E nurse. Emergency Nurse 6(1): 26–9.

Lockhart T (1997) Problem drinkers in A&E: health promotion initiatives. A&E Nursing 5(1): 16–21.

McConnell D (1997) Health promotion for A&E practice (role of the nurse practitioner). Emergency Nurse 5(7): 19–22.

McKenna G (1994) The scope for health education in the A&E department. A&E Nursing 2(2): 94–9.

References

Farquhar M (1990) The use and misuse of paediatric casualty. Nursing Standard 26(4): 34–5.

Jones G (1990) A&E Nursing: A Structured Approach. London: Faber & Faber.

Lane M, Beales J (1998)Health promotion in relation to domestic violence. Emergency Nurse 6(1): 26–9.

Latter S, Macleod M, Clark J, Wilson Barnett J, Mabean J (1992) Health education in nursing: perceptions of practice in acute settings. Journal of Advanced Nursing 17: 164–72.

McConnell D (1997) Health promotion for A&E practice. Emergency Nurse 5(7): 19–22.

McKenna A (1993) The scope for health education in the A&E. A&E Nursing 2: 94–9.

The New Oxford Dictionary of English (1998) Oxford: Clarendon Press.

Walsh M (1985) A&E Nursing: A New Approach. Oxford: Butterworth-Heinemann.

Walsh M (1996) A&E Nursing: A New Approach, 3rd edn. Oxford: Butterworth-Heinemann.

Watson J, Royle J (1991) Medical-Surgical Nursing and Related Physiology, 3rd edn. London: Baillière Tindall.

World Health Authority (1996) Ottawa Charter for Health Promotion. Copenhagen: WHA.

World Health Organisation (1991) Health of the Nation. London: HMSO.

World Health Organisation (1993) Health of the Nation: One Year On. London: HMSO.

Chapter 19
The Role of the A&E Nurse in Dealing with Bereavement

Nancy Fontaine

Introduction

Death is an inevitable part of the human experience, a powerful enigma, leaving the greatest of pain in its wake. Birth and death are the most obvious boundaries of human freedom as set by universal order, and for the most part society uneasily avoids the subject of death. The progress of medicine has increased life expectancy and changed patterns of mortality, allowing a contemporary belief that death has been conjured away and that when it does strike it will be 'a tame death' (Aries, 1983). Many deaths occur with some warning, allowing the process of 'anticipatory' grief prior to the loss (Lindemann, 1944). Anticipatory grief allows purposeful psychological preparation for death, thereby providing the adaptive function of protecting the dying and assisting the survivors to resume effective functioning more rapidly.

However, sudden death occurs without warning, in the form of sudden infant death syndrome, suicide and trauma. Sudden death allows no psychological preparation and the shock alone prolongs the grief (Lundin, 1984). When sudden death occurs, a significant and meaningful relationship has been lost, exerting the most tragic sense of loss.

Sudden death has been shown to have a major impact upon families, producing ill health, poor coping behaviour and disturbed social functioning. Studies have indicated that those who have experienced sudden death have significantly more somatic and psychiatric illnesses than those who experience an anticipated death. There is also an increased likelihood of morbidity during the first two years of bereavement amongst those who have suffered a sudden loss

(Lundin, 1984). The cognitive and behavioural responses after sudden death include social withdrawal, persistent bewilderment, discontent and protest, to which Parkes (1975) ascribed the term 'unexpected loss syndrome'. This cluster of symptoms is so severely debilitating that maladaptive grief is inevitable.

The sudden death experience means that survivors are denied the necessary time for anticipatory grief. Accident and emergency (A&E) nurses have to utilize the turbulent moments preceding a patient's death to begin preparation for the traumatic aftermath. The lack of anticipatory preparation means that survivors not only have to comprehend the loss as a reality, but they also have to reconcile a 'normal' grief reaction. This appears unlikely when sudden loss is a tragedy unequalled by any other, and is reported to be as psychologically traumatic as a severe burn or wound is physiologically traumatic (Engel, 1961). A&E nurses are acutely aware that breaking bad news and bereavement support are distressing and emotionally fraught tasks. As harbingers of bad news nurses must inflict pain, a concept alien to them and one they are ill prepared to deal with, mainly through lack of death education and training. Nurses feel great anxiety when faced with a task that they cannot perform adeptly and often resort to repressive coping techniques which may be viewed as ambivalence by the bereaved. In order to cope, manage and fully understand death, nurses have formulated an adaptive protection that sanitizes death, thereby negating its emotional impact. Although in the short term this adaptation may provide the nurse with adequate protection, the long-term effects may include depersonalization, poor job satisfaction and emotional isolation (Fontaine, 1996).

This chapter aims to provide psychological, cultural and practical information on the enigma of sudden death. It will briefly outline religious and cultural differences, knowledge of which is integral to meeting the needs of our multicultural client groups. Advice on the provision of an optimal environment for the bereaved and strategies for breaking bad news will be addressed. Finally, the importance of staff counselling and support will be discussed. The scope of the chapter precludes detailed discussion of paediatric death, miscarriage and organ donation. With greater insight it is hoped that A&E nurses will be able to employ appropriate psychosocial skills in order to assist themselves, their colleagues and the survivors to rationalize sudden death, thereby minimizing the likelihood of maladaptive grief and coping.

Conceptualization of Death

In order for nurses to be instrumental in guiding survivors toward an adaptive grief process they must have an understanding of the inter-relationship between death and bereavement. They must also be aware of the ensuing effects of perception and cognition of death, which ultimately affect the person, his/her life and those around him/her. Western culture continues to perpetuate a social avoidance of mortality, banishing the notion of death from both its language and daily life. Medical developments have assisted society in this avoidance, allowing technology to depersonalize the relationship between death and the individual. However, death is inevitable and it is essential that Western society endorses the humanist element of death and bereavement, rather than relegating death to the status of a social taboo. Inability to accept the reality of death may exacerbate the stages of disbelief and denial, thereby predisposing the survivors to maladaptive grief. Furthermore, the use technology, particularly in the A&E department, suggests that the deceased had been denied the tranquillity of a 'tame' death. Conversely, sudden death may be perceived by others as the ideal demise as it allows no time for fear or prolonged suffering (Raphael, 1984).

Human existence demands that relationships are formed and attachments made. Indeed, the strongest emotions, whether associated with joy or pain, are displayed during the course of attachment-related events. Death disrupts these attachments, leaving the survivors to cope with the pain caused by that loss. Bereavement is the survivors' response to that loss and is an essential transitional process, allowing the survivors to reconcile their separation from the deceased. Once the loss of this relationship has been accepted, the survivors should emerge from this transitional state and successfully reintegrate into society.

Bowlby (1977) suggested that humans have a tendency to make strong and affectionate bonds with others, with emotional turmoil inevitable when the bonds are threatened or terminated: the 'attachment theory'. Any situations that endanger these bonds will precipitate specific and sometimes extreme reactions including anger and weeping, which represent the first phase of mourning as the individual attempts to recover the 'lost' person and the relationship. Therefore, even during bereavement when the search for the person is fruitless, a separation anxiety is provoked. Parkes (1975) applied an attachment model to observations on the course of grief. These included denial, numbing, searching for the lost object, anger, guilt, mitigation and defence.

The links between attachment, loss and grief are fourfold:

- childhood experiences – these shape ideas about security and trust, thereby assisting self-identity. The quality and vicissitudes of these childhood relationships are determinants of personality development and mental health (Bowlby, 1977);
- the process by which parental attachment invokes the need for attachments in adulthood;
- the way in which these adult attachments become so firmly embedded in one's outlook on life that their loss initiates grief;
- grieving, by which this traumatic loss of meaning is rectified (Marris, 1992).

Grief work appears to support liberation, accommodating strong, genuine emotions that may have been previously suppressed. This hypothesis emphasizes that all nurses must understand and acknowledge the psychological implications of grief and be prepared to manage and support these emotional reactions. In particular the A&E nurse has a fundamental role in assisting the bereaved to accept the reality of the loss, which is a pivotal step in the mourning process.

Religious and Cross-cultural Aspects of Bereavement

Grief is universal. However, within each culture and religion there is a diversity of spiritual observance and belief. Therefore, although the meaning of life and death may be universal, it cannot be assumed that expression of grief will be uniform. Furthermore, the spiritual dimension of each individual is inherently personal and may become more pronounced during times of distress, whether or not that person belongs to a designated faith group. Sudden death, in particular, may even challenge beliefs that previously offered comfort and strength and may raise issues concerning self-worth, the purpose of existence and the need for forgiveness. Irrespective of whether individuals belong to specific faith groups, it is dangerous to make assumptions and the only way to ascertain the needs and wishes of the survivors is to ask. It is subsequently imperative that A&E nurses endeavour to promote a secure environment which can accommodate a diversity of practices.

Generally, both full- and part-time religious advisers are available via the hospital switchboard and the family may also have their own minister or priest whom they would rather contact. This is a useful link as such religious advisers may also be able to offer continued support to the survivors within the community.

The following is a brief summary of different religious practices and rituals that take place at the time of, and after, the death.

Church of England

Baptism may be requested for critically ill adults and children. Nurses, midwives and parents can also baptise. This information should be clearly documented in the nursing notes.

Roman Catholic

The Roman Catholic chaplain may administer 'The Blessing of the Sick' when the patient's condition becomes terminal or the 'Sacrament of Baptism' for a critically ill infant.

Free Churches

The Free Churches comprise the following Protestant groups: Methodist, Baptist, Evangelical, Congregational, Pentecostal, Quaker, Salvation Army, United Reformed and some other smaller churches. No one doctrine is universally accepted by all groups.

Islam

When Muslims are about to die they may request to lie facing Mecca and it is general practice for those around the patient to recite from the Koran. Once the patient has died, non-Muslims should not touch the deceased and nurses should therefore take care to wear disposable gloves. The family will wash and prepare the body, continuing to recite verses from the Koran. The body is clothed in white and covered in a white sheet with the head turned to the left shoulder so that the body can be buried facing Mecca, which is generally in a south-easterly direction (Speck, 1978). In Islam, Allah has made life sacred and a person is not considered the owner of his/her body. For this reason there must be no attempt to harm or destroy any part of that body. Muslims, therefore, are opposed to post-mortems and cremation and the subject of organ donation must not be raised. In addition, suicide is a particularly sensitive and distressing issue because it suggests that an individual has taken his/her life unjustly, a life that Allah had made sacred.

Hinduism

Human life is perceived as cyclical: after death the soul leaves the body and is reborn in the body of another person, animal or mineral. For a dying Hindu, the best procedure would be to call a Hindu priest to perform specific rites such as sprinkling blessed water from the Ganges on the patient and reading from the sacred Sanskrit books. The priest will tie a thread around the neck or wrist of the patient, indicating that a blessing has been given, and this must not be removed. Hindu women may wear a nuptial thread around their neck and a red mark on the forehead. Men may wear a sacred thread around their arm, symbolizing adult religious status that again should remain *in situ*. There is no ritual washing, but nurses should therefore ensure that jewellery and sacred objects remain intact and that the body is wrapped in a plain sheet. The eldest son is responsible for the funeral arrangements and cremation is usual. There is no objection to post-mortems or organ donation.

Sikhism

Sikhism is a combination of Hinduism and Muslim beliefs. If a dying patient is unable to recite prayers a priest or relative should be contacted to recite appropriate verses from the Holy Scripture. Sikhs share the Hindu belief in transmigration and favour cremation. There is no objection to nursing staff handling the body, although any traditional religious symbols worn should not be removed.

These include:

- kesh – long, uncut hair;
- kanga – a comb to keep the hair in place and symbolize discipline;
- kara – a steel bangle worn on the right wrist to symbolize strength and unity;
- kirpan – a sword, often worn as a brooch, which symbolizes authority and justice;
- kachj – a pair of shorts worn to symbolize spiritual freedom (Owen-Cole, 1973).

Judaism

In Judaism there is a specific structure to the ritual of death. The family may wish to be present at death, particularly to perform closure of the eyes, and a Rabbi should be informed. The body of the Jewish patient is sacrosanct and only co-religionists may touch it. All body fluids, bandages, catheters and tubing are considered part of the body and should be left *in situ* and buried with the body. The family may wish to prepare the body themselves or send a member of their community to do so. If no family is available, then the local Jewish undertaker should be contacted for advice. Burial should occur within twenty-four hours of death. Cremation is forbidden and post-mortem is regarded as the highest form of insult to the deceased as it is seen as mutilation of the corpse. There is no objection to organ transplants. Overt expression of grief is encouraged within Judaism and in particular the tearing of clothes is a visible sign of being inwardly rent with grief.

Buddhism

For a Buddhist a calm, clear and hopeful state of mind at death is essential for passing into the next life. Some Buddhist patients may therefore refuse analgesia in order to ensure clarity of mind, and their views should be respected. There is no strict protocol following the death of a Buddhist and most Western and Tibetan Buddhists insist on cremation, although traditional Chinese Buddhists generally prefer burial (Rinpoche, 1992).

Bereavement Management in A&E

Bereavement care must encompass the survivor's physiological needs in addition to psychological well-being. Ideally the bereaved should be taken to a private room adjacent to the resuscitation room, which avoids having to escort distressed relatives through the A&E department. It should have a tranquil ambience, with dimmed lighting, a sofa and comfortable chairs. The relatives should have access to a direct telephone line; tissues and tea-making facilities should be available.

Strategies for Survivor Support

Although bereavement management is acknowledged to be one of the central facets of A&E provision, relatives are frequently dissatisfied with the failure in human terms rather than procedural aspects. One study reported that up to 50% of people contacting a CRUSE support group did so because of feelings of anger, anxiety and frustration originating from the attitudes of health professionals (Ewins and Bryant, 1992). The paucity of effective bereavement care in A&E includes failure to provide a support nurse to care solely for the relatives (RCN and BAA&EM, 1995). Survivors have subsequently reported lack of opportunity to express their fears and anxieties with an appropriately trained health professional. The fact that the grief process may be inhibited because of inadequate staffing levels is cause for concern and it is advocated that bereavement training and education be mandatory for all A&E nurses, to ensure that both the physical and psychological morbidity for survivors is reduced.

Sudden death is a crisis-inducing event, necessitating structured management. Survivors are often helpless, their usual coping strategies are no longer successful and they become reliant upon the support of others and susceptible to their responses. Thus, in order to avoid maladaptive grief, effective intervention must be initiated in A&E. Communication and interpersonal skills are at the crux of all nursing interventions and bereavement care is no exception. It is therefore imperative that the strategies used for breaking news of sudden death are optimal. The bereaved should be given licence to express unrestricted emotions, to verbalize their need for answers, to be prepared for the final proof of death (viewing the body) and should be given unconditional support. This process requires that A&E nurses are familiar with the responding techniques of empathy and non-directive interventions, thereby allowing the survivors to impart their distress.

Contacting the Family

Using the telephone to inform the family/partner/friends that a patient is seriously ill or has died is a tremendously harrowing task. There is no way of knowing how they will react and, if there is a maladaptive outcome, what the next approach should be. As this is such an agonizing and delicate component of bereavement care it is advised that the nurse making the call should be as experienced as possible. The nurse must identify him- or herself clearly, stating the name of the hospital and department and the name of the family member. In most instances, for example when a resuscitation attempt is occurring, the survivors should be informed that their relative is seriously ill or injured and that they should attend the hospital immediately. Someone other than the immediate family member should drive whenever possible.

Generally it is accepted practice that news of the death should not be communicated over the telephone, because of the potential complications of violent grief reactions in a situation where the relative may endure prolonged shock and isolation. However, there are exceptions, particularly when the family live a significant distance from the hospital. In such situations the nurse should ascertain whether there is another relative or friend available to offer support and comfort and then break the news slowly, giving the relative time to adjust. It is always worth broaching the subject by offering an introductory warning of the impending news: 'I'm telephoning because I have some upsetting news for you...'. If interrupted by the anxious relative, the narrative approach should be used to confirm the death. Whenever possible, further contact numbers and names should be offered since these may offer some comfort and an essential link.

Arrival of the Relatives/Significant Others

A designated A&E nurse should always meet the relatives and escort them to a private waiting room, introducing him/herself. The relatives may not remember the nurse's name, but hearing distressing news from an unacquainted third party makes the news even harder to accept. The nurse must ascertain precisely which relatives are present and ascertain vital information about the patient's medical history and recent physical state. While the patient remains alive or throughout the resuscitation attempt, the nurse must keep the survivors informed of any changes in the patient's condition. The nurse must harness these moments in order to initiate the preparatory process of breaking bad news. If the nurse is able to be honest and tell the relatives that the prognosis is poor then any false hopes can be dismantled, aiding acceptance of the death.

The most overt preparation for the death of a relative is through the medium of witnessed resuscitation. This topic is highly controversial and deserving of a chapter in itself. However, its inclusion is central to the theme of bereavement care. Generally the presence of parents during paediatric resuscitation is accepted practice. However, for adult resuscitation the fears and reservations of the health professionals appear to provide a significant barrier to instigation of such a practice. From a medical perspective, the main issues include physical or verbal interference from distressed relatives, and medico-legal repercussions (Doyle et al., 1987). Nursing resistance may stem from feelings of inadequacy regarding bereavement education, dealing with critical incidents effectively and an individual's own perceptions of death. However, grief theories suggest that for some survivors witnessed resuscitation may provide the necessary visual evidence to negate maladaptive denial or perhaps avoid protracted 'searching' for the deceased during bereavement.

Although procedural aspects of bereavement can easily be categorized, strategies for breaking the news of death are merely guidelines and there is no infallible prescription.

Notification of Death

Breaking the news of a sudden death requires particular skill and sensitivity as the grief process commences immediately after such a tragic announcement and may evoke acute grief reactions such as anger, blame, guilt and denial. Grief expression may manifest as a hysterical outburst, inconsolable sobbing or a detached, silent demeanour. Survivors solicit licence for unrestricted expression of grief and assistance with decision-making, express a desire for detailed information and often disclose personal memories of the deceased. Skilled, empathic intervention may assist with adaptation and help survivors to participate in closure activities, therefore enabling them to progress through the differing stages of grief.

Proximity is paramount when attempting to convey news of death and health professionals should ensure that they and the family are sitting down in order to promote a more secure and congruent environment. They should ensure that they convey the impression that time is no object and that they will remain as long as the relatives need them. The allocated nurse must establish the identity of each attending relative in order that the news is confirmed to the closest member. The nurse originally dedicated to the relatives may be the most appropriate individual to inform the relatives of the death, particularly if he/she is experienced in bereavement care. However, the relatives may also want to hear a medical explanation of the death and so the family should be given the opportunity to hear from the physician and to ask further questions.

A recommended strategy for breaking bad news is to utilize the narrative approach by establishing how much the family knows and continuing with an outline of the events immediately preceding the death. However, the prime task is to convey news of the death. The survivors may not recall much of this information and reiteration should be expected. Essential components of this narrative may include emphasizing that the patient was oblivious to pain and discomfort and that every conceivable resuscitation attempt was employed. It is imperative that there is no ambiguity and so the use of euphemisms such as the terms 'moved on' or 'passed away' must be avoided. The phrase 'is dead' can sound harshly detached whereas ' he has died' may sound better. This formative information lays down a fundamental basis for cognitive appraisal of the death and provides an integral framework enabling 'normal' grief work to commence.

The Grief Response

Commonly the reaction described is one of complete numbness or bewilderment, characterizing the initial stage of the bereavement process (Parkes, 1975). An icy silence often ensues and it will be tempting for the nurse to feel that he/she should apologise for the death or perhaps offer a sympathetic platitude. However, silence can be therapeutic and one should never say something just to break the silence, because the nurse is invariably only doing so for his/her own benefit. Even if the nurse has experienced death of a close relation it is impossible to sympathize with another

ings. Empathic responses are therefore the most
ntion during this traumatic time: 'this must be over-
ou'.

common and disturbing reaction to death, often
ealth professionals for failing to preserve life. This
emotion ... be associated with the issue of unfinished business or
unexpressed feelings towards the deceased such as resentment or
abandonment. Although disconcerting for those present, it is imperative that such overt expressions are sanctioned in this protected
environment rather than suppressed. Similarly, survivor guilt is
frequently cited following sudden death, particularly the idea of a
relative or close friend having not being present or that the death
should have been anticipated. Without demeaning the survivor's
fears, the nurse must attempt to allay irrational guilt that may
complicate the bereavement process further.

Although it is accepted that nurses are not trained in formal
person-centred counselling (Rogers, 1980), the use of responding
techniques such as paraphrasing is a skill that A&E nurses could
utilize. The person-centred approach has been used extensively in
training health professionals because it advocates the safer supportive process of entering the survivor's perceptual world without
making interpretation or probing the unconscious (Corey, 1991). Its
simplicity enables people with limited experience to translate
congruence, empathy and unconditional positive regard to devas-
tated survivors.

The use of touch frequently poses a dilemma and can make
some nurses feel uneasy. There are no specific guidelines, although
the introductory handshake may have already bridged the gap.
Similarly, the issue of nurses demonstrating their emotion overtly
causes concern and appears to defy the archetypal coping martyr-
dom of nursing sub-culture. Expression of emotion by nursing staff
can dismantle the rigidity of the professional/lay relationship,
thereby enhancing the empathic rapport. Disbelief as an initial
reaction to bereavement is common and invariably transient. Its
incidence is more prevalent amongst those who were not present at
the time of the death and studies suggest that viewing the body may
ameliorate protracted denial (Cathcart, 1988; Schmidt and Tolle,
1990).

Viewing the Body

The opportunity to view the body should be broached by the nurse, referring to the deceased by name. However, the relatives should not be made to feel obliged to do so and if they decline the nurse must be prepared to alleviate any guilt that may arise from this refusal. It is essential that the nurse views the deceased in advance to ensure that there have been no untoward incidents such as fluid leakage. The family must be forewarned of any disfigurements, skin colour changes and any medical equipment left *in situ*, to avoid further distress.

Viewing the deceased is a form of closure for the survivors and this delicate and indelible experience should be made as dignified as possible. It is good practice to provide a secluded, peaceful area where the relatives may spend time with their loved one. The hands of the deceased, where possible, should be left accessible. The survivors may be reluctant to touch the body and the nurse may need to give the family affirmation and encouragement that it is acceptable to hold or touch the deceased. The family may appreciate a moment of privacy. It may be necessary to allow children to view the deceased, but it is advocated that they be accompanied and that a nurse is available to provide additional support.

The procedure varies if the death is that of an infant. The infant should be wrapped in a shawl and placed in a Moses basket or, if requested, in a parent's arms. They may appreciate a photograph of the child or perhaps a lock of hair. In some cases the parents may prefer a hand- or footprint from the child.

The Process of Closure

After viewing the survivors may have further questions surrounding the death, which will need addressing in order to prevent morbid preoccupation. Definitive information must be disseminated to the relatives regarding procedures after the death. The possibility of a post-mortem should be discussed, particularly if the death was unexpected, violent or caused by an accident, in which case a post-mortem is mandatory. Many hospitals now provide printed leaflets in several languages delineating the practical aspects that have to be addressed after a death, including obtaining the death certificate, registering the death and subsequent funeral arrangements. The hospital policy will outline any specific procedures and some hospitals may arrange for the survivors to meet the patient affairs officer on the next working day, who will return any clothing and valuable effects, clarify bereavement procedures and advise on details regarding a post-mortem. Furthermore, he or she usually informs the general practitioner of the death unless the A&E department has already done so.

Although seemingly unimportant, the return of valuables can have a major impact on the survivors' memories of the death. Ashdown (1985) reported that relatives consistently remarked unfavourably about the 'plastic bin liner' that contained the possessions of the deceased. Before discarding any soiled, cut clothing it is therefore worth asking the survivors for their preference as some items may be of great significance. Taking time to fold the clothes neatly also signifies a mark of caring and respect.

The final action of leaving the deceased is enmeshed within the issue of closure. The survivors may need to be reassured that it is acceptable to leave as they may perceive departure as abandoning the deceased. The nurse offering his/her name and a contact number, thereby providing both professional support and a perceptual link with the deceased, may help ameliorate such bewilderment. The relatives may be offered transport home and, as a formal closure, the supporting nurse should escort the relatives to the car.

Strategies for Staff Support

Nurses are often ill equipped to assimilate the aftermath of crisis and it is suggested that recurrent exposure to death may precipitate deep emotional anxiety and psychological distress similar to that experienced in post-traumatic stress disorder. Nurses are used to stifling expression of emotional pain because despair is seen as unacceptable. They may be unable to recall negative events because of their ability to 'block them out'. The use of humour often emerges as a method of coping with death yet actually represents a refined form of avoidance, incorporating both cognitive and emotional responses to a stressful situation (Fontaine, 1996). However, suppression of anxiety/sadness or flippancy may be interpreted as ambivalence by the relatives. It may be concluded that this emotional suppression parallels the survivor's reactions through withdrawal from pain and loss. This psychological detachment appears to indicate a normal defence mechanism against constant exposure to highly emotional and harrowing circumstances, although repeated exposure to death does not inoculate nurses from psychological or emotional turmoil (Menzies, 1960).

The inadequacy of staff support measures has been cited (Mood and Larkin, 1979) and correlates with data suggesting that nurses have difficulty discussing death and consequently reject the idea of peer support. Additionally, the suppression of emotional stress increases the likelihood of dysfunctional staff interactions and dismantles team cohesion. It is suggested that nurses may perceive formal debriefing sessions as a threat, fearing self-exploration and self-disclosure, and data do imply that there is a fear of loss of professional credibility (Hansell, 1976; Booth and Faulkner, 1986).

Nurses must be given the opportunity and continuing support to work through death experiences to prevent emotional desolation, low morale and a loss of concern for the bereaved. Furthermore, the need for debriefing in A&E is heightened owing to the shock of sudden death and the subsequent severity of the grief reactions. It is therefore imperative that nurses learn to recognize their own unresolved grief and anxiety using the process of debriefing. Critical Incident Debriefing is a means to confronting the distress of sudden death, and is not intended to replace professional counselling but merely to lessen the impact of negative stressors. The use of debriefing has been shown to provide immediate crisis intervention, enhance staff support and improve communication (Rubins, 1990).

Conclusion

An understanding of bereavement theories and an awareness of specific precursors of maladaptive grief are integral to effective bereavement care within the accident and emergency setting. With increased bereavement education it is hoped that A&E staff will not only be better equipped to facilitate grieving, but will also have an enhanced ability to understand and acknowledge both their own feelings and those of their colleagues.

Suggested Further Reading

Buckman R (1992) How To Break Bad News. A Guide for Health-Care Professionals. London: Pan Macmillan.

Raphael B (1984) The Anatomy of Bereavement: A Handbook for the Caring Professions. London: Hutchinson.

RCN and British Association of Accident and Emergency Medicine (1995) Bereavement Care in A&E Departments: Report of the Working Group. London: Department of Health.

References

Aries P (1983) The Hour of Death. Aylesbury: Peregrine Books.

Ashdown M (1985) Sudden death. Nursing Mirror 18(161): 22–4.

Booth K, Faulkner A (1986) Problems encountered in setting up support groups in nursing. Nurse Education Today 6: 244–51.

Bowlby J (1977) The making and breaking of affectional bonds. British Journal of Psychiatry 130: 201–10.

Cathcart F (1988) Seeing the body after death. British Medical Journal 297: 997.

Corey G (1991) Theory and Practice of Counselling and Psychotherapy, 4th edn. Pacific Grove, CA: Brooks Cole.

Doyle C, Post H, Burney R (1987) Family participation during resuscitation: an option. Annals of Emergency Medicine 16(6): 107–9.

Engel G (1961) Is grief a disease? Psychosomatic Medicine 23: 18–22.

Ewins D, Bryant J (1992) Relative comfort. Nursing Times 88(52): 61–3.

Fontaine N (1996) A naturalistic enquiry into nurses' perceptions of bereavement in an accident and emergency department. Unpublished thesis, University of East London.

Hansell N (1976) The Person in Distress: Bio-social Mechanics of Adaption. New York: Plenum Press.

Lindemann E (1944) Symptomatology and management of acute grief. American Journal of Psychiatry 101(September): 141–8.

Lundin T (1984) Long-term outcome of bereavement. British Journal of Psychiatry 145: 424–8.

Marris P (1992) Grief, loss of meaning and society. Bereavement Care 11(2): 18–22.

Menzies I (1960) A case study in the functioning of social systems as a defence mechanism against anxiety: a report on a study of the nursing service of a general hospital. Human Relations 13(2): 95–121.

Mood DW, Larkin BA (1979) Attitudes of nursing personnel towards death and dying. Research in Nursing and Health 2(2): 53–60.

Owen-Cole W (1973) A Sikh Family in Britain. Norwich: Religious Education Press.

Parkes CM (1975) Determinants of outcome following bereavement. Omega 6(4): 303–23.

Raphael B (1984) The Anatomy of Bereavement: A Handbook for the Caring Professions. London: Hutchinson.

RCN and British Association of Accident and Emergency Medicine (1995) Bereavement Care in A&E Departments: Report of the Working Group. London: Department of Health.

Rinpoche S (1992) Tibetan Book of the Living and Dying. London: Rider.
Rogers C (1980) A Way of Being. Boston: Houghton Mifflin.
Rubins J (1990) Critical incident stress debriefing: helping the helpers. Journal of
    Emergency Nursing 16 (July/August): 4.
Schmidt TA, Tolle SW (1990) Emergency physicians' responses to families following
    patient death. Annals of Emergency Medicine 19: 125.
Speck P (1978) Loss and Grief in Medicine. London: Baillière Tindall.

Chapter 20
Violence in A&E

Andrew Carter

Introduction

Violence within the accident and emergency (A&E) setting is an issue that will not go away. Society over recent years has become more violent and volatile. As A&E departments are the interface between the hospital and the community, this may go some way to explain the increase in violent incidents in our working environment. A&E will, in essence, reflect society.

This chapter will explore the history and incidents of violence in A&E nursing. It will ask 'what is' and even 'who are' responsible? Factors that may influence aggressive behaviour will be highlighted and management strategies will be developed.

History

Society has always been violent but hospitals historically appeared relatively safe, owing to the fact that they were there for the greater good and were respected for what they were offering the community.

This situation has changed dramatically and hospital employees have increasingly become the victims of aggression and violence. Table 20.1 shows the number of incidences healthcare workers are now experiencing.

What has caused the rise in violence within healthcare and A&E departments? Expectation has changed dramatically over the years since 1948 when the modern NHS was formed. These expectations rose again with the publication of *The Patient's Charter* (DoH, 1992), which set standards of care predominantly based on time. It was this

Table 20.1 Incidence of violence to healthcare workers

Occupation	Incidents per 10,000 workers
Medical practitioners	762
Nurses and midwives	580
Other health-related occupations	830
All subjects surveyed	251

Note: Violence includes: wounding, common assault, robbery and theft while staff were at work, not domestic related incidents.
Source: Home Office Research and Statistics Directorate, British Crime Survey, 1996.

factor that turned the tide against the A&E departments as they faced increasing complaints regarding waiting times. Have the raised public expectations of the service increased intolerance and caused the escalation of violence in A&E?

Close contact with people in many and varied circumstances when they are anxious, agitated and in pain will lead to more aggressive and potentially violent episodes. Some members of the public that A&E staff deal with are naturally violent but responses to pain, long waits and fear may manifest as violence in others who would normally be calm and collected. Working practice or simply just the role that we are in can have an important part to play in why violence occurs. Violence can be traced back to opportunity. If staff allow themselves to work alone in the A&E department they make themselves more vulnerable. Offering a service that has an open-door policy, as all A&Es do, provides more opportunity for violence to erupt. Dealing with emotionally charged incidents such as deaths, physical assaults and patients who are affected by drink, drugs and mental illness increases the risks. Exercising authority can result in aggressive encounters. A&E nurses deal with these emotions and situations daily.

Violence in A&E now affects 50% of staff and nursing had been labelled the most dangerous profession in the UK, with 34% of nurses being attacked while on duty (Saines, 1999). This contrasts with the Health Services Advisory Committee (HSAC) survey of 1987 when the highest incident of violence in the nursing profession occurred in the psychiatric setting. This was followed by violence to staff working with the elderly mentally ill and people with learning disabilities. General hospital incidents were placed fourth in the list. However, this survey concluded that within general hospitals A&E

nursing was a problem area with 1.8% of staff reporting major injury.

The Royal College of Nursing survey on the frequency and types of abuse experienced by nurses concluded that:

- 47% of respondents had been physically attacked in the previous year. This included slaps, punches and being spat at;
- patients themselves had carried out 98% of attacks;
- 85% of nurses had been verbally abused;
- 48% of nurses reported that patients' relatives were abusive;
- over 80% of those who responded felt that aggressive incidents had increased from when they started nursing;
- 78% believed that attacks were 'part of the job' (Kydd, 1998).

This demonstrates that the problem of violence in nursing is real and increasing. With A&E departments bearing the brunt of the dissatisfaction, staff are at considerable risk if they fail to act positively.

What constitutes violence and aggression? Before discussing methods of dealing with violence and aggression in A&E nursing one must first define what it is. Baron and Richardson (1994) defined aggression as a form of behaviour that is intended to injure someone physically or psychologically. Whittington (1998) stated that any violent incident could be considered along a number of dimensions such as:

- nature: physical or verbal;
- target: self, others or objects;
- perpetrator: patient, relative, visitor or colleague;
- injury: none, minor or major.

The HSAC (1997) definition is clear: 'Any incident in which a person working in the healthcare sector is verbally abused, threatened or assaulted by a patient or visitor in relation to his/her work'.

Why do groups of patients become aggressive? What can be done to prevent these incidents and do any factors act as a catalyst?

Influences

Many studies have highlighted common factors surrounding violent outbursts in hospitals (Hammond, 1995; Brennan, 1997; HSAC,

1997; Patterson et al., 1997; Whittington, 1997). Table 20.2 outlines the most common associated factors accompanying violent episodes. These factors seem to fall into two broad categories:

(1) provocation, i.e. poor information;
(2) the individual's ability to rationalize, i.e. alcohol.

Lanciotti and Hopkins (1995) termed the first of these categories frustration aggression, which may be a normal response to annoying stimuli, and the second the social learning theory, which proposed that this response was learnt just like any other response.

If staff are able to highlight the possible risk factors involved in violence in A&E departments, they must put together strategies to reduce those they can influence and to manage those they cannot.

Table 20.2 Most common factors associated with violent episodes

Reduction of rational thought
Alcohol, drugs, psychiatric illness, mental disability, pain, injury, fear, anxiety, medical conditions, acute confusion, poor coping mechanisms (social learning theory)

Provocation
Poor communication, poor departmental layout, poor departmental seating, poor departmental environment (too hot, too cold, too dark, flickering lights), inner city department, unexplained waits, poor clinical practice, triage, police/security, children in pain, long waits, staff response, queue jumping

Management of Violence in A&E

The NHS and the individual hospital Trusts have a duty of care under the Health and Safety at Work Act (1972) to ensure, so far as is reasonably practicable, the health, safety and welfare of their employees. This includes the prevention and monitoring of violent episodes. The Management of Health and Safety at Work Regulations (HMSO, 1992) highlighted the importance of prevention and protective measures. The employer's duty is to assess the risks to the health and safety of the employees and to identify measures to enable compliance with their duties under the legislation. The Trust is responsible for establishing and implementing procedures for serious and imminent danger and associated danger areas. Under the

Reporting of Injuries, Diseases and Dangerous Occurrences Regulations (HMSO, 1995) it is a statutory requirement for the organization to record, report and investigate accidents and incidents that fall within RIDDOR. These are a death at work, over three days' sickness following injury including violence and completion of accident report forms. But what about the psychological effects of verbal and non-verbal threats and violence? These are as damaging to the morale and therefore effectiveness of the individual concerned and the environment that all A&E nurses work in but within present legislation may be neglected.

Management of violence in A&E departments must therefore take place in a variety of ways to ensure the safety of staff, patients and visitors. By dividing the management of violence in A&E into three distinct areas one can ensure that all associated factors are highlighted and addressed:

(1) advance preparation;
(2) reporting;
(3) debriefing.

Advance Preparation

This section is multifaceted, as it must encompass departmental assessment, staff training, community liaison and the development of Trust-approved working policies.

Departmental Assessment

This should include department structure and also working practice.

Departmental Structure

The layout of the department can go a long way to create feelings of insecurity and vulnerability in both patients and staff. A department that is divided into many small rooms and corridors is not only very difficult to manage effectively but will create many occasions when staff are tending patients alone. Those designing A&E departments must balance the need for privacy and confidentiality with the need for support and observation. Large, open-plan designs may also contribute to safety by reducing patient anxiety and frustration. Frustration can result from lack of information and patients' inability to see staff at work. Therefore a well-designed department will ensure that staff cannot be segregated from colleagues and also that patients can see activity or ask questions. Dark, oppressive departments may generate feelings of depression and agitation, thus creating problems for staff to deal with that may not have arisen with bright, thoughtfully decorated departments. If people are comfortable they may be more amenable to a wait for treatment than those in uncomfortable departments with limited amenities. Information on departmental practice, triage, the emergency nurse practitioner system and departmental clinics is vital to ensure patients and visitors do not become agitated and challenging as a result of what they see as unfair treatment.

Closed circuit television (CCTV) may be built into the fabric of the A&E department. This must have a recording facility. CCTV may act as a deterrent if made highly visible. Large television screens facing the entrance, showing staff and visitors entering the building that they are being filmed and recorded, will give the message that anyone causing an affray will be identified. CCTV can, however, irritate and cause confidentiality issues to arise. Therefore surveillance in public access areas is the favoured option with CCTV within clinical areas being reserved for special circumstances.

The development of restricted zones in the department will provide staff with the ability to politely question members of the public in areas clearly not intended for their access. This may be facilitated by having colour-coded areas (Table 20.3). One area may be open to public access, for example the waiting room, refreshment machines and general toilets. The clinical areas may be colour coded to denote controlled or restricted entry only. Staff rest areas, offices and storerooms may be coded to signify no entry. This will prevent members of the public denying any knowledge of where they are permitted within the unit.

Table 20.3 Colour-coded areas

Public Notice	
Red Area	No Public Access
Blue Area	Restricted Access
Green Area	Public Area

The above restrictions are in place to protect our patients and the general public using this department

The colour-coding system can be implemented by displaying a large notice in the waiting area of the department. To reinforce this notice, doors to areas or even the floor can be colour coded to denote the area entered.

The facilities within the A&E department can improve the quality of the patient's wait and therefore may reduce violent outbursts. As people get bored their tolerance of noise, other patients, children, the environment and the length of time spent in the department reduces. This means that a confrontational episode is more likely to arise. Facilities to occupy the patient and relatives during the waiting period may help. Up-to-date reading materials for all ages may be a source of information and entertainment if the material is a mix of educational literature and popular press. In many A&E departments the introduction of a television has helped occupy both the young and old. However, very loud background noise or the nature of the programmes on view may irritate some patients. If a video player is available educational videos may help to inform. There are many organizations that have information on video, which could be used to occupy the patients' waiting time with viewing material changed regularly throughout the day. The A&E department may make its own information video to describe the nature of the work in the department. This may be undertaken using media studies students at local colleges and universities, thus keeping costs to a minimum.

Fish tanks are popular as a calming influence but they can also pose a safety risk if not appropriately positioned and maintained. The fish tank must be in a position that prevents children and other members of the public interfering with it. The tank may also need to be made out of laminated glass or plastic to avoid injury if it is damaged.

Activities in the waiting room may act as a stimulus and divert attention away from 'clock watching'. It may be appropriate for the A&E department to develop close links with health promotion agencies and provide space throughout the year for them to run roadshows. During no-smoking week, diabetes week and child accident prevention week, for example, staff from local groups may wish to set up displays and answer questions on relevant issues for patients and visitors attending the department. This will provide an interactive department and an improved waiting environment for patients and their relatives. Interactive activities may reduce complaints as the patients can be occupied and also reduce inappropriate attendance in the long term by educating those waiting.

Suitable space is the limiting factor when arranging displays within many A&E departments, as can be the local enthusiasm. If the public get involved in activities within the A&E department the community attitude may slowly change.

All A&E departments need to provide refreshments for waiting relatives and members of the public. The facilities need to be well stocked and maintained if of the vending type and open appropriately if run by catering services within the hospital or the Women's Royal Voluntary Service (WRVS). It must be emphasized around the department, however, that the patient should check with the triage nurse prior to taking any refreshments. The patient and relatives must also have access to a telephone, as the ability to contact other members of the family and friends will reduce anxiety and agitation.

Working Practice

It is easy to say that new and well-designed departments will solve many of the violent incidents in A&E but few Trusts can afford the luxury of new departments or expensive upgrade work. So how can things be improved in the departments that currently exist? Assessing working practice and the risks associated with different tasks may help. This assessment needs to be undertaken by all staff, not just the managers, and during both the day and night shifts. Safe practice during the day may become markedly unsafe during the night when staffing levels reduce.

For example, when suturing a patient's head at night, the nurse is positioned at the head of the A&E trolley. Does this place the patient between the nurse and the exit? By simply turning the trolley round and suturing the patient's head with the nurse positioned near the exit of the cubicle the member of staff has immediately reduced the chance of injury should the patient become violent, with no cost implications and only minimal planning.

Assessing the risks in all clinical practice, which is a requirement of Health and Safety legislation, will enable a modified approach to many basic tasks, therefore reducing the risks to those performing them.

Triage

Effective, informative and consistent assessment may help to reduce anxiety, answer questions and keep the patients and their relatives informed of delays. The triage nurse must be in a position to see and assess the waiting area repeatedly but being the focus of attention will mean that an anxious and unhappy patient or relative may aim any outburst at him/her. Triage must occur in an area where sensitive questions can be asked and answered. The need for privacy may have the potential to put the triage nurse at risk. The triage area itself needs to be safe, but private. Effective curtaining may help to provide some privacy but will not prevent conversations being overheard. A more formal screen may provide better soundproofing, but as formal partitions or walls are built the nurse becomes more isolated. Panic buttons and two entrances/exits must be provided. Equipment that has the possibility of being used as a weapon must be avoided. Simply redesigning the seating in the waiting area may take the focus off the assessment and treatment areas and therefore reduce the frustration of the patients waiting. Providing areas of seating that focus on different activities can do this. Some seats could face the television, and for those patients not wishing to watch television other seats could face health posters.

Pain assessment and adequate analgesia administered at triage may also help reduce anxiety and therefore intolerance. Following recognized guidelines and local standing orders may improve the assessment of pain and empower the triage nurse to intervene effectively and make the wait for definitive care more tolerable. If these standing orders include paediatric simple analgesia parental anxieties may also reduce, resulting in fewer outbursts by unhappy and agitated parents.

Patient Movement in A&E

Does the department design force patients to make repeated unnecessary trips: from reception to the waiting area, to the triage nurse, to the doctor, to X-ray, to the nurse, to the waiting area, to the doctor etc? The list goes on, and as tiresome as this is to read it is more tiresome for the patient to do, especially if in pain or if explanations are poor and signs difficult to follow. By assessing the flow of patients within the department staff will be able to re-engineer the processes and may reduce the frustration that such pointless movement produces.

Good clear signs will help patients. Staff may be of the opinion that patients do not read the signs, but why is this? A patient entering the hospital for an X-ray of his/her wrist, for example, will be looking for the X-ray department, not radiology. It may be that the example set by the paediatric wards and hospitals in removing the words from signs should be followed. It would be far simpler for the patient going to X-ray to follow the pictures of bones painted on the floor and/or walls. The patient going to pharmacy could follow the medicine bottles and the patient going to the pathology laboratory could follow the syringes. This work may be done using local art students who need to complete projects for their examinations and will again enhance the department's relationships with the local community. By using local students to help with such projects the cost is also minimized. If signs to and from A&E departments are improved, this will help to reduce both patient and visitor frustration.

Staff Training

Nurses are committed to a Duty of Care, therefore some measures to protect A&E staff may conflict directly with their Code of Conduct. One such measure that some nurses find difficult to justify is the teaching of breakaway techniques, as this may seem to go against all that has been taught regarding patient care. Indeed, when tackling violence in A&E, prevention is better than cure. All staff must be trained to recognize warning signs and body language which may indicate that a violent outburst is imminent (Paterson et al., 1997). A calm and helpful approach may defuse a situation. An even temper and careful eye contact will demonstrate a desire to assist. The nurse should try to remove the perception of him/herself as an aggressor or victim. Through a confident and considerate approach the likelihood of an escalation of the conflict is reduced. Defusing violent situations prior to any verbal or physical threats results in far less stress, time wasted and injury than meeting force with force. However, some incidents will occur without warning and therefore other methods of protecting staff and patients may be needed. Personal security alarms may give the individual staff member improved confidence and also hasten support should a violent incident occur. Personal alarms can alert other staff and/or security officers to an emergency. Alternatively, audible personal alarms may shock an attacker momentarily thus providing valuable time for the staff member to escape to safety and summon assistance.

Advice from the local police force is essential to discuss the needs and weaknesses of individual departments. All police stations will have training officers who are skilled in unarmed defence techniques, and these experts may be available to educate regarding common and criminal law confines. This training may include self-defence techniques aiming to create space between the healthcare professional and the assailant.

Security officers effectively trained and managed within the department may be seen as an integral part of the team. Staff managed well within the A&E department will adopt a role effective for the client population and respond well to incidents, working with the clinical and clerical staff. The main role of security officers must be to act as a deterrent and they can display the security message of the hospital just by being present in the department. However, the presence of security officers, especially those wearing uniforms resembling those of the military or police, may promote a violent incident. This may be caused by a patient or relative reacting negatively to their presence, because of either the perceived provocation that an official uniform may cause or the individual's inability to rationalize the situation he/she is in. This may be the individual's learned response to authority or the fact that alcohol, drugs, pain, fear or grief affects him/her. It may be more appropriate for the security officers to wear less imposing clothing with appropriate name badges. Security officers need structured education on their role within the A&E department, and this must be tailored to each department's need. Common elements should be criminal and common law; the role of A&E; and interpersonal skills, commonly known as customer care courses. Security officers must be educated in confidentiality and how it is related to their role. Education in the management of violence and aggression to ensure that security officers are able to intervene, thus calming hostile situations rather than escalating them, is essential. Security officers must feel valued members of the A&E team. One way to draw them into the team may be to employ security officers in a multifunctional role, including portering. This will develop a team of A&E dedicated porters with security skills. It may also help to reduce the feelings of provocation that some patients adopt towards security officers and enable the individual officer to play a more supportive and subtle role should an incident arise.

Community Liaison

Establishing the role of the police is essential in fostering good security within the A&E environment, and a start can be made by inviting the local Crime Prevention Officer to assess the department. This officer will highlight and advise on areas of concern, and will be able to provide detailed statistics on the nature of crime in an individual A&E department's area. He/she will also provide the department with the names of contacts within the local police force to enhance relationships.

Many A&E departments already have good working relationships with local police officers. These can be developed by the local community police officer visiting the department regularly and/or being based within the department. The ideal site for such a community police office would be adjacent to the waiting area. This office could also be utilized by other police officers on business in the department. They could write their reports and complete paperwork within this office. An on-site police office will ensure a constant police presence within the department and thus the local community will become aware of this liaison very quickly.

In addition to the role of the police within the department, the local community can have a tremendous part to play in improving the department's public relations. Involving the department in cor imunity projects with schools, youth centres and sports clubs and bringing students to the department to enhance the departmental fabric will engender ownership of the department by the community it serves. Over time this may mean that the department is being visited by patients who have been actively involved and are therefore more tolerant of some of the practices that occur.

Trust Policies

As well as departmental training, education and practice, a policy must be drawn up for the management of violence and aggression. All staff should be encouraged to contribute to this document and the final draft must be discussed prior to ratification. This policy must outline the department's and therefore the hospital's responsibilities under current legislation. The policy must also state the role of individual members of staff regarding the reporting of incidents and their conduct during dangerous or threatening events. The policy should cover the incidents that will be classified as violent episodes within the department concerned. It should also state the actions the department and the hospital intend to take should an incident arise. Such policies must emphasize to departmental staff the importance placed on their safety, thus improving staff morale. In addition to the departmental policy on security, a general notice to the public placed on display within public access areas will inform them of the importance the hospital places on staff protection (Table 20.4). Such a notice must be endorsed by the Trust chief executive.

Table 20.4 Staff protection

Important Notice
Our staff work hard to provide you with the best possible care. Please help them by giving them the courtesy and cooperation they deserve. We will not tolerate verbal or physical abuse to our staff, or damage to our property. All such incidents will be treated seriously and may lead to the prosecution of the individuals involved.

Reporting

Incident reporting must be an integral part of the management of violence and aggression in A&E. Without accurate reporting it is not possible to evaluate the effectiveness of control measures. A reporting system must be robust and easy to complete. Clinical governance and risk management have meant that all hospitals must have incident report forms in place. These may be suitable for data collection and the subsequent evaluation of violent incidents. However, existing forms and databases may not enable the appropriate information to be recorded and it may be necessary for the A&E department to work closely with the risk manager and the clinical audit department to develop separate reporting forms that can uniquely identify violent occurrences. A simple form must be developed that is unambiguous and easy to complete. The nature of the incident must be specific if management strategies are to be effective. Specific words must describe the nature of the incident: for example, verbal abuse, verbal threats, physical threats and actual physical attack. This will facilitate an accurate review of the problems staff face. Time of day must be included because if incidents are occurring at specific times other management strategies, including increasing the level of staff on duty, may need to be instituted. The actual location of the incident, such as 'A&E waiting area', not just 'A&E' is essential to assist management to isolate specific problem areas. Areas of the department that would not necessarily be regarded as problem areas may over time become the focus of attention and therefore resources.

Incident reports must be critically reviewed regularly. It is not enough to make a report and not act on the information given or the trends demonstrated, and there must be time to reflect on events and decide on future developments to target the issues identified. Departmental managers must insist that report forms are completed accurately. If issues are tackled and addressed by the department this will encourage all staff to complete the forms. A robust and reactive reporting system again may improve morale and confidence in the department. All documentation must enable Health and Safety legislation to be followed; thus involvement of the hospital legal advisers and Health and Safety advisers may be necessary.

Debriefing

Following any violent or aggressive incident within the A&E department it is essential to re-evaluate the processes in place. Risk assessments need repeating. Management strategies need to be modified. Staff must be given the time to express their concerns and feelings regarding the incident. The role of critical incident debriefing has had mixed reviews recently (Chadda, 1998). A debrief must occur soon after the event to prevent staff experiencing the traumatic event for a second time. Providing time for staff to raise their concerns in a protected environment with peers may be appropriate for some staff. Other staff may need referral to occupational health for the chance to discuss feelings and issues remaining. The A&E management must be sensitive to the different reactions of individuals and not underestimate the impact that violent events may have on staff morale and confidence. If the violent incident is ignored and not dealt with the department may suffer from increasing sickness and absenteeism, which will increase the workload and stresses upon remaining staff. With reduced staffing levels there may be an increased risk of more violent events occurring as a result of increased dissatisfaction with the service provided.

Conclusions

Violence and aggression will not go away from society or, therefore, the A&E environment. Assessment of the problem and reporting of incidents is the first stage in building strategies to manage violent and aggressive events and protect staff. Regular review of incidents will provide detailed information, which will enable specific situations to be targeted for action. It may highlight the need to change clinical practice or modify practice at different times of the day or night. Regular review and action will demonstrate to staff a commitment towards their well-being.

Involving community police will improve liaison and the feelings of safety. If staff work on local community projects this will have the dual benefit of engendering community spirit regarding the role of the A&E department and educating the public on the appropriate use of emergency resources.

A&E departments must value their staff and actively demonstrate this to the public. Notices highlighting the seriousness with which violence is tackled by the A&E management must be displayed and enforced.

To retain and recruit staff the management of violence in A&E must be high on both the local and the national agenda.

Suggested Further Reading

HSAC (1997) Violence and Aggression to Staff in the Health Services. Guidance on Assessment and Management. Norwich: HSE Books.
NHS Executive (1997) Effective Management of Security in A&E. London: AEA Technology, Department of Health.

References

Baron RA, Richardson DR (1994) Human Aggression, 2nd edn. London: Plenum Press.

Brennan W (1997) Pressure points. Nursing Times 93(43): 29–32.

Chadda D (1998) When it's time to call in CID. Health Service Journal (29 January): 15.

Department of Health (1992) The Patient's Charter. London: Department of Health.

Hammond P (1995) I'm a doctor, hit me. Nursing Times 91(44): 48.

Health Services Advisory Committee (HSAC) (1987) Violence to Staff in the Health Service. London: HMSO.

Health Services Advisory Committee (HSAC) (1997) Violence and Aggression to Staff in the Health Services. Norwich: HMSO-HSE Books.

HMSO (1972) Health and Safety at Work Act. Norwich: HMSO-HSE Books.

HMSO (1992) The Management of Health and Safety at Work Regulations. Norwich: HMSO-HSE Books.

HMSO (1995) Reporting of Diseases and Dangerous Occurrences Regulations. Norwich: HMSO-HSE Books.

Home Office Research and Statistics Directorate (1996) British Crime Survey (unpublished).

Kydd P (1998) Pinpointing the problem of violence. Emergency Nurse 6(8): 8–10.

Lanciotti L, Hopkins A (1995) Breaking the cycle. Nursing Standard 10(11): 22–3.

Paterson B, Leadbetter D, McCormish A (1997) De-escalation in the management of aggression and violence. Nursing Times 93(36): 58–61.

Saines J (1999) Violence and aggression in A&E. Accident and Emergency Nursing 7: 8–12.

Whittington R (1997) Violence to nurses: prevalence and risk factors. Nursing Standard 12(5): 49–54.

Whittington R (1998) Violence to nurses: prevalence and risk factors. Emergency Nurse 5(8): 31–7.

Chapter 21
Major Incidents

MELANIE HOUSE

Introduction

Anybody who has seen media coverage of disasters and large-scale tragedies over recent years will have an idea of what constitutes a major incident. However, in health service terms it is viewed in a very broad context that reflects the ability of services to cope with a huge disruption, not only over a matter of hours but also over the following days and even weeks. A major incident for one emergency service, therefore, may not be so for another. The Home Office (Department of Health, 1994) subsequently defined a health service major incident as any occurrence which presents a serious threat to the health of the community, disruption to the service or causes (or is likely to cause) such numbers or types of casualties as to require special arrangements to be implemented by hospitals, ambulance services or health authorities.

This chapter aims to give a brief overview of current trends and associated rationale for major incident planning.

Overview

Major incidents may be either natural or man-made. Natural disasters are produced by the violence of nature (e.g. earthquakes, floods, hurricanes or drought) and the death toll from such disasters can sometimes increase dramatically during the aftermath. For example, 900,000 people died during flooding when the Yellow River in China burst its banks in 1887, whilst a million more died from resultant famine and disease. Natural disasters or war may further compound any major incident response through damage to vital infrastructure (e.g. in January 1994, the Los Angeles earthquake left many hospitals without water, power or communications and some had to be evacuated).

The list of man-made disasters is very diverse, but the common link is the large number of dead and injured casualties that may be generated.

For example, in the UK:

- Sporting:
  1985   Bradford City Football stadium
  1989   Hillsborough Football stadium
- Terrorist:
  1993   Warrington bombing
  1996   Manchester bombing
- Industrial:
  1988   Explosion on Piper Alpha oil rig

Planning for Potential Incidents

Health authorities are required to maintain and establish an effective emergency response for a broad spectrum of scenarios involving both immediate casualties and those that pose a threat to public health. Effective planning is therefore paramount if this requirement is to be met and guidelines have been laid down by the Department of Health (DoH, 1990) who recommended that an 'all-hazards' approach should be adopted within any emergency planning, that all hospitals should have an emergency plan and that training is essential to prepare for a major incident. The guidelines also state that all staff involved should use action cards. However, Carley and Mackway-Jones (1996) concluded that out of 142 major incident plans analyzed, only 119 used subsequent action cards and of these only 65 were deemed comprehensive enough to include all staff who were likely to be involved.

Effective planning may be difficult to achieve owing to the infrequent occurrence of such incidents coupled with their diversity, but it is possible to anticipate key individual roles when dealing with large numbers of potential casualties. Following the Manchester bombing in 1996, a casualty profile was developed and the authors advocated that similar documents be produced for a variety of potential incidents to ensure that adequate staff training, equipment provision and support services could be facilitated (Carley and Mackway-Jones, 1997).

Any hospital plan should be fully integrated with other emergency services and should also incorporate voluntary support services including the Red Cross, St John's Ambulance and the WRVS. Hospital and accident and emergency (A&E) department plans should be reviewed and updated regularly to reflect any changes in specialities, staffing levels and any recommendations made following scenario practice. The plan must be worded clearly, outlining a quick chain of command to facilitate decision-making and listing the members of the hospital coordination team with their relevant roles and responsibilities.

Members should include:

- a medical coordinator;
- a chief triage officer – to ensure that the casualty reception area is prepared and to carry out the initial re-triage of casualties upon their arrival;
- a senior hospital manager – to coordinate all non-clinical areas and their subsequent requirements;
- a senior nurse manager – to ensure that all clinical areas are prepared to receive casualties and that appropriate staffing is achieved (Hodgetts and Mackway-Jones, 1995).

A cascade telephone system can be effective to alert off-duty staff, as can a broadcast appeal through the local media (Walsh, 1989). Any plan should subsequently outline where staff report to and who is responsible for the allocation of staff to both A&E and the other areas of the hospital. If staff not normally acquainted with A&E work are allocated to that area, it is recommended that key A&E personnel are made readily identifiable by wearing labelled fluorescent tabards.

Arrangements need to be made for the clearance of the A&E department to allow for the influx of casualties and for urgent discharges from wards, a task that is particularly important because hospitals often run at 100% bed occupancy. Arrangements must also be made for the replenishment of stock to prevent vital resources from running out.

Communication is a vital component of a hospital major incident plan, with the ultimate goal of transmitting the right information to the right people at the right time in an understandable and effective form (Cummings, 1987). Lines of communication will need to be set up between the hospital and the site of the incident, and for the police documentation team that will be based at the hospital. Staff should be cautious about relying on cellphones during an incident as the network may become blocked very quickly, particularly by members of the press. Indeed, in many inquiries following incidents the most common failing is that of communication, yet it is clearly a key achievable factor in their effective management.

Mobile Medical Teams

As well as a major incident plan, all listed hospitals are required to provide a mobile medical team, either to assist with trapped casualties or to assist with triage and treatment at the casualty clearing station. These teams usually consist of two doctors and two nurses who will remain responsible to the medical incident officer (who may be either a hospital-based doctor or an immediate care doctor). There is no official guidance as to the composition, equipment or training of these teams and so the standard is variable. The team should have knowledge and expertise in initial assessment and resuscitation, ideally with advanced life support and trauma qualifications. This may mean that A&E staff are involved and therefore a mobile team may be dispatched from a hospital some distance from the scene of the incident so as not to deplete valuable staff in the receiving hospitals.

Personal and Medical Equipment

Personal protective equipment is essential as individuals with incorrect attire will not be allowed near the scene, and clothing should conform to Department of Health and international specifications. Wellington boots should be oil and acid resistant. Jackets and over-trousers should be made of high-visibility, fire-retardant materials and have clear identification. Helmets should be fitted with visors and be made of high-specification material (e.g. Kevlar composite). Heavy-duty gloves should also be available to protect staff from glass and shrapnel. Team members should be aware of the size of clothing they require so that time is not wasted. Thought should also be given to suitable personal underclothing for cold-weather conditions.

Medical equipment is a matter for decision by individual A&E departments in conjunction with the ambulance service to ensure that appropriate equipment is provided whilst avoiding duplication. When deciding on equipment it is useful to consider what treatment is likely to be needed and then plan accordingly.

For example:

- Life-saving first aid:
  - airway: chin lift, jaw thrust, c-spine immobilization;
  - breathing: mouth-to-mouth/mouth-to-nose ventilation;
  - circulation: control of external haemorrhage.

- Advanced procedures:
  - airway: oropharyngeal and nasopharyngeal airways, endotrachreal intubation, surgical airway;
  - breathing: mouth-to-mask and bag-valve-mask ventilation, needle thoracocentesis, chest drain insertion;
  - circulation: peripheral and central venous access, intravenous infusion, defibrillation.

Equipment must then be stored in durable and easily transportable containers, for example large boxes and/or rucksacks, that are clearly labelled with the name of the hospital. As with major incident plans, all clothing and equipment must be checked on a regular basis.

Training

As stated earlier, training is essential when preparing for a major incident plan. The Department of Health (NHS Executive, 1996) recommended that staff receive regularly updated training to prepare them to handle major incidents.

The recommendation advocated:

- that medical staff who are likely to form part of the mobile teams receive appropriate training (e.g. ATLS, Immediate Care Course);
- that nursing staff who are likely to form part of mobile teams be experienced A&E nurses with the ENB 199 and ATLS qualifications;
- that appropriate staff should receive training in the use of emergency communication equipment;

- that all staff should participate in regular exercises on all or part of the major incident procedure.

Major Incidents involving Chemicals or Radiation

Incidents involving hazardous materials are often complex, may involve large numbers of specialist agencies and local authorities and planning is of the utmost importance. Major incident plans should therefore be expanded and adapted to ensure that necessary precautions are in place and that channels of communication exist.

The Fire Service usually undertakes decontamination but this is not always the case and A&E departments should be prepared to receive contaminated casualties. All patients should consequently be treated as if contaminated unless stated otherwise. Figure 21.1 highlights the ideal principal circuit for the movement of contaminated casualties.

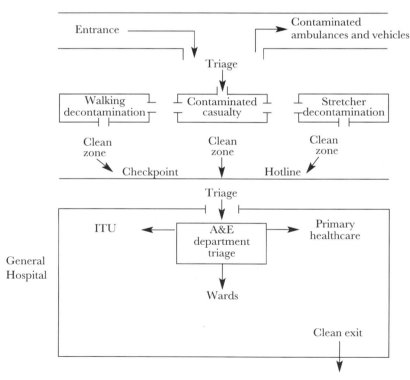

Figure 21.1 Ideal plan for movement of contaminated casualties (Wheeler, 1998).

Decontamination should ideally take place outside the department or in an allocated area that is both separate and well ventilated. Decontamination of chemical substances is carried out by gentle washing with soap and water or by showering for 20 minutes, taking care to avoid further chemical spread. Clothing should be placed in clear plastic bags and labelled accordingly. Decontamination of radioactive materials should be undertaken using swabs moistened with saline or Hibiscrub, with gentle irrigation of small areas. It is important to avoid the spread of the contaminant at all times and levels of contaminant should be recorded before and after decontamination. A radiation protection adviser should subsequently check all personnel before moving into the clean zone.

In the case of chemical incidents, gloves and gowns are usually sufficient, although skin or mucosal contact with the casualty and his/her clothing should be avoided. Staff who will come into contact with radioactive contaminant should be provided with theatre scrubs, long plastic aprons, caps, boots or overshoes and two pairs of gloves (with the inner pair being taped to the sleeves). It is important to remember that although the emphasis is to remove the contaminant and limit its spread, the first priority remains that of life-saving interventions.

Counselling and Debriefing

Towards the end of an incident a period of reflection will take place and this is usually when the full extent of what has happened is realized. Medical/nursing staff are used to dealing with distressed relatives on a day-to-day basis but perhaps not on such a large scale, and this can take its toll. Effective counselling and debriefing can subsequently help all those involved to cope with the experience of surviving a disaster and enable them to function in the following weeks or months.

In the early stages of an incident, victims are often stunned or dazed by what has happened. They may be anxious or upset about their injuries or about the condition or whereabouts of loved ones. It is less common for A&E personnel to exhibit such signs of distress at this point as they should be working within a coordinated structure. In the later stages following an incident it is important that all individuals involved are aware of how to gain access to debriefing and counselling support. This may involve social workers, GPs and community psychiatric nurses having to make special arrangements to cope with increased workloads.

Debriefing may be evident quite early on in the form of colleagues talking during a rest break or as the incident winds down, or it can be formal within an organized and structured meeting soon after the event. There is a positive view amongst healthcare professionals about debriefing as it provides a good opportunity to discuss events or incidents with others who have shared the same experience, and also allows examination of clinical judgement and decisions.

It is important to recognize that some individuals may wish to use their own coping mechanisms and choose not to discuss their feelings openly within the group setting. Timing is also important as debriefing within 24 hours to 48 hours may be acceptable for some but not for others. Formal help may be needed if signs of post-traumatic stress disorder (PTSD) begin to show as these symptoms may continue for many years if left untreated and can seriously affect a person's ability to continue with his/her normal daily routine.

Conclusion

This chapter has given an overview of current trends regarding major incidents. However, it cannot be over-emphasized that careful planning, responsive to both national and local needs, with frequent practices and subsequent critical evaluation and review, is the only way to ensure that departments are best prepared for the unexpected. Of course, no plan can ensure a perfect response to such a wide range of possible scenarios but safety, communication and effectively rehearsed teamwork are all advocated as key elements for success.

Suggested Further Reading

Hodgetts TJ, Mackway-Jones K (1995) Major Incident Medical Management and Support. Plymouth: BMJ Publishing Group.
NHS Executive (1996) Emergency Planning in the NHS: Health Service Arrangements for Dealing with Major Incidents. London: Department of Health.

References

Carley S, Mackway-Jones K (1996) Are British hospitals ready for the major incident? Analysis of hospital major incident plans. British Medical Journal 313: 1242–3.

Carley S, Mackway-Jones K (1997) The casualty profile for the Manchester bombing 1996: a proposal for the construction and dissemination of casualty profiles from major incidents. Journal of Accident and Emergency Medicine 14: 76–80.

Cummings H (1987) Disaster planning for hospitals. Nursing Management 18(9): 106–8.

Department of Health (1990) Emergency Planning in the NHS: Arrangements for Dealing with Major Incidents, 2nd edn. London: Department of Health.

Department of Health (1994) Dealing with Disaster, 2nd edn. London: Home Office Publications.

Hodgetts TJ, Mackway-Jones K (1995) Major Incident Medical Management and Support. Plymouth: BMJ Publishing Group.

NHS Executive (1996) Emergency Planning in the NHS: Health Service Arrangements for Dealing with Major Incidents. London: Department of Health.

Walsh M (1989) Coping with catastrophe. Nursing Times 85(19): 27–31.

Wheeler H (1998) Major incident planning: particularly those including chemicals. Emergency Nurse 6(1): 12–16.

Index

dopamine 38, 124, 195
Down's syndrome 130
dyspareunia 128
dyspnoea 25, 37, 70, 123
   asthma 61, 64
dysrhythmia 153, 154, 157, 159, 165,
   166
dysuria 117

ear, nose and throat (ENT) conditions
   355–80
ears 356, 364–70, 411
   foreign bodies 364–6
   injury to pinna 366–8
   vertigo 368–70
eating problems 212, 214
economy class syndrome 69
ecstasy (MDMA) 145
eczema 62
elbow fractures 239–40
electrical burns 262, 268, 269–70, 272,
   274, 278–9
electrocardiograph (ECG) 18–19, 26–8,
   296, 370
   aortic aneurysm 89
   burns and scalds 274, 281, 283
   cardiac emergencies 18–19, 23–4,
     26–9, 31–3, 36, 39, 43
   CO poisoning 164, 283
   CPR 48, 52
   gastrointestinal bleeds 93
   lower limb fractures 248–9
   panic attacks 219
   respiratory conditions 70, 74, 81
   status epilepticus 199
   TSS 124
   unconscious patient 157, 163–4, 166,
     169, 170
electrolytes 40, 188, 195, 198
   burns and scalds 281, 282
   paediatric care 305–6
   unconscious patient 149–50, 153,
     155, 168, 170
   see also urea and electrolytes
electro-mechanical dissociation (EMD)
   53
embolectomy 71
embolism 21, 102, 103–4

orthopaedics 230, 246, 252
   strokes 201, 203
   see also pulmonary embolism (PE);
     thromboemboli
emergency nurse practitioner (ENP) 392,
   396–408, 459
emphysema 77–8, 161, 267, 345, 361
empyema 379
encephalitis 158
encephalopathy 149, 150
endocrine disorders 149, 153–6
endometriosis 124
endoscopy 94
enophthalmos 345
Entonox 255, 256
environment and exposure 196, 199,
   296, 297
environmental conditions 392, 457,
   458–63
epididymitis 106–7, 108
epiglottitis 72, 289, 373–6
epilepsy 152–3, 196–201
   neurological emergencies 187, 189,
     196–201, 205
   paediatric care 302
   unconscious patient 149, 152–3
epinephrine 51, 54, 55, 67, 83–4, 195
   paediatric care 295, 296
epistaxis 72, 356–9, 360, 361
Epstein-Barr virus (EBV) 376
erosion of mucosa 92–3
erythema 264, 269, 273, 277–8, 374
erythromycin 75
escharotomy 270, 280, 282
Escherichia coli 192
ethambutol 77
ethylene glycol (antifreeze) 159
exercise 21–2, 25, 40, 72, 151, 154, 161
   osteoporosis 233
extracorporeal membrane oxygenation
   (ECMO) 194
eyepads and patches 347, 350
eyes 147, 271, 341–53
   burns and scalds 262, 270–1, 275,
     278, 345, 351–2

Family Reform Act (1969) 311
fasciotomy 255

X-rays 307, 316, 462–3
    acute respiratory conditions 66, 71,
        75, 81
    ENP 398, 400, 406
    ENT 362, 364, 373
    neurological emergencies 187–8, 198

ophthalmic injuries 346, 350
orthopaedics 230, 232, 234, 239–42,
    244, 247–9, 252, 254–7
surgical conditions 88, 101
    unconscious patient 161–3, 168

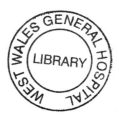